Jorge G. Burneo · Bart M. Demaerschalk
Mary E. Jenkins
Editors

Neurology

An Evidence-Based Approach

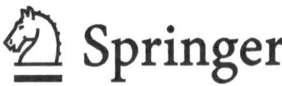 Springer

Editors
Jorge G. Burneo, MD, MSPH
London Health Sciences Centre
Department of Clinical Neurosciences
University of Western Ontario
339 Windermere Road
London Ontario, N6A 5A5, Canada
jorge.burneo@lhsc.on.ca

Bart M. Demaerschalk, MD, MSc, FRCPC
Department of Neurology
Mayo Clinic
5777 East Mayo Boulevard
Phoenix, AZ 85054, USA
demaerschalk.bart@mayo.edu

Mary E. Jenkins, MD, FRCPC
London Health Sciences Centre
Department of Clinical Neurosciences
University of Western Ontario
339 Windermere Road
London Ontario, N6A 5A5, Canada
mary.jenkins@lhsc.on.ca

ISBN 978-0-387-88554-4   e-ISBN 978-0-387-88555-1
DOI 10.1007/978-0-387-88555-1
Springer New York Dordrecht Heidelberg London

Library of Congress Control Number: 2011936746

Printed on acid-free paper

Springer is part of Springer Science+Business Media (www.springer.com)

Neurology

To our families, with love.

Foreword

"Errors in judgment must occur in the practice of an art which consists largely of balancing probabilities" opined William Osler. Fortunately, since he wrote these words, we can balance probabilities better, thanks to the emergence of evidence-based medicine. Although evidence for the diagnosis, management and rehabilitation of neurological disease is growing, challenges remain: The evidence is scattered and hardest to judge by those who need it most medical students, primary care physicians and trainees, and practitioners in internal medicine, neurology and neurosurgery to whom this book is addressed.

This volume deals with the major neurological problems systematically and boils down the evidence in two useful headings "Bottom lines" and "Summary," each with key references for the overwhelmed medical students, trainees and busy practitioners. Although the main aim of the book is practicality, the evidence revised is of high quality and can also serve those who want to review the most relevant publications in a given area.

The editors and contributors emphasize that the level of evidence for different aspects varies, and for some decisions we have no evidence at all. These limitations of the evidence-based approach are acknowledged and addressed and pragmatic alternatives suggested.

An attractive feature is that the three editors are in the ascending limb of their careers, close enough to their training days to know the needs of their audience and far enough along in their own fields to have mastered what is known.

Knowing what evidence to apply depends on knowing what is wrong with the patients in the first place. Brain imaging and other modern techniques have made diagnosis easier in many ways, but more difficult in other ways. Test profusion leads to confusion and often the answer is not reflected in the tests. In such cases, it is well to remember Gordon Holmes advice "More puzzles are solved by taking a second history than by doing all the tests."

May this comprehensive, yet concise and practical book enjoy the broad readership that it deserves.

London, ON, Canada   Vladimir C.M. Hachinski

Preface

The concept of this book arose from a perceived need for a comprehensive review of the current best evidence in the practice of neurology. Our goal was to present the evidence in a user-friendly and easily accessible manner. We hope we have achieved our objective.

The three co-editors are linked in their passion for evidence-based clinical practice in the clinical neurological sciences, connected to a common historical origin at the University of Western Ontario (UWO), London, Ontario, Canada, influenced directly by Evidence-Based Medicine teachings of McMaster University, Hamilton, Ontario, Canada, and two of them trained by a terrific mentor, Samuel Wiebe. Mary Jenkins and Bart Demaerschalk completed neurology residency at UWO, and Jorge Burneo trained in Epidemiology at the University of Alabama at Birmingham, and later joined UWO as faculty. All three co-editors are actively involved in teaching and practicing evidence-based neurology at their respective institutions, UWO and Mayo Clinic. Their common link, initially in training and now teaching in evidence-based neurology, fueled their desire to complete this book.

Dr. Burneo was initially approached by Springer Publishing regarding the concept of this book. He then included Dr. Jenkins and Dr. Demaerschalk and the editing team was born. We thank the publishers at Springer publishing for bringing the three of us together in this project.

We would like to extend our thanks to each of the talented authors who worked so diligently on their respective chapters. As editors, we were fortunate to work with an amazing group of skilled and determined evidence-based neurologists. We would also like to thank Connie Walsh from Springer Publishing who guided us through this journey and kept us on our course.

May you find the contents of this book helpful to you, the reader, in the management of patients in your individual practices, your personal education and training, and in your mentorship and instruction of those more junior to you.

Enjoy.

London, ON, Canada   Jorge G. Burneo
Phoenix, AZ   Bart M. Demaerschalk
London, ON, Canada   Mary E. Jenkins

Contents

Contributors

Maria I. Aguilar, MD Neurology Department, Mayo Clinic, Phoenix, AZ, USA

Khurram Bashir, MD, MPH Division of Neuroimmunology and Multiple Sclerosis, Multiple Sclerosis Center, Department of Neurology, University of Alabama at Birmingham, Birmingham, AL, USA

Jorge G. Burneo, MD, MSPH Neurology, Biostatistics and Epidemiology, Clinical Neurological Sciences, The University of Western Ontario, London, ON, Canada

Miguel Bussière, MD, PhD, FRCPC Neurology and Interventional Neuroradiology, The Ottawa Hospital, Ottawa, ON, Canada

Brian A. Crum, MD Neurology Department, Mayo Clinic, Rochester, MN, USA

Kirk R. Daffner, MD Division of Cognitive and Behavioral Neurology, Brigham and Women's Hospital, Boston, MA, USA

Neurology, Harvard Medical School, Boston, MA, USA

Bart M. Demaerschalk, MD, MSc, FRCPC Neurology Department, Mayo Clinic, Phoenix, AZ, USA

Rajat Dhar, MD Neurology Department, Washington University School of Medicine, St. Louis, MO, USA

Esma Dilli, BSc, MD, FRCPC Neurology Department, Mayo Clinic, Phoenix, AZ, USA

Elliot L. Dimberg, MD Department of Neurology, Mayo Clinic, Jacksonville, FL, USA

Michael N. Diringer, MD, FCCM, FAHA Neurology Department, Washington University School of Medicine, St. Louis, MO, USA

David W. Dodick, MD Neurology Department, Mayo Clinic, Phoenix, AZ, USA

Mohamed B. Elamin, MBBS Knowledge and Evaluation Research Unit, Department of Medicine, Division of Endocrinology, Mayo Clinic, Rochester, MN, USA

Yngve Falck-Ytter, MD Department of Medicine, Case and VA Medical Center, Case Western Reserve University, Cleveland, OH, USA

Elizabeth Finger, MD Clinical Neurological Sciences, University of Western Ontario, London, ON, Canada

Brent P. Goodman, MD Neurology Department, Mayo College of Medicine, Mayo Clinic, Scottsdale, AZ, USA

Gordon H. Guyatt, MD, MSc, FRCPC Department of Medicine, McMaster University, Hamilton, ON, Canada

Department of Clinical Epidemiology and Biostatistics, McMaster University, Hamilton, ON, Canada

Vladimir C. M. Hachinski, MD, FRCCP, DSc, Dr hon. causa Clinical Neurological Sciences, London Health Sciences Centre, University of Western Ontario, London, ON, Canada

Mary E. Jenkins, MD, FRCPC Clinical Neurological Sciences, University of Western Ontario, London, ON, Canada

Nicholas L. King, MD Clinical Neurology, Indiana University School of Medicine, Indianapolis, IN, USA

Robert C. Knowlton, MD, MSPH Associate Professor Director, UAB Epilepsy Program, Department of Neurology University of Alabama at Birmingham, Birmingham, Alabama, USA

Lawrence Korngut, MD, FRCPC Department of Clinical Neurosciences, Rockyview Hospital, Calgary, AB, Canada

Janis M. Miyasaki, MD, Med, FRCPC Division of Neurology, Medicine Department, University of Toronto, Toronto, ON, Canada

The Movement Disorders Centre, University Health Network, Toronto Western Hospital, Toronto, ON, Canada

Victor M. Montori, MD, MSc Knowledge and Evaluation Research Unit, Department of Medicine, Division of Endocrinology, Mayo Clinic, Rochester, MN, USA

Devon I. Rubin, MD Department of Neurology, Mayo Clinic, Jacksonville, FL, USA

Oksana Suchowersky, MD, FRCPC, FCCMG Professor of Medicine & Medical Genetics, Toupin Research Chair in Neurology, University of Alberta Hospital, Edmonton, Alberta, Canada

Dean M. Wingerchuk, MD, MSc, FRCPC Neurology Department, Mayo Clinic, Scottsdale, AZ, USA

Part I
Basics of Evidence-Based Clinical Practice

Chapter 1
Evidence-Based Clinical Practice and the Neurosciences

Jorge G. Burneo, Bart M. Demaerschalk, and Mary E. Jenkins

Keywords Evidence-based medicine • Evidence-based clinical practice • Neurology • Critically appraised topics • Medical education

What Is Evidence-Based Clinical Practice?

The Principles of EBCP

Evidence-based clinical practice (EBCP) is the conscientious, explicit, and judicious use of current best external evidence in making decisions about the care of individual patients [1, 2]. This is, in contrast to the traditional way of learning and teaching medicine, which is based on personal clinical experience, with an authoritarian way to deliver [3, 4].

The practice of neurology has shifted from a rich, descriptive discipline, to one of increasing, diagnostic and therapeutic interventions. Every day we are faced with the pressure to apply the best evidence to our patients, and when this happens in a suboptimal way, we witness large variations in the way we practice. Furthermore, there is lots of information from different sources and we cannot keep up with it. EBCP allows clinicians to tap directly into clinical research results, assess their validity and usefulness, and keep up-to-date [5].

It is important to keep in mind two principles that have been fundamental in EBCP: Hierarchy of Evidence and Clinical Decision Making [4].

J.G. Burneo (✉)
Neurology, Biostatistics and Epidemiology, Clinical Neurological Sciences,
The University of Western Ontario, 339 Windermere Road B10-118, London,
ON, Canada N6A 5A5
e-mail: jorge.burneo@lhsc.on.ca

J.G. Burneo et al. (eds.), *Neurology: An Evidence-Based Approach*,
DOI 10.1007/978-0-387-88555-1_1, © Springer Science+Business Media, LLC 2012

Hierarchy of Evidence

A hierarchy of evidence has been proposed by Guyatt et al. [4] and accepted widely.

Hierarchy of evidence
1. N-OF-1 randomized trial
2. Systematic reviews of randomized trials
3. Single randomized trial
4. Systematic review of observational studies
5. Single observational study
6. Physiologic studies
7. Clinical observations

Guyatt et al. also mentioned that this hierarchy is not absolute, meaning that some studies of lower hierarchy can provide better evidence [4]. Nonetheless, a clinician should look for the best evidence from that hierarchy when trying to answer a specific question regarding a specific patient.

Clinical Decision Making

"Each patient is different" is a common phrase that we hear in neurology, and that is true, particularly when a physician is trying to apply the best evidence. The preference of each particular patient will play an extremely important role not only in the decision-making process but also in the outcome of his/her condition. Picture for instance a patient diagnosed with medically-intractable temporal lobe epilepsy due to mesial temporal lobe sclerosis. He may decide not to pursue surgical treatment even though the evidence points to it [6].

Challenges and Limitations

Practicing EBCP is a very time-consuming process. A busy clinician may not have time to search the literature exhaustively to find the best evidence. That is why there are international efforts to synthesize whatever information is available and present it in a user-friendly manner. The best example of this is the Cochrane Database of systematic reviews. There are other sources available for the neurosciences (see below).

Another challenge is that sometimes there is no evidence or the evidence is not relevant. This is particularly seen in highly specialized areas such as Neurology. Then, one has to resort to the next available evidence, even though sometimes it is difficult to extrapolate.

Neurology and EBCP

The Role of EBCP in Neurology

Quality and effectiveness of healthcare means "providing the right care to the right patient at the right time and getting it right the first time," according to the Agency for Healthcare Quality and Research [7]. Miyasaki reminded all practitioners of neurology that the agency's mission is to conduct and support health services research that "reduces the risk of harm from health care services by using evidence-based research and technology to promote the delivery of the best possible care; transforms research into practice to achieve wider access to effective health care services and reduce unnecessary health care costs; and improves health care outcomes by encouraging providers, consumers, and patients to use evidence-based information to make informed choices and decisions." [8] Miyasaki proclaims that EBCP plays, and will continue to play, a crucial role in improving health care quality and encourages every neurologist to master EBCP skills in order to provide patients with the best possible care [8].

Who in Neurology Should Partake in EBCP?

Traditionally, the field of clinical neurosciences has been slower to recognize, adopt, practice, and teach EBCP [9], but through initiatives like those of the American Academy of Neurology, other national clinical neurological associations, and those of individual universities, that has improved over time. Every neurology provider can participate in EBCP in one mode or another. "Doers" of EBCP (frequently those with training in EBCP and clinical epidemiology) take on the whole process step by step. "Users" of EBCP seek, evaluate, appraise, and incorporate into their practice the prepackaged best-evidence summaries produced and published by others. "Replicators" of EBCP may only have time to rely on distilled best-evidence summary information from respected opinion leaders in the field [10]. Busy neurologists need not tackle all the EBCP steps from scratch. Nonetheless, they must still know how to efficiently locate high-quality, valid, and useful summaries of the best evidence, to interpret them, and to apply them to their patients.

What EBCP Resources Are Available for Neurologists?

EBCP resources for neurologists are plentiful. For those interested in acquiring all the tools necessary to teach and practice, the American Academy of Neurology EBM Toolkit Workgroup has developed an EBM Toolkit. The EBM Toolkit and all of its modules have been offered to the faculty and trainees of neurology residency training programs. The American Academy of Neurology develops clinical practice guidelines to assist all of its members in clinical decision making related to the prevention, diagnosis, treatment, and prognosis of neurologic disorders. Each guideline makes specific practice recommendations based upon a rigorous and comprehensive evaluation of all available scientific data [11, 12]. Journals, such as The Neurologist and the Canadian Journal of Neurological Sciences regularly publish critically appraised topics, concise summaries of the current best evidence that addresses a specific clinical question [13–15]. Many of the references in the list, below, offer recommendations of high-yield internet resources for neurologists who wish to access evidence-based medicine information [16].

How Do We Practice Evidence-Based Neurology?

The practice of evidence-based neurology begins with a clinical problem; the type of problem that we encounter daily in our neurology clinic. What is the optimal treatment for early Parkinson's disease? What is the best test to diagnose a patient with multiple sclerosis? What risk factors predict longer survival in motor neuron disease?

To answer these questions, we rely on the principles of evidence-based neurology. The practice of evidence-based neurology is an explicit, rigorous, and structured approach to guide us through the application of these principles. The practice of evidence-based neurology involves the following steps (1) developing an answerable question, (2) searching the literature for the best-available evidence, (3) critically appraising the evidence, and (4) applying this knowledge to the management of the patient [17].

Developing the Answerable Question: Use of PICO Format

We start first with the patient and the clinical problem. From the problem, we construct a focused, answerable question using a standard format. In evidence-based neurology, the answerable question is divided into four components – Patient, Intervention, Comparison, and Outcome [17]. This is termed the PICO format.

PICO format – the answerable question	
P = Patient	Age, sex, situation, comorbid conditions
I = Intervention	Treatment, investigation, exposure
C = Comparison	Another medication, placebo, gold standard investigation
O = Outcome	Survival, improvement in morbidity, time to recover

For example, we start with a treatment question about Parkinson's disease. It is important to better define all components of PICO – Patient, Intervention, Comparison, and Outcome. Each of these components may lead to a complete separate question to be answered. The patient's age, comorbid conditions, and cognitive function are all important to consider. The treatment you are interested in may be dopamine agonists, rasagiline, amantadine etc. The comparison may be placebo (no treatment) or a standard "older" treatment such as levodopa. Finally the outcome of interest may be improvement in motor function, improvement in cognitive function, or risk of adverse events. As you can see these details will lead to very different questions and very different answers!

Once you have developed your PICO question, you are ready to move to searching the literature. For our example, we have chosen the following PICO elements – P(patient)–50-year-old, man, no other comorbid features; I (intervention)–Dopamine agonist; C (comparison) – Levodopa; O (outcome) – Improvement in motor function, risk of adverse affects. The clinical question is developed from the PICO components – *In the treatment of a 50-year-old man with Parkinson's disease, are dopamine agonists more effective in improving motor function and limiting side effects than levodopa.*

Searching the Literature

Now that the question has been defined, the next step is to search the literature for the best-available studies. There are a number of search engines used, although Medline is the site most commonly used in North America. Medline is available free through Pubmed [18] and Sumsearch [19].

Other sites include Embase [20], which is European based. The Cochrane Library [21] provides meta-analysis on some topics.

Once you choose a search engine, the next step is to develop search terms or key words. The key words come out of the PICO question. In our case, the terms could include *Parkinson's AND dopamine agonist AND levodopa*. More terms may be added later to refine or narrow the search. Limits, such as "meta-analysis" or "randomized controlled trial," can be applied to narrow the search to obtain the highest level of evidence available (see above).

The search will reveal a list of articles that are manually screened for relevance to the clinical question. This list of articles is then screened to obtain the highest level of evidence available (e.g., meta-analysis or randomized controlled trial for a treatment article). The best one or two articles are chosen for critical appraisal.

Critical Appraisal of the Literature

The guidelines for critical appraisal of the literature were first published in a series of articles by Guyatt and Sackett in JAMA from 1993 to 2000. These are now available in one publication [22] and on the web [23]. Many of these guidelines have been adapted and are available on other websites [24]. Using a systematic approach,

Table 1.1 Guidelines for appraisal of therapy article (randomized controlled trial)

Are the results of this single therapeutic trial valid?
  Did the authors address a focused clinical question?
  Was the assignment of patients to treatment randomized?
  Was the randomization list concealed?
  Was the follow-up of patients sufficiently long?
  Were all patients analyzed in the groups to which they were randomized? (intention-to-treat)
  Were patients and physicians kept blind to which treatment was being received?
  Were groups treated equally, apart from the experimental treatment?
  Were the groups similar at the start of the trial?

What were the results and are they important?
  What are the overall results of the study? (Number needed to treat, odds ratio, relative risk,
    absolute risk reduction)
  How precise were the results? (*p* value, 95% confidence intervals)

Will the results help me in caring for my patients?
  Are the patients in this trial similar to my patient?
  Were all clinically important outcomes considered?
  Is the treatment feasible?
  What are the potential benefits and harm? Are the benefits worth the harm and costs?

Table from http://www.uwo.ca/cns/ebn/

the guidelines are a series of questions that guide you through appraising or evaluating the article (see Table 1.1 for an example). The key three areas addressed are (1) validity – is this a well-designed and carefully administered study? (2) strength of the results – how large and precise is the treatment effect? and (3) applicability – are the study results applicable to my patient? Guidelines have been developed to assess different types of articles including therapy (randomized controlled trials and meta-analysis), diagnosis, prognosis, harm. Table 1.1 is an example of these guidelines from the University of Western Ontario EBN website [24].

Through the application of the guidelines to your chosen article, areas of strength and weakness are identified. There is no perfect study, but you must decide if the study design is sufficiently valid and the results are sufficiently strong and precise to be accepted as "good evidence."

Applying the Evidence to Your Patient

This is the most important step in the application of evidence-based medicine. The "evidence" is only one element in the clinical decision-making process. Two other key elements must be considered (1) the clinical judgment of the physician and (2) the values and preferences of the patient [22, 25]. Once you have completed the appraisal of the evidence, it is important to go back to the clinical case. For instance, the patient may have a comorbid illness that precludes starting the treatment that is deemed "the best evidence." The patient may not wish to start medical treatment even though you may feel that is indicated. The patient may agree that one treatment is ideal, but cost may be factor. The evidence, clinical judgment, and the patient preferences must all be taken into account. This last step is the most critical in determining your patient management.

How the Book Is Arranged

The book is organized around three parts. Part I: The Basics of Evidence-Based Clinical Practice, Part II: The Common Neurological Diseases, and Part III: Teaching Evidence-Based Neurology.

Part I: The Basics of EBCP

This section introduces the principles and practice of EBCP including some of the challenges and limitations. The role of EBCP in the neurosciences is discussed. The mechanics of practicing EBCP including levels of evidence and use of guidelines are reviewed. Resources used in EBCP are presented.

Part II: The Common Neurological Diseases

The second section is composed of clinical subspecialties and the main neurological diseases. Each chapter is arranged with a clinical case, clinical question, and search strategy that the authors used to determine the best evidence. The best available evidence is summarized in the subsections of epidemiology, diagnosis, treatment, and prognosis for each disease. At the end of each of these subsections are Clinical Bottom Lines that highlight the most important points of evidence for this subsection.

Part III: Teaching Evidence-Based Neurology

The final section includes the Evidence-Based Neurology Curriculum and other resources to facilitate development of an evidenced-based neurology program within your own setting.

Intended Audience

This book should provide a shelf-reference for neurologists, neurosurgeons, primary care physicians, and internists. The book might also serve as a potential study source for neurology and neurosurgery residents studying for certification examinations.

References

1. Sackett DL. Evidence-based medicine, how to practice and teach EBM. London: Churchill Livingstone; 1997.
2. Demaerschalk BM, Jenkins ME, Wiebe S. Evidence-based neurology: an innovative curriculum for post-graduate training in the neurological sciences. 2001. http://www.uwo.ca/cns/ebn. Accessed 13 July 2010.
3. Burneo JG, Jenkins ME, Bussiere M. Evaluating a formal evidence-based clinical practice curriculum in a neurology residency program. J Neurol Sci. 2006;250(1–2):10–9.
4. Guyatt G et al. Users' guides to the medical literature: a manual for evidence-based clinical practice. 2nd ed. Chicago: McGraw Hill; 2008.
5. Wiebe S. The principles of evidence-based medicine. Cephalalgia. 2000;20 Suppl 2:10–3.
6. Wiebe S et al. A randomized, controlled trial of surgery for temporal-lobe epilepsy. N Engl J Med. 2001;345(5):311–8.
7. Available at http://www.ahrq.gov/about/highlt07.htm. Accessed 24 Aug 2010.
8. Miyasaki JM. Using evidence-based medicine in neurology. Neurol Clin. 2010;28:489–503.
9. Wiebe S, Demaerschalk B. Progress in clinical neurosciences: evidence based care in the neurosciences. Can J Neurol Sci. 2002;29:115–9.
10. Strauss SE, McAlister FA. Evidence-based medicine: a commentary on common criticisms. CMAJ. 2000;163:837–41.
11. Invited Article: Lost in a jungle of evidence: we need a compass. Neurology. 2008;71:1634–8.
12. Invited Article: Practice parameters and technology assessments: what they are, what they are not, and why you should care. Neurology. 2008;71:1639–43.
13. Demaerschalk BM, Wingerchuk DM. The MERITs of evidence based clinical practice in neurology. Semin Neurol. 2007;27:303–11.
14. Wingerchuk DM, Demaerschalk BM. Critically appraised topics: the evidence based neurologist. The Neurologist. 2007;13(1):1.
15. Tartaglia MC, Pelz D, Burneo JG, Jenkins ME. Critically appraised topic – cerebral angiography and diagnosis of CNS Vasculitis. Can J Neurol Sci. 2009;36:93–4.
16. Al-Shahi R, Sandercock PAG. Internet resources for neurologists. JNNP. 2003;74:699–703.
17. Straus SE, Richardson WS, Glasziou P, Haynes RB. Evidence-based medicine: how to practice and teach EBM. 4th ed. London: Churchill Livingstone; 2005.
18. http://www.ncbi.nlm.nih.gov/sites/entrez?db=pubmed.
19. http://sumsearch.uthscsa.edu.
20. http://www.embase.com.
21. http://www.theCochraneLibrary.com.
22. Guyatt G, Rennie D. Users' guides to the medical literature. Chicago: AMA; 2002.
23. http://www.userguides.org.
24. http://www.uwo.ca/cns/ebn.
25. Sackett DL, Rosenberg WM, Gray JA, Haynes RB, Richardson WS. Evidence based medicine: what it is and what it isn't. BMJ. 1996;312(7023):71–2.

Chapter 2
The Hierarchy of Evidence: From Unsystematic Clinical Observations to Systematic Reviews

Mohamed B. Elamin and Victor M. Montori

Keywords Evidence-based medicine • Hierarchy of evidence • Study design

Any observation in nature is evidence [1]. The human brain is infinite in its ability to draw cause-and-effect inferences from these observations. Unfortunately, these inferences are open to cognitive errors. The scientific method, a method that relies on observations in nature and on evidence, has evolved to minimize error, both random (or due to chance) and systematic error or bias. A key principle of evidence-based medicine is the recognition that not all evidence is similarly protected against error, and that decisions that rely on evidence would be more confident when the evidence is more protected against bias by virtue of the methods used [2]. Thus, a fundamental principle of evidence-based medicine is the recognition of a hierarchy of evidence.

In this chapter, we will review the different approaches the scientific method has evolved to protect evidence from bias. We will then review the evolution of how methodologists have built hierarchies of evidence and note the limitations and merits of these approaches. While this field continues to move forward, we will finish describing what we think represents the state-of-the-art approach to hierarchies of evidence at the time of writing this chapter.

What Is a Hierarchy of Evidence?

To the extent that the evidence is protected against bias it would lead to more confident decision making [2]. Using "risk of bias" as an organizing principle results in a hierarchy of evidence that places studies with better protection against bias at the

V.M. Montori (✉)
Knowledge and Evaluation Research Unit, Department of Medicine,
Division of Endocrinology, Mayo Clinic, Rochester, MN, USA
e-mail: kerunit@mayo.edu

J.G. Burneo et al. (eds.), *Neurology: An Evidence-Based Approach*,
DOI 10.1007/978-0-387-88555-1_2, © Springer Science+Business Media, LLC 2012

top and less-protected evidence at the bottom. "Risk of bias" may not be the only desirable organizing principle of all available hierarchies, but we will focus on it and on the ability to apply evidence to the care of the individual patient when we discuss the position of different forms of evidence on a hierarchy of evidence.

Unsystematic Observations

Imagine that you are seeing a patient diagnosed with multiple sclerosis (MS). One of your clinical preceptors recommended using cyclophosphamide in the treatment of these patients. He had seen many patients improve on this drug and considered the drug both greatly efficacious and quite safe given the patients' dilemma.

Indeed, prior to the advent of evidence-based medicine, unsystematic personal observations from experienced clinicians carried great weight in shaping the practice and teaching of medicine. These observations are the subject of a number of biases introduced by psychological and cognitive processes that make recall and summary of one's experiences suspect. Clinicians interested in exploring these biases can review the work of Kahnemann and Tversky, and of Gigerenzer and colleagues [3–6]. These biases were recognized in research practice prior to clinical practice and the need for methods that will limit the possibility of error, both random and systematic, arose. Indeed, in many hierarchies, unsystematic personal observations often take the lowest or least trustworthy position and are often mistakenly considered "expert opinion." Opinions about observations should not be confused with the observations themselves (evidence), and experts can derive their opinions from any level of the hierarchy of evidence. Thus, expert opinion should not be part of any hierarchy of evidence.

Moving from your memories of what your teacher may have indicated, you seek to look at the body of scientific studies about the risk and benefits of available therapies. As a part of this effort, you decide to search for evidence investigating the use of cyclophosphamide in patients with MS and you find some studies describing the basis by which cyclophosphamide exerts its effect on MS.

Physiology and Mechanistic Studies

Physiology studies, both descriptive and experimental, provide us with the support we need to understand why, for instance, cyclophosphamide and other immunosuppressive regimens might help ameliorate MS symptoms. Searching for physiology studies, you find one of many mechanistic studies published that may potentially help you understand the pathogenesis of MS. This study found increased levels of interleukin-12 in patients with progressive MS compared to controls [7]. How strong is the evidence from physiology studies to support clinical treatment decisions?

There are multiple experiences in which mechanistic explanations have failed to predict outcomes in patients. Trying to answer a question of whether clofibrate in men without clinically evident ischemic heart disease will affect mortality, a before–after physiology study examined the effect of clofibrate on total cholesterol [3]. Patients were given 750–1,500 mg of the drug for 4 weeks after which a significant reduction in total cholesterol level was achieved in 30 out of 35 treated patients. Moreover, the tolerance to the drug was excellent and was not associated with any observed side effects. The positive expectation suggested by these results was shattered by the results of a randomized trial in men randomized to receive either clofibrate or placebo. After a mean follow-up of 9.6 years, the drug increased the risk of death by 25% ($P < 0.05$) despite reducing cholesterol levels and the risk of ischemic heart disease (20%, $P < 0.05$) [4].

Case Reports and Case Series

Case reports describe individual patients who showed an unusual or an unexpected event, either favorable or unfavorable. These cases may lead to new clinical hypotheses and further clinical care research. Furthermore, case reports and case series are extremely useful in documenting rare events, which may have been obscured in other study designs, as we will discuss later. This makes them of particular importance in studies of harm i.e., unwanted events, which could not be readily studied in an intentional manner, or because of their rarity cannot be studied prospectively.

In your literature search, you stumble over a case report describing a 48-year-old woman, similar to your patient, describing complete remission of MS with a dose of 3,800 mg of cyclophosphamide, which interestingly was given accidentally to that patient [5]. At this point, you were impressed with the results of that case report and how it fits with the biological understanding of both the disease and the medication. Because case reports describe individual patients with no comparison, it is difficult to know that this patient improved *because* of this treatment. This makes case reports highly susceptible to erroneous cause and effect inferences and does not protect against possible confounders, including the passage of time (e.g., spontaneous waxing and waning of disease manifestations over time).

You also find a series of five patients with MS who are not responding to multiple treatments [6]. These patients were given monthly pulse intravenous cyclophosphamide at a dose of 1 g/m^2 unlike the treatment described in the case you read previously. The authors conclude that "aggressive immunosuppressive therapy may be useful in some rapidly deteriorating refractory patients and further controlled studies should be considered in order to full evaluate this type of treatment as a potential therapy in MS." Evidence of large treatment effects in patients who have not responded to therapy and who otherwise have stable or deteriorating disease is often compelling, with some residual uncertainty associated with patient expectations (placebo effects), natural history of the disease, and other potential explanations. The search to decrease this residual uncertainty must then continue to ensure that your decision making gains in confidence.

Case-Control Study Design

Case-control studies are best used when conditions are rare and investigators are interested in identifying risk factors for their development. These studies enroll a group of patients with a given outcome or condition. The investigators aim to identify risk factors in a retrospective fashion. These studies identify risk factors as those characteristics that are more common among those with the outcome than in those without the outcome (protective factors can be identified with the inverse association). The key determinants of the validity of these study designs rely on the nature of the comparison group (e.g., do these only differ in their outcome status?), and in the quality of the ascertainment of both exposures and outcomes.

In your patient's medical record you find a history of infectious mononucleosis (IM). You look for studies, which might have reported an association between MS and IM. You find a case-control study of 225 patients with MS and 900 controls matched for age and gender [7]. The researchers compared the mean rates of IM infection per patient in different period of times preceding the onset of MS symptoms. They found that a history of IM was significantly associated with the risk of MS compared to the controls (odds ratio 5.5, 95% CI 1.5, 19.7). This information may help you explain why the patient developed MS. Of interest, observational studies of this nature may have explored many different exposures (a key advantage of case-control studies) and only published the statistically significant associations, some of which may have occurred by chance. Other studies that may have found no association with IM, may not have been published, leaving the reader with the impression that IM *causes* MS. Furthermore, the temporary sequence almost always (perhaps with the exception of genetic risk factors) is difficult to establish such that the risk factor may or may not have occurred prior to the development of the disease, a concern that is further worsened by recall bias. Also, difficult to measure or unexpected risk factors or factors associated with those which were measured or assessed may not be accounted for and as a result these studies could mislead.

Cross-sectional studies seeks coexistence of factors at a point in time and – unlike other observational studies that follow individuals over time – cross-sectional studies report what is present or not at a fixed time period, e.g., prevalence of a condition. Indeed, one of the studies you find is a cross-sectional study of the association between MS-related fatigue and treatment. This study was conducted on 320 patients with MS, of which half of them had a complaint of fatigue [8]. After controlling for several factors, the investigators found no significant association between use of immunosuppressive or immunomodulatory drugs and MS-related fatigue. While these studies suggest that cyclophosphamide may not improve fatigue, you

Table 2.1 Criteria that strengthen causal inferences

Analogy
Plausibility
Consistency
Dose–response
Reversibility
Specificity
Strength
Temporality
Adapted from Hill [9]

must remember that cross-sectional studies do not accurately establish causal relationship between exposures and outcomes with multiple explanations for the presence or absence of association. Consider, for instance the fact that one cannot establish the order in which exposure and outcome occurred when sampling at one point in time – can treatment improve in some patients *and* cause fatigue in others? Can those on treatment report fatigue differently than those on different or no treatment? Studies that follow patients over time may better deal with temporal relationships – it is key to establish that an exposure preceded an outcome in order to make causal inferences. Table 2.1 describes criteria that strengthen causal inferences set forth by Bradford Hill [9].

Cohort Study Designs

A cohort study design, in general, enrolls individuals characterized by their exposure status (as oppose to case-control studies which enroll individuals by their outcome status) and follows them for a period with the expectation that some of them will develop the outcomes of interest. These then allow the investigator to measure the incidence or risk of developing the outcome and compare this risk among those exposed and those unexposed. When the investigator plans the study after the participants have started follow-up, then the cohort study is said to be retrospective (the longitudinal follow-up happened in the past); when the investigator sets up the study before the individuals start follow-up, the cohort study is said to be prospective. The nature of the cohort study, prospective or retrospective, does not determine the quality of the cohort study, although prospective cohort studies offer the investigator greater control over the ascertainment of exposure and outcomes and the opportunity to limit the introduction of bias.

Cohort studies can be setup to follow patients for a long time, which makes them suitable for the study of the natural history of disease and for the detection of uncommon harms of treatment or consequences of disease that occur after long exposures (i.e., postmarketing surveillance). Well-conducted cohort studies may occupy top positions in some hierarchies, as we will discuss later.

Among the many limitations of observational studies is that the exposure (i.e., to the treatment vs. no treatment) occurs by choice rather than by chance. This means that when treatment is associated with outcome, it is not only the treatment but also the reasons the patient received the treatment that are associated with the outcome. For instance, women receiving estrogen were found to have lower cardiovascular risk in prospective cohort studies. Importantly, these women were also of higher socioeconomic status, had better access to healthcare, had healthier habits, and took better care of themselves than women who did not receive estrogen therapy. The ability of these observational studies to account for these factors associated with both treatment and outcome (also known as confounders), was limited and only the randomized trials (which assigned exposure by chance rather than by choice) were able to elucidate the lack of cardiovascular protection afforded by estrogen preparations. Many comparisons have shown, however, that observational studies and randomized controlled trials (RCTs) often agree [10]. The trick here is that sometimes they do not and there is no way to know until the randomized trials are performed.

Two examples vividly reflect the importance of the residual uncertainty that exists when inferences drawn from the results of observational studies (with results supported by strong, often post hoc, biological rationale) go unchecked in a randomized trial. Consider an observational study based on secondary analysis of data obtained from a randomized trial data [11], which found that high-dose aspirin (650–1,300 mg daily) given to patients undergoing carotid endarterectomy was associated with 1.8% risk of perioperative stroke and death compared to 6.9% after low-dose aspirin (0–325 mg daily). Later, the randomized trial showed that high-dose aspirin was associated with an 8.4% risk of stroke, myocardial infarction, or death compared to only 6.2% risk in patients receiving low-dose aspirin ($P=0.03$) [12]. Or consider an observational study assessing the effect of extracranial to intracranial bypass surgery on altering the risk of ischemic stroke, a pre–post examination of 110 patients undergoing the bypass was performed. Stroke rate was 4.3% in 70 patients with transient ischemic attacks undergoing the bypass compared with a rate between 13% and 62% in transient ischemic patients who have not undergone surgery and were reported in other published literature. After a 3-year follow-up of all the 110 patients, stroke rate was 5% [13]. The readers would conclude that extracranial to intracranial bypass led to improvement in the symptoms of all patients. In contrast to this conclusion, an RCT of 1,377 patients studying whether bypass surgery benefits patients with symptomatic atherosclerotic disease of the internal carotid artery, found a 14% increase in the relative risk of stroke in patients undergoing surgery over those treated medically [14].

Randomized Trials

In all previous designs, the exposure was not under the control of the investigator and is thus considered observational. This is in contrast with randomized trials in which investigators randomly assign participants to either intervention or control.

Thus, obligatorily these studies are executed prospectively (making it redundant to describe these as "prospective randomized trials"). A well-conducted trial limits any opportunity for patients, clinicians, or investigators to choose to which arm of the trial the participant will be assigned. This feature (randomization) limits bias by not allowing for selecting patients with different prognosis to go to different trial arms. To protect randomization, trials conceal the allocation sequence from participants and investigators, particularly from investigators assessing the eligibility of patients. The most common form to conceal the allocation sequence is central randomization (by computer or phone, at the pharmacy). Enough participants allow chance to also achieve another goal of randomization (in addition to preventing selection bias), which is to create groups with the same prognosis. This allows the investigators to draw causal inferences linking treatment or control to the different prognoses of these arms at the end of the trial. In addition to having two groups with similar prognosis at baseline, blinding of participants, clinicians, and investigators prevents the introduction of cointerventions that would differ between the arms and offer alternative explanations to the findings of these studies. To preserve this balance in prognosis, it is important that these studies follow the intention to treat principle [15]. This principle states that patients should stay in the arm to which they were randomized throughout the study conduct and analyses. Thus, intention-to-treat trials do not have patients unavailable to ascertain their outcomes (loss to follow-up), do not allow unplanned cross over, and seek to have patients receiving as much of their planned exposure for as long as possible. This will provide an unbiased estimate of the treatment effect.

You find a multicenter, placebo-controlled randomized trial studying the effect of cyclophosphamide and other treatments in patients with MS [16]. After at least 12 months of follow-up, the effects of cyclophosphamide given to MS patients did not statistically differ from patients receiving placebo (35% of treatment failures with cyclophosphamide vs. 29% with placebo). You realize, however, that other randomized trials are available and that they have found different results.

Individual-patient randomized trials can only be used to evaluate the effect of treatment in individual patient with stable conditions for which the candidate treatment can exert a temporary and reversible effect. Individual patient randomized trials (also known as n-of-1 trials) require the clinician and patient to use a random sequence to determine treatment order. The patient starts the trial with either the intervention or a matching placebo prepared by a third party, a pharmacist for example. The patient and clinician record the effect of the intervention and ensure patients go through a random sequence of exposure to treatment or placebo, typically 3 times [2]. At the end of the trial, both the physician and the patient will have evidence to determine whether the intervention was beneficial or not. An example of such a study design was an n-of-1 study conducted with a patient diagnosed with chronic inflammatory demyelinating polyradiculopathy [12]. Although showing initial improvement of symptoms with subsequent remission and relapses, treatment with prednisolone and azathioprine did not stop the slow disease progression. Evaluation of the use of intravenous immunoglobulin (IVIG) was commenced in a blinded placebo-controlled trial with four treatment cycles, consisting of four infusions, two IVIG (0.4 g/kg) and two albumin infusions as placebo. Each infusion was given once every 3 weeks over a period of 48 weeks. The neurological outcomes of interest were time to walk 10 m, maximum number of squats in 30 s, and maximum range of ankle dorsiflexion, all of which failed to find a clear treatment effect.

Systematic Reviews and Meta-analyses

Evidence-based medicine requires that decisions be made taken into account the body of evidence, not just a single study [2]. Thus, clinicians should be most interested in studies that systematically and thoroughly search for studies that would answer a focused review question. Candidate studies are assessed using explicit eligibility criteria and those selected are subject to evaluation regarding the extent to which they are protected from bias. Investigators then systematically extract data from these studies and summarize it. When these summaries involve statistical pooling, we then say that the systematic review included a meta-analysis. Of note, meta-analyses could also be conducted on an arbitrary collection (i.e., biased selection) of studies; thus the key methodological features is that evidence collections are systematic and that assess the quality of the included studies; meta-analyses do not improve the quality of the studies summarized and will also reflect any biases introduced in the study-selection process. Thus, clinicians should not look for meta-analyses but for systematic reviews (preferably those that conduct a meta-analysis).

Systematic reviews offer evidence that is as good as the best available evidence summarized by the review [2]. For example, for a given research question, high-quality systematic reviews including high-quality trials would yield stronger inferences than systematic reviews of lower quality trials or well-conducted observational studies. Stronger inferences will also be drawn when the studies in the review show consistent answers or when the inconsistency can be explained (often through subgroup analyses). Thus, systematic reviews contribute by improving the applicability of the evidence, and through meta-analyses, by increasing the precision of the estimates of treatment effect. What systematic reviews and meta-analyses do not achieve is the amelioration of any biases present in the studies summarized.

Another key limitation of systematic reviews is that they often rely on published evidence. The published record is subject to bias to the extent that some studies get published later or never and in obscure journals depending on their results, a phenomenon called publication bias. To minimize the possibility of publication bias, the reviewers can search thoroughly and systematically and contact experts in the field. When the studies are published but select the outcomes that received full attention in the manuscript on the basis of their results, a similar phenomenon, reporting bias, takes place. To minimize reporting bias, reviewers contact authors of these studies to verify the data collected and to ask for pertinent data that may have been omitted in the original publication.

You found a systematic review of RCTs studying the efficacy of cyclophosphamide in patients with MS [17]. The systematic review in general was well conducted; the search was thorough, study selection and data extraction was done in a duplicate manner, and authors of primary studies were contacted for missing data. The trials included in the study, although randomized, had serious study design limitations. Data regarding the Expanded Disability Status Scale score was extracted from eligible trials to measure the course of the disease. Pooled results showed that, compared to placebo or no treatment, intensive immunosuppression with cyclophosphamide in patients with progressive MS did not significantly prevent progression to long-term disability as defined as evolution to a next step in the disability score. After reading this review, you conclude that cyclophosphamide is not your best treatment option and you start looking for different approaches to treat your patient.

RAND Methodology

This technique is used to combine evidence with expert opinion [18, 19]. It starts by summarizing available evidence addressing a specific issue, usually by conducting systematic reviews. Evidence is then synthesized and distributed to a panel of experts in the field under investigation. The panel members rate predefined indicators first, and then arrange for a face-to-face meeting where deliberations are held. After the meeting, the panel members may change their previous ratings based on the discussions they had.

The strengths of the RAND technique is that it allows panelists to rate indicators based on a systematic summary of the evidence, and that they meet together in order for an open discussion to occur. Potential drawbacks may include possible intimidation of some panel members by more influential members. For practical reasons the panel may not be as large as one would prefer and it would not include patients' participation.

This overview of the different study designs should begin to configure a hierarchy of evidence in the reader's mind. Several elements reviewed here could help configure such a hierarchy: protection against biased inferences of cause and effect, consistency and precision of the estimates, and applicability of the findings. We will now review how the notion of a hierarchy of evidence has evolved. To approach this topic, we will focus mostly on hierarchies for prevention and treatment.

History of the Modern Hierarchy of Evidence

Methodologists, early in the evolution of practice guidelines, thought of designing a guide to different levels of evidence in the form of hierarchies that would link the quality of the evidence to the strength of the recommendations in the guidelines. To our knowledge, the first published modern hierarchy of evidence appeared in the year 1979, authored by the Canadian Task Force on the Periodic Health Examination (Table 2.2) [20].

Table 2.2 The Canadian Task Force's hierarchy of evidence

I.	Evidence obtained from at least one properly RCT.
II-1.	Evidence obtained from well designed cohort or case-control analytic studies, preferably from more than one center or research group.
II-2.	Evidence obtained from comparisons between times or places with or without the intervention. Dramatic results in uncontrolled experiments.
III.	Opinions of respected authorities, based on clinical experience, descriptive studies or reports of expert committees.

Table 2.3 U.S. Preventive Services Task Force's hierarchy of evidence

I.	At least one well-conducted RCT
II-1.	Controlled trials without randomization
II-2.	Well-designed cohort or case-control studies, preferably from multiple sites
II-3.	Multiple time-series with or without intervention
III.	Expert opinion

Adapted from Atkins et al. [21]

Table 2.4 The American College of Chest Physicians' hierarchy of evidence

I.	Evidence from randomized trials with a statistically significant effect.
II.	Evidence from randomized trials with a statistically insignificant effect.
III.	Evidence from nonrandomized concurrent comparisons.
IV.	Evidence from nonrandomized comparisons between current patients who received therapy and former patients.
V.	Evidence from case series without a control group.

This first classification of evidence depended mainly on study design (as a surrogate for the quality of evidence) regardless of the quality of the actual studies. It placed RCT, of any quality, at the top of its hierarchy. It also considered opinions from experts as a level of evidence, though, as we discussed earlier, opinions are not forms of evidence. One can see elements of this first hierarchy in some contemporary ones, including the one used until recently by the US Preventive Services Task Force (Table 2.3) [21–23].

Sackett et al. added to study design the precision of the results (in the hypothesis testing framework) in his hierarchy of evidence in 1989 [24].

When the American College of Chest Physicians drafted its antithrombotic guidelines, they correctly excluded expert opinion as a form of evidence and added meta-analyses (rather than meta-analyses within systematic reviews) to their hierarchy (Table 2.4) [24]. Other hierarchies have used this one as a template (see for instance those by Cook et al., Guyatt et al., and Wilson et al.) [25–28].

In 2000, Guyatt et al. introduced a new hierarchy for studies of therapy (Table 2.5) [1]. For the first time, this hierarchy considered *n*-of-1 trials at the top

Table 2.5 Hierarchy of evidence for treatment decisions

I.	Evidence from n-of-1 randomized trial.
II.	Evidence from systematic reviews of randomized trials.
III.	Evidence from single randomized trials.
IV.	Evidence from systematic reviews of observational studies.
V.	Evidence from single observational studies.
VI.	Evidence from physiological studies.
VII.	Evidence from unsystematic observations.

Table 2.6 The American Academy of Neurology's hierarchy of evidence

I.	Randomized, controlled clinical trial with masked or objective outcome assessment in a representative population. Relevant baseline characteristics are presented and substantially equivalent among treatment groups or there is appropriate statistical adjustment for differences. The following are required: (a) concealed allocation, (b) primary outcome(s) clearly defined, (c) exclusion/inclusion criteria clearly defined, and (d) adequate accounting for drop-outs (with at least 80% of enrolled subjects completing the study) and cross-overs with numbers sufficiently low to have minimal potential for bias.
II.	Prospective matched group cohort study in a representative population with masked outcome assessment that meets b–d above OR a RCT in a representative population that lacks one criteria a–d.
III.	All other controlled trials (including well-defined natural history controls or patients serving as own controls) in a representative population, where outcome is independently assessed, or independently derived by objective outcome measurement.
IV.	Studies not meeting Class I, II or III criteria including: consensus, expert opinion or a case report.

Adapted with permission from the American Academy of Neurology [27]

of the hierarchy. In this hierarchy, systematic reviews of randomized trial and of observational studies were included as separate levels of evidence. These modifications indicate that in addition to bias protection and precision, now applicability (enhanced in both *n*-of-1 trials and systematic reviews) became a guiding principle of these hierarchies.

Different organizations adopted or modified preexisting hierarchies [25]. Others, in addition to evidence of treatment studies, added evidence levels for prognostic, diagnostic, and economic analytic studies [26]. The American Academy of Neurology (ANA) adopted its own classification of evidence (Table 2.6) [27]. ANA classified evidence into four classes (I through IV). RCTs were given the highest level of evidence, but with certain requirements. Expert opinions were included at the bottom of the hierarchy, perpetuating the error of the earlier hierarchies. Again, this hierarchy includes elements of bias protection, precision, and applicability.

The state-of-the-art approach to describe the quality of evidence was recently released by the Grades of recommendation, assessment, development, and evaluation (GRADE) working group. The GRADE system and guidelines will be discussed later in Chap. 3.

Practical Applications

The term evidence-based medicine first appeared in 1991 in an article by Gordon Guyatt in the American College of Physicians' Journal Club [28]. Since then, the concept of practicing and teaching evidence-based medicine has exploded. The fundamental principles of evidence-based medicine are (1) the better the quality of the evidence, the more confident the clinical decision making, and (2) evidence alone does not tell us what to do, but decisions should also incorporate patient preferences and values as well as the patient's clinical and personal context. The central role of the hierarchy of evidence in the practice of evidence-based medicine indicates that it is key when considering policies for clinicians: evidence-based policy makers should rely on the highest quality of evidence.

Professional organizations have embarked on the task of developing clinical practice guidelines to provide helpful recommendations to practicing clinicians, to improve quality of care, and to enhance patient outcomes. By producing guidelines, these organizations seek to emphasize their academic credentials and assert their leadership in areas of primary concern. Given the policy and legal implications of guidelines, state-of-the-art guideline developers should follow rigorous and transparent procedures for formulating recommendations for or against a particular diagnostic or therapeutic intervention [2]. Key to their success is the expectation that clinicians will deliver better care for their patients if they follow guideline recommendations. To achieve this goal, the strongest recommendations should result from considering the highest quality of evidence; the higher the level of evidence, the stronger the recommendations. This can be seen in ANA's classification of recommendations based on the level of evidence into four levels (Table 2.7) [27].

Table 2.7 AAN classification of recommendations for therapeutic intervention[a]

A. Established as effective, ineffective or harmful (or established as useful/predictive or not useful/predictive) for the given condition in the specified population. (Level A rating requires at least two consistent Class I studies.)[b]

B. Probably effective, ineffective or harmful (or probably useful/predictive or not useful/predictive) for the given condition in the specified population. (Level B rating requires at least one Class I study or at least two consistent Class II studies.)

C. Possibly effective, ineffective or harmful (or possibly useful/predictive or not useful/predictive) for the given condition in the specified population. (Level C rating requires at least one Class II study or two consistent Class III studies.)

U. Data inadequate or conflicting; given current knowledge, treatment (test, predictor) is unproven. (Studies not meeting criteria for Class I–Class III.)

Adapted with permission from the American Academy of Neurology [27]
[a]Please refer to Table 2.6 for classification of studies
[b]In exceptional cases, one convincing Class I study may suffice for an "A" recommendation if (1) all criteria are met, (2) the magnitude of effect is large (relative rate improved outcome >5 and the lower limit of the confidence interval is >2)

Conclusion

The recognition of hierarchies of evidence is a key principle of evidence-based medicine. We have discussed here how the need to protect inferences against error has guided the sophistication of the scientific method from unsystematic observations to very large rigorous experiments. We have also reviewed how policy makers have refined the idea of a hierarchy of evidence that initially set forth risk of bias as the sole organizing principle to current strategies that also consider risk of random error (precision), applicability or directness, publication and reporting bias, and consistency in results across studies as additional features of the evidence base to consider. This increased sophistication has set aside reliance of judgments only at the study level moving to making judgments at the "body of evidence" level. Finally, it has also corrected the initial mistake of confusing opinion (of an expert, of a panel, or otherwise) with the observations (evidence) that support such opinions.

It is helpful also to remember that the recognition of hierarchies of evidence is not the only principle of evidence-based medicine. As such, the application of the evidence into clinical decision making and policy making requires consideration of context as well as the values and preferences of the patients because the evidence alone is never sufficient to inform a clinical decision.

References

1. Guyatt GH, Haynes RB, Jaeschke RZ, et al. Users' Guides to the Medical Literature: XXV. Evidence-based medicine: principles for applying the Users' Guides to patient care. Evidence-Based Medicine Working Group. JAMA. 2000;284(10):1290–6.
2. Guyatt G, Rennie D, Meade MO, Cook DJ. User's guide to the medical literature: a manual for evidence-based clinical practice. 2nd ed. London: AMA; 2002.
3. Delcourt R, Vastesaeger M. Action of atromid on total and beta-cholesterol. J Atheroscler Res. 1963;3:533–7.
4. A co-operative trial in the primary prevention of ischaemic heart disease using clofibrate. Report from the Committee of Principal Investigators. Br Heart J. 1978;40(10):1069–118.
5. de Bittencourt PR, Gomes-da-Silva MM. Multiple sclerosis: long-term remission after a high dose of cyclophosphamide. Acta Neurol Scand. 2005;111(3):195–8.
6. Gobbini MI, Smith ME, Richert ND, Frank JA, McFarland HF. Effect of open label pulse cyclophosphamide therapy on MRI measures of disease activity in five patients with refractory relapsing-remitting multiple sclerosis. J Neuroimmunol. 1999;99(1):142–9.
7. Marrie RA, Wolfson C, Sturkenboom MC, et al. Multiple sclerosis and antecedent infections: a case-control study. Neurology. 2000;54(12):2307–10.
8. Putzki N, Katsarava Z, Vago S, Diener HC, Limmroth V. Prevalence and severity of multiple-sclerosis-associated fatigue in treated and untreated patients. Eur Neurol. 2008;59(3–4): 136–42.
9. Hill AB. The environment and disease: association or causation? Proc R Soc Med. 1965;58:295–300.
10. Benson K, Hartz AJ. A comparison of observational studies and randomized, controlled trials. N Engl J Med. 2000;342(25):1878–86.
11. Taylor DW, Barnett HJ, Haynes RB, et al. Low-dose and high-dose acetylsalicylic acid for patients undergoing carotid endarterectomy: a randomised controlled trial. ASA and Carotid Endarterectomy (ACE) Trial Collaborators. Lancet. 1999;353(9171):2179–84.

12. Hankey GJ, Todd AA, Yap PL, Warlow CP. An "n of 1" trial of intravenous immunoglobulin treatment for chronic inflammatory demyelinating polyneuropathy. J Neurol Neurosurg Psychiatry. 1994;57(9):1137.

13. Popp AJ, Chater N. Extracranial to intracranial vascular anastomosis for occlusive cerebrovascular disease: experience in 110 patients. Surgery. 1977;82(5):648–54.

14. Failure of extracranial-intracranial arterial bypass to reduce the risk of ischemic stroke. Results of an international randomized trial. The EC/IC Bypass Study Group. N Engl J Med. 1985;313(19):1191–200.

15. Montori VM, Guyatt GH. Intention-to-treat principle. CMAJ. 2001;165(10):1339–41.

16. The Canadian cooperative trial of cyclophosphamide and plasma exchange in progressive multiple sclerosis. The Canadian Cooperative Multiple Sclerosis Study Group. Lancet. 1991;337(8739): 441–6.

17. La Mantia L, Milanese C, Mascoli N, D'Amico R, Weinstock-Guttman B. Cyclophosphamide for multiple sclerosis. Cochrane Database Syst Rev. 2007(1):CD002819.

18. Brook RH, Chassin MR, Fink A, Solomon DH, Kosecoff J, Park RE. A method for the detailed assessment of the appropriateness of medical technologies. Int J Technol Assess Health Care. 1986;2(1):53–63.

19. Campbell SM, Braspenning J, Hutchinson A, Marshall M. Research methods used in developing and applying quality indicators in primary care. Qual Saf Health Care. 2002;11(4):358–64.

20. The periodic health examination. Canadian Task Force on the Periodic Health Examination. Can Med Assoc J. 1979;121(9):1193–254.

21. Atkins D, Eccles M, Flottorp S, et al. Systems for grading the quality of evidence and the strength of recommendations I: critical appraisal of existing approaches The GRADE Working Group. BMC Health Serv Res. 2004;4(1):38.

22. Harris RP, Helfand M, Woolf SH, et al. Current methods of the US Preventive Services Task Force: a review of the process. Am J Prev Med. 2001;20(3 Suppl):21–35.

23. Woolf SH, Battista RN, Anderson GM, Logan AG, Wang E. Assessing the clinical effectiveness of preventive maneuvers: analytic principles and systematic methods in reviewing evidence and developing clinical practice recommendations. A report by the Canadian Task Force on the Periodic Health Examination. J Clin Epidemiol. 1990;43(9):891–905.

24. Sackett DL. Rules of evidence and clinical recommendations on the use of antithrombotic agents. Chest. 1989;95(2 Suppl):2S–4.

25. Guyatt G, Schunemann H, Cook D, Jaeschke R, Pauker S, Bucher H. Grades of recommendation for antithrombotic agents. Chest. 2001;119(1 Suppl):3S–7.

26. Oxford Centre for Evidence-based Medicine Levels of Evidence. http://www.cebm.net/index. aspx?o=1025. Accessed Feb 2009.

27. Edlund W, Gronseth G, So Y, Franklin G. Clinical practice guideline process manual, 2004 Edition, Appendix 9. The American Academy of Neurology. http://www.aan.com/globals/axon/assets/3749.pdf. Accessed Feb 2009.

28. Guyatt G. Evidence-based medicine. ACP J Club (Ann Intern Med). 1991;114(Suppl 2):A-16.

Chapter 3
Guidelines: Rating the Quality of Evidence and Grading the Strength of Recommendations

Yngve Falck-Ytter and Gordon H. Guyatt

Keywords Quality of evidence • Strength of recommendation • Rating • Grading • Guidelines • Methodology • Evidence-based medicine

Introduction

Clinical experts and organizations providing recommendations in the form of clinical practice guidelines have not always carefully considered the quality of the available evidence [1]. For decades, dose-adjusted i.v. unfractionated heparin was routinely recommended and administered to patients with acute stroke despite the lack of evidence for a long-term reduction in unfavorable outcomes. In 2002, the American Academy of Neurology (AAN) Guideline Development Committee finally called for an end to this practice [2].

The proliferation of guidelines over the last decade has provided welcome assistance to practitioners – as well as patients and policy makers – in decision making about appropriate health care. Still, for clinicians to most effectively apply guideline recommendations to patient care requires an understanding of the underlying evidence and the trade-offs between benefits and downsides (harms, burden, and cost). However, the variability in quality of clinical practice guidelines has compromised their possible positive impact on clinical practice. Of particular importance is their clarity and explicitness. Increasingly, guideline authors realize that providing graded recommendations helps them succeed in delivering a consistent message that clinicians find useful.

Y. Falck-Ytter (✉)
Department of Medicine, Case and VA Medical Center,
Case Western Reserve University, 10701 East Blvd.,
Cleveland 44106, OH, USA
e-mail: yngve.falck-ytter@case.edu

J.G. Burneo et al. (eds.), *Neurology: An Evidence-Based Approach*,
DOI 10.1007/978-0-387-88555-1_3, © Springer Science+Business Media, LLC 2012

It is, therefore, not surprising that a large number of evidence rating schemes have been developed. Almost all are based on a hierarchy of clinical study designs (with randomized controlled trials (RCTs) or meta-analysis on top and case series or observations of experts at the bottom), usually as the sole basis to determine whether the evidence is high or of low quality. The proliferation of grading systems [3, 4] has confused health care providers, consumers, and policy makers. For instance, consulting international guidelines whether patients with rheumatic mitral valve disease and atrial fibrillation should use long-term warfarin treatment for stroke prevention, clinicians face an array of letters and numbers: the American Heart Association (AHA) rates the evidence as "B" and its recommendation is "Class I" [5]; the Scottish Intercollegiate Guideline Network (SIGN) rates the evidence as "IV" and its recommendation is "C" [6]; and the American College of Chest Physician (ACCP) rates the evidence as "A" and its recommendation is "1" [7]. Because a common and systematic approach to rating the quality of evidence and strength of management recommendations has the potential to minimize bias and aid interpretation in the development of guidelines, this chapter illustrates recent developments in this area.

At the outset, the Grades of Recommendation, Assessment, Development and Evaluation (GRADE) working group conducted a review [8] of existing grading systems. The review found that no single system was completely satisfactory. The five most important shortcomings were the following:

- *The lack of a distinct separation between quality of evidence and strength of recommendation*: Almost always, highest level of evidence automatically meant highest grade of recommendations.
- *The lack of explicit criteria how the overall quality of evidence is rated across outcomes*: The overall evidence level was based on the anticipated benefit only, often ignoring the quality of evidence for risks.
- *The lack of transparency about judgments*: Most of the time, the evidence systems were not explicit about when, why, and to what extent the level of evidence had to be adjusted for methodological shortcomings, size of effect, or precision.
- *The lack of balancing expected benefits as well as downsides in the rating process*: Rating the strength of a recommendation falls short if only the expected benefits but not all downsides are considered.
- *The lack of explicit acknowledgement of values and preferences*: Past systems did not explicitly consider patient's values and preferences as factors in the formulation of recommendations.

Understanding the variety of flawed systems to which neurologists are exposed is neither an efficient nor realistic use of clinicians' time. Abandoning formal schemes to grade the quality of evidence and strength of recommendations is, however, problematic. Clinicians need concise summaries to tell them whether recommendations are strong or weak. Moreover, medicine faces major challenges that stem from the introduction of pay-for-performance schemes that require criteria for what constitutes acceptable performance. Developing these criteria involves decisions regarding both quality of evidence and the balance of desirable and undesirable consequences of alternative management strategies.

A universal, methodologically sound, and widely accepted methodology to support guideline development could help to lay the framework for international collaboration and to effectively use limited resources [9]. The GRADE working group aims to achieve just that. The GRADE approach is simple, yet methodologically sound [10–13]. It has been adopted by a large number of organizations, such as the ACCP, the WHO, the American College of Physicians, the American Thoracic Society, the American Endocrine Society, UpToDate, the Cochrane Collaboration, and many other international organizations (for a full list and additional information on GRADE, see http://www.gradeworkinggroup.org/).

Grading Recommendations in Guidelines

A separation of quality of evidence and strength of recommendations recognizes that although the underlying quality of evidence usually (though not always) has a defining influence on the strength of recommendation, the magnitude of benefits versus downsides (harms, inconvenience, and cost) is at least equally important. For instance, symptomatic patients with 50–69% carotid stenosis may benefit from carotid endarterectomy with a number needed to treat of 22 to prevent one ipsilateral stroke over 5 years, but at a cost of perioperative morbidity and mortality with a number needed to harm of 14 for perioperative stroke or death within 30 days [14]. Because patients have different values and preferences and, therefore, see the trade-off differently, the close balance between desirable and undesirable consequences precludes, despite the high-quality evidence, a strong recommendation for or against carotid endarterectomy in these patients.

GRADE classifies recommendations either as strong or weak. The strength of recommendations is a continuum; nevertheless, ease of understanding, ease of implementation, and clearly defined implications associated with only two grades of recommendations make this dichotomy useful (Table 3.1).

The strength of a recommendation reflects the extent to which we can, across the range of patients for whom the recommendations are intended, be confident that desirable effects (such as a reduction of morbidity and mortality or improvement in quality of life) of a management strategy outweigh undesirable effects (such as treatment risks, burdens, and cost). In selecting a strong recommendation for an intervention, we are confident that almost all patients, fully informed, would choose to undergo treatment. In general, strong recommendations are appropriate if high-quality evidence that provides precise estimates of benefits as well as downsides is available. However, an unequivocal balance in favor (or against, for that matter) of the benefit compared to the downsides is also crucial in defining a recommendation as strong.

If evidence is of low or very low quality and uncertainty regarding the magnitude (or even the presence) of benefits and harms exists, strong recommendations are seldom warranted. In addition, whether or not evidence is of high or low quality, a close balance between desirable and undesirable consequences mandates a weak recommendation. Table 3.2 summarizes the four factors that guideline panels must consider in deciding whether a recommendation is strong or weak.

Table 3.1 GRADE's binary classification of strength of recommendations provides clear direction to patients, clinicians, and policy makers

Strength of recommendation	Implications		
	For patients	For clinicians	For policy makers
Strong	Most individuals in this situation would want the recommended course of action and only a small proportion would not Formal decision aids are not likely to be needed to help individuals make decisions consistent with their values and prefer-ences, but could help with implementation	Most individuals should receive the intervention There is no need to spend time ascertaining if the recommendation is consistent with patients' values and preferences	The recommendation can be adopted as policy in most situations Adherence to this recommendation according to the guideline could be used as a quality criterion or performance indicator
Weak	The majority of individuals in this situation would want the suggested course of action, but many would not Decision aids may be useful in helping individuals make decisions consistent with their values and preferences	Examine the evidence or a summary of the evidence yourself Work with patients to ensure that decisions are consistent with their values and preferences	Policy making requires substan-tial debates and involvement of many stakeholders

Table 3.2 Factors that affect the strength of a recommendation

Factor	Examples that are likely to lead to strong recommendations	Examples that are likely to lead to weak recommendations
Quality of evidence	Many high-quality randomized trials have demonstrated a mortality reduction of statins in patients at risk for stroke	Only case series have examined the utility of a ketogenic diet for the treatment of epilepsy
Uncertainty about the balance between desirable and undesirable effects	Penicillin for the treatment of meningococcal infections is highly effective with acceptable undesirable effects and relatively low cost	Warfarin in low-risk patients with atrial fibrillation results in small stroke reduction but increased bleeding risk and substantial inconvenience
Uncertainty or variability in values and preferences	Younger patients with mesial temporal sclerosis and temporal lobe epilepsy place a higher value on seizure control offered by surgery over treatment risks	Older patients with mesial temporal sclerosis and temporal lobe epilepsy may not place a higher value on seizure control offered by surgery over treatment risks
Uncertainty about whether the intervention represents a wise use of resources	The low cost of aspirin as prophylaxis against stroke in patients with transient ischemic attacks	The high cost of clopidogrel and of combination dipyridamole and aspirin as prophylaxis against stroke in patients with transient ischemic attacks

Performance measures are increasingly used to guide clinicians in best care practices. GRADE provides clear guidance in choosing performance measures: only strong recommendations are candidates. When evidence is of lower quality or benefits and downsides are more closely balanced, performance measures must focus on whether clinicians have ensured that the chosen treatment is consistent with the patient's values and preferences.

Rating the Quality of Evidence

Sources of evidence to guide recommendations are diverse and may include basic science research to case reports, observational evidence, and randomized, controlled trials. Interpreting such a wide variety of evidence can be challenging.

For example, considerable epidemiological evidence from large, prospective cohort studies demonstrates that a 25% lower blood homocysteine level is associated with a 19% lower risk of stroke [15]. The perception that treatment with vitamin B_{12} and folate not only effectively lowers homocysteine levels, but would also have virtually no readily apparent downsides, sparked early and wide adoption of vitamin supplementation to lower the risk of cardiovascular events. Some authors suggest an 80% reduction in cardiovascular disease by combining folate with other established medications in the form of a "Polypill" [16]. However, several large, well-designed, randomized, controlled trials, including VISP [17], NORVIT [18], and more recently WENBIT [19] and the WAFACS [20], have failed to show any effect of vitamin B supplementation in the prevention of cardiovascular events. Moreover, vitamin supplementation, such as folate, may lead to an increased risk of advanced colorectal neoplasia [21].

GRADE is about supporting an informed choice between two clinical management options. It is, therefore, helpful to frame the clinical question accordingly and the PICO approach has been proven successful: "P" for population with a certain condition; "I" for the intervention in question; "C" for the comparison (which may be to do nothing (or placebo) or usual care or an alternate management approach); and "O" for outcomes. Once all focused clinical questions for a particular recommendation have been clearly defined, it is useful to categorize those outcomes as critically important or important, but not critical for decision making.

GRADE is not about rating the quality of individual studies. Rather, GRADE is outcomes-centric, and the quality of evidence is always rated for each outcome across all available studies. Evidence should be summarized in rigorous systematic reviews that provide summary estimates for inclusion in GRADE evidence profiles (Table 3.3 shows an example of such a profile).

GRADE defines quality of evidence as our confidence in the estimates of effect – whether benefit or downsides – to support management decisions. Although quality of evidence is a continuum, a finite number of levels of quality have the advantage of increased clarity and simplicity. The GRADE system places evidence into one of four categories: high, moderate, low, or very low. The GRADE quality of evidence rating process starts with an assessment of study design and then moves the quality rating down – or up – according to a number of other criteria. For management

Table 3.3 GRADE Evidence Profiles

GRADE Evidence Profile

Author(s): Holger Schünemann

Date: 4/28/2006

Question: Should warfarin vs placebo or no treatment be used for patients with nonvvular atrial fibrillation?

Patient or population: Patients with nonvvular atrial fibrillation

Settings: Long-term outpatient management

Systematic review: Aguilar and Hart[33] and Van Walraven et al[34]

Quality assessment						Summary of findings		Effect			
						No of patients					
No of studies	Design	Limitations	Consistency	Directness	Other considerations	Warfarin	Placebo or no treatment	Relative (95% CI)	Absolute (95% CI)	Quality	Importance
Disabling or fatal stroke (ischemic and hemorrhagic) (Neuroimaging or autopsy[a] follow-up: Mean: 1.5 years)											
5	Randomized trials	No limitations[b,c]	No important inconsistency	No uncertainty	Strong association[d]	18/1,154 (1.6%)	39/1,159 (3.4%)	RR 0.46 (0.27–0.81)	20/1,000 (30 fewer/ 1,000–10 fewer/1,000)	⊕⊕⊕⊕ High	9[e]
Intracranial hemorrhage (Clinical diagnosis confirmed by CT or postmortem follow-up: Mean follow-up: 1.5 years)											
5	Randomized trials	No limitations	No important inconsistency	No uncertainty	Imprecise or sparse data (−1)[f]	5/1,154 (0.4%)	2/1,159 (0.2%)	RR 1.87 (0.51–6.82)	3/1,000 (0 more/ 1,000–10 more/1,000)	⊕⊕⊕○ Moderate	8
Extracranial hemorrhage (Transfusion or invasive procedure requirement[g] follow-up: 1.9 years)[b]											
6	Randomized trials	No limitations[b]	No important inconsistency	No uncertainty	None	85/1,939 (4.4%)	52/2,113 (2.6%)	RR 1.71 (1.21–2.41)	18 more/ 1,000 (1 more/ 1,000–30 more/1,000)	⊕⊕⊕⊕ High	7

All cause mortality[i,j] (Direct patient follow-up: 1.5 years)

| 5 | Randomized trials[k] | No limitations | No important inconsistency | No uncertainty | None | 69/1,225 (5.6%) | 99/1,236 (8%) | RR 0.70 (0.52–0.95) | 20/1,000 (40 fewer–1 fewer/1,000) | ⊕⊕⊕⊕ High | 9 |

Vascular death[l] (Death due to stroke, heart disease, and hemorrhage and sudden death follow-up: 1.5 years)

| 5 | Randomized trials[k] | No limitations | No important inconsistency | No uncertainty | None | 43/1,154 (3.7%) | 51/1,159 (4.4%) | RR 0.85 (0.57–1.26) | 1/1,000 (3 fewer/ 1,000–1 more/ 1,000) | ⊕⊕⊕⊕ High | 9 |

All ischemic stroke (Neuroimaging or autopsy[a,m] follow-up: 1.5 years)

| 5 | Randomized trials[b,n] | No limitations | No important inconsistency | No uncertainty | Strong association (+1)[o] | 22/1,154 (1.9%) | 69/1,159 (6%) | RR 0.32 (0.20–0.51) | 40/1,000 (60 fewer/ 1,000–20 fewer/1,000) | ⊕⊕⊕⊕ High | 7 |

[a]Follow-up for this outcome was less than 100%

[b]In two studies (CAFA; SPINAF), patients and outcome assessors were blind to OAC administration while in the remaining trials, treatment was given open label with outcomes verified by those unaware of treatment assignment

[c]Loss to follow-up not reported in AFASAK I and CAFA, ranged from 0 to 3% in other studies

[d]Strong association present: RR 0.46

[e]Importance is rated on a scale from 1 to 9. 1 represents least important (not important for decision making) and 9 most important (for decision making)

[f]Only 17 events in the OAC and 16 events in the control group

[g]Required transfusion of two or more units of red blood cells, hospitalization, or invasive procedures to control bleeding, and those that resulted in death or permanent functional impairment (e.g., blindness) were included

[h]Data from systematic review by van Walraven (control is aspirin therapy)

[i]All cause mortality: Death from any cause (vascular and nonvascular) within 30 days from onset of stroke symptoms. For this outcome, results of published data, which included about 6% of patients with prior stroke or TIA, were used

[j]From Fig. 10 of Aguilar and Hart

[k]Lack of blinding in two trials of lesser concern

[l]The diagnosis of MI was usually based upon electrocardiographic changes, elevation of enzymes or postmortem examination. These consisted of death due to stroke, heart disease and hemorrhage and sudden deaths of unknown cause

[m]Ischemic stroke was an identified outcome in all trials, with the ischemic nature confirmed by neuroimaging or autopsy in the majority of cases

[n]Methodological quality was not downgraded because the lack of blinding in some studies did not have important impact on the results

[o]Strong association present: RR 0.32

Guyatt G, Rennie D, Meade M, Cook D. Users' Guides to the Medical Literature: essentials of Evidence-Based Clinical Practice. 2nd edition (JAMA and Archives Journals). McGraw-Hill. Professional, 2008.

Table 3.4 Grading the quality of evidence for each important outcome. Has the outcome been studied in randomized controlled trials or observational studies?

a) Evidence from **randomized controlled trials**: Start as high quality, then rate down to moderate, low or very low quality

Check list:	*What to look for:*
Study limitations	Major limitations, such as lack of allocation concealment, lack of blinding, large loss of follow-up, no intention-to-treat analysis, and terminated early for benefit
Inconsistency of results	Widely differing estimates of the treatment effect (variability in results or heterogeneity)
Indirectness of evidence	Indirect comparisons: e.g., no head to head comparison of two interventions
	Population: e.g., differences in age, gender, medical condition
	Intervention: e.g., differences in dose, alternative agent in same class
	Comparator: e.g., differences in dose of the active comparator
	Outcomes: e.g., use of surrogates, short-term vs. long-term
Imprecision	Wide confidence intervals / small sample size / few events that make the result uninformative
Publication bias	High probability of failure to report studies (usually because no effect was observed)

b) Evidence from **observational studies**: Start as low quality, then rate up to moderate or high quality

Check list:	*What to look for:*
Large magnitude of effect	RR > 2 or RR< 0.5
	Two or more observational studies, direct evidence, no plausible confounders, no threats to validity, sufficiently precise estimate
Very large magnitude of effect	RR > 5 or RR< 0.2
	Two or more observational studies, direct evidence, no plausible confounders, no threats to validity, sufficiently precise estimate
Dose-response	Presence of a dose-response gradient, (e.g., between INR and risk of gastrointestinal bleeding in patients on warfarin for stroke prevention)
Plausible confounders	Unaccounted, plausible biases from observational evidence that moves the result in the direction of underestimating the apparent treatment effect

RR = relative risk, INR = international normalized ratio

decisions (whether it is a procedure, medication, or a clinical management question that involve a test, such as a screening question), RCTs provide, in general, significantly stronger evidence than observational studies. Well-designed cohort and case-control studies provide stronger evidence than uncontrolled case series. There are five additional factors that guideline panels need to consider in determining the final quality of evidence for each outcome (Table 3.4).

Rating the Quality of the Evidence: Rating Quality Down

Methodology limitations: When assessing the quality of evidence, serious methodological flaws in the design and execution of RCTs, such as lack of allocation concealment; losses to follow-up that are large in relationship to the event rate; failure to adhere to the intention-to-treat analysis; as well as stopping early for benefit may lead to rating down the quality of evidence. Lack of blinding constitutes another important threat to validity. For instance, Noseworthy and colleagues elegantly demonstrated in the Canadian cooperative trial of cyclophosphamide, prednisone, and plasma exchange to improve the outcome of multiple sclerosis that the apparent significant treatment effect was eliminated when outcome assessors were sufficiently blinded to the treatment assignment [22]. When utilizing Cochrane reviews as an evidence source, the new Cochrane risk of bias tool is helpful in the judgment whether study limitations are present.

Inconsistency of results: Our confidence in the estimate of benefits and downsides is lower if studies show large differences in estimates of the magnitude of and/or direction of effect (heterogeneity). For example, a recent Cochrane systematic review compared surgical endarterectomy with endovascular treatment in symptomatic carotid artery stenosis [23]. Although the safety analysis showed no difference in neurological or vascular complications or death within 30 days of surgery, there were large differences in the direction and magnitude of effect of the included trials. This significant heterogeneity of trial results would likely lead to rating down the quality of the evidence from high to moderate (Fig. 3.1).

Indirectness of evidence: The quality of evidence is lower when comparing the efficacy of two interventions if no head-to-head trials exist (e.g., trials have compared duloxetine versus placebo and pregabalin versus placebo in diabetic peripheral neuropathic pain, but no direct comparisons between the two drugs are available); if the study population is very different to the patients in question (e.g., we may be interested in treating patients with alcoholic cirrhosis and seizures, but efficacy trials of a new antiepileptic drug excluded patients with cirrhosis); if the intervention differs (e.g., we want to know about levetiracetam as a treatment of refractory status epilepticus, but available randomized trials have only used older antiepileptic drugs); if the comparator differs (e.g., we are interested in less neurological adverse effects of newer neuroleptic agents, but the comparator was only fixed high-dose (20 mg) haloperidol – not a dose that is usually used in practice); or the outcome differs from that in which we are interested (e.g., surrogate outcomes, such as carotid intima-media thickness on ultrasound instead of cardiovascular events in studies of lipid-lowering agents for stroke prevention).

Imprecision: When studies include few patients and few events and thus have wide confidence intervals, the quality of the evidence is lower because of resulting uncertainty in the results. For example, a well-designed and rigorously conducted RCT addressed the use of nadroparin, a low-molecular-weight heparin, in patients with cerebral venous sinus thrombosis [24]. Of 30 treated patients, four had a poor outcome, as did six of 29 patients in the control group. The investigators' analysis suggests a 36% relative risk reduction of a poor outcome, but the result was not statistically significant.

Publication bias: The quality of evidence may be downgraded if there is good evidence that trials may not have been reported (typically, those that show no effect).

Study or subgroup	Endovascular n/N	Surgery n/N	Odds Ratio M-H,Random,95% CI	Weight	Odds Ratio M-H,Random,95% CI
BACASS 2006	0/10	1/10		6.8 %	0.30 [0.01. 8.33]
CAVATAS-CEA 2001	28/252	73/253		22.5 %	0.31 [0.19. 0.50]
EVA-3S 2006	53/265	33/262		22.5 %	1.73 [1.08. 2.78]
Kentucky 2004	23/53	9/51		20.0 %	3.58 [1.45. 8.82]
Leicester 1998	5/11	0/12		7.7 %	21.15 [1.01. 445.00]
SAPPHIRE 2004	10/167	17/167		20.6 %	0.56 [0.25. 1.27]
Total (95% CI)	**758**	**755**		**100.0 %**	**1.16 [0.41, 3.24]**

Total events: 119 (Endovascular). 133 (Surgery)
Heterogeneity: Tau^2 = 1.17; Chi^2 = 41.46, df = 5 (P<0.00001): I^2 =88%
Test for overall effect: Z = 0.28 (P = 0.78)

0.01   0.1   1   10   100
Favours endovascular   Favours surgery

Fig. 3.1 Death or neurological or vascular complications within 30 days of treatment of symptomatic stenosis with either endovascular treatment or surgical endarterectomy. From [23]. Reprinted with kind permission from BMJ Publishing Group Ltd

This can be seen, for example, in situations where only small trials are available, all of which are industry funded. A collection of evidence for a particular outcome can suffer from more than one of these limitations, and the greater the limitations, the lower the quality of the evidence. When systematic reviews of randomized trials uncover serious limitations in three or more of these areas, very low quality of evidence would result.

Rating the Quality of the Evidence: Rating Quality Up

When several well-done observational studies yield large or very large, consistent and precise estimates of treatment effects, we may be confident that a substantial treatment effect exists. While observational studies are at risk of overestimating (usually) or underestimating (less common) the true effect and when effects are very large and the observational studies are well-done, bias is unlikely to explain the apparent effect. Thus, despite the general lower quality of evidence from observational studies, under these circumstances we are confident that the effect exists.

Table 3.4 shows how the magnitude of the effect in these studies may move the assigned quality of evidence from low to moderate or, on rare occasions, to high. For instance, a meta-analysis of observational studies showed that bicycle helmets reduce the risk of head injuries in cyclists by a large margin (odds ratio 0.31, 95% CI 0.26–0.37) [25]. This large effect suggests that rating up to moderate-quality evidence is reasonable. An even larger effect was found in a meta-analysis of 37 observational studies evaluating the impact of warfarin prophylaxis in cardiac valve replacement: The relative risk for thromboembolism with warfarin was 0.17 (95% CI 0.13–0.24) [26] – a very large effect, justifying rating up the quality of evidence from low to high.

On occasion, all plausible, residual biases in observational data may be moving the result in the direction to underestimate an apparent treatment effect. For example, a rigorous systematic review of observational studies, including a total of 38 million patients, demonstrated higher death rates in private-for-profit versus private-not-for-profit hospitals [27]. One conceivable confounder relates to different disease severity in patients in the two hospital types. It is likely, however, that patients in the not-for-profit hospitals were sicker than those in the for-profit hospitals. Thus, to the extent that residual confounding existed, it would bias results against the not-for-profit hospitals. In addition, because for-profit hospitals are likely to admit a larger proportion of well-insured patients than not-for-profit hospitals, the less well-insured patients may benefit from a "spillover" effect of resources available to the well-insured; the bias is once again against the not-for-profit hospitals. Since these plausible confounders would all reduce the demonstrated treatment effect, the true effect could potentially be even larger and one might consider the evidence from these observational studies as moderate rather than low quality.

Another reason for rating up the quality of evidence from observational studies is the presence of a dose–response gradient. For instance, result from observational studies show that the higher the international normalized ratio (INR) values the higher the risk of bleeding in patients on warfarin. The observed dose–response gradient between the INR and the risk of hemorrhage increases our confidence in the causal relation between warfarin and bleeding, and rating up the quality of evidence may be justified [28].

Defining the Overall Quality of Evidence Across Outcomes

Recommendations are usually informed by a body of evidence that includes several studies that address each of the outcomes in question. Traditionally, guideline developers have not explicitly addressed how to arrive at an overall quality of evidence when the quality differs across important outcomes. In the past, guideline developers have usually based the overall quality of evidence on the primary beneficial outcome alone. However, since treatment decisions should be based on a balance between benefits and risks of an intervention, and quality of evidence regarding harms may be low, this one-dimensional approach becomes problematic. For example, the AAN recommends natalizumab monotherapy as effective treatment for patients with relapsing–remitting multiple sclerosis ("Class I – Level A") because two randomized controlled trials have shown its efficacy and large treatment effect [29]. The quality of evidence on the risk of developing progressive multifocal leukoencephalopathy (PML) as a result of natalizumab treatment is less clear and because only case reports exist, the evidence of harm is of moderate quality. A guideline panel should consider an overall quality of evidence that reflects this lower-quality evidence. The GRADE system, therefore, specifies that the overall quality of evidence is based on the lowest quality of evidence of all outcomes that are critical for decision making. If the outcome for which evidence is of lower quality is important but not critical, the GRADE approach suggests an overall rating reflecting the higher-quality evidence from the critical outcomes.

Presentation of Summary Results

To aid guideline panels in producing a comprehensive, but condensed, display of all relevant evidence related to a clinical question, the working group has developed GRADE evidence profiles (see Table 3.3). These evidence profiles contain all important outcomes necessary for clinical decision making, including detailed evaluation of the study quality by outcome (across studies) and the associated relative and absolute effects. These profiles can then be used by guideline developers to develop recommendations. The example (see Table 3.3) from the management of atrial fibrillation with oral vitamin K antagonists show how guideline panelists might work through the issues that influence the quality of evidence and strength of a recommendation.

Applying GRADE

If high-quality RCTs are available, additional results from observational studies are not likely to increase our confidence in the true effect of that intervention. However, not infrequently, high-quality data regarding efficacy from RCTs does not include sufficiently precise estimates of associated risks and/or downsides. In these situations, well-done observational trials may contribute valuable information regarding those undesirable effects. On occasion, even putative harms from only a few observations may need to be included if the underlying biology is compelling. For example, only five patients out of over 20,000 patients treated with natalizumab have developed PML, but because the postulated mechanism of effect of natalizumab makes the occurrence of certain infections more likely, these rare but plausible events become important.

Values and Preferences

Given that the choice between two treatment options always demonstrates advantages and disadvantages, how a guideline panel values benefits, risks, and other downsides is critical to any recommendation. If guideline authors are uncertain about or find evidence of large variability of values and preferences regarding the relative desirability (or undesirability) of particular outcomes, the strength of a recommendation may be downgraded from strong to weak. Unfortunately, a paucity of studies has carefully examined patients' values and preferences. However, some

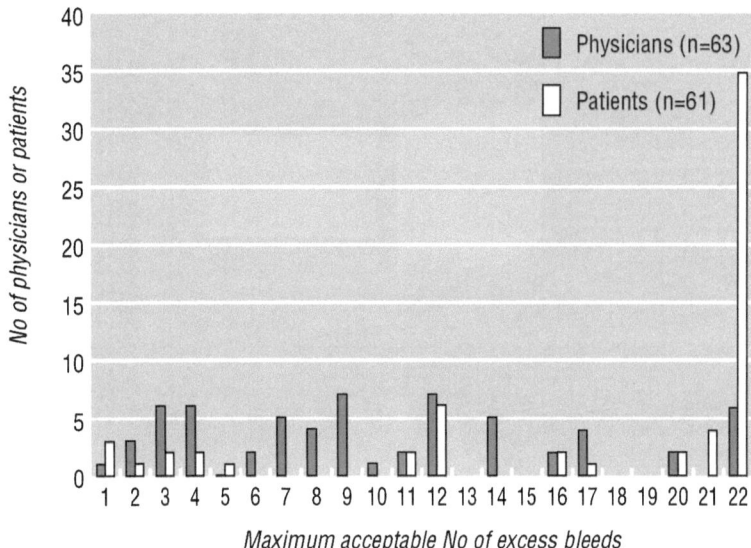

Fig. 3.2 Varying thresholds of major gastrointestinal bleeding found acceptable by patients and physicians for the prevention of eight strokes in 100 patients (From Devereaux et al. [30]. Reprinted from British Medical Journal with kind permission from BMJ Publishing Group Ltd.)

data is available and clinicians' experience with patients may provide additional insight. For example, the use of warfarin may reduce the risk of stroke in patients with nonvalvular atrial fibrillation by approximately 65%, but at the expense of an increased risk of major gastrointestinal (GI) bleeding. A study by Devereaux et al. [30] investigated the number of GI bleeds 61 patients and 63 physicians would tolerate in a theoretical population of 100 patients and still be willing to take or prescribe warfarin to prevent eight strokes (four minor and four major) in those patients. Figure 3.2 shows that, while physicians gave a wide variety of responses, most patients placed a high value on avoiding a stroke and were ready to accept a bleeding risk of 22% to reduce their chances of having a stroke by 8%. Nevertheless, because of the variability in values and preferences among the patients, these data suggest that only in patients at high risk of stroke would a strong recommendation for warfarin treatment be warranted.

Resource Use

Recommendations inevitably involve judgments about the allocation of resources, judgments commonly referred to as costs. Because cost can be extremely different depending on the health care setting, resource use questions are always addressed after all other factors have been considered. Because the judgment of the quality of

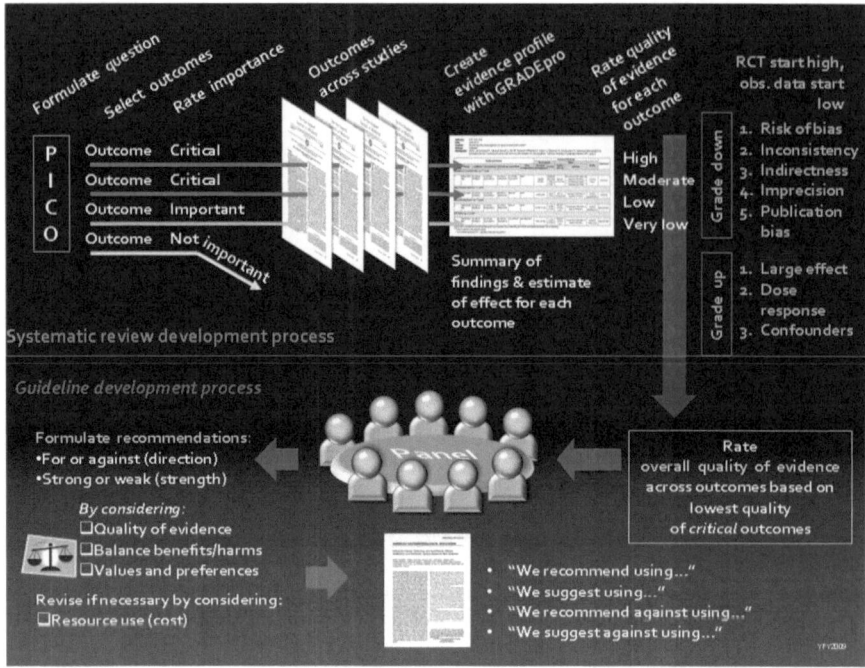

Fig. 3.3 Summary of the GRADE rating process: Starting by formulating a PICO question (PICO = patients, intervention, comparison, outcomes) to the selection of important outcomes; the extraction of study outcomes from systematic reviews; the creation of GRADE evidence profiles that display the quality of evidence rating for each outcome; to the rating of the overall quality of evidence across all critically important outcomes; to the formulation of recommendations by considering the quality of evidence, balance of benefit and downsides, as well as values and preferences and resource use

evidence of studies that deal with resource use adds additional layers of complexity, readers interested in further guidance should refer to other publications by the GRADE working group [31].

Wording of Guidelines

When guideline authors disseminate their findings, the appropriate choice of words may become important. For example, a recent AAN guideline makes the following recommendation: "Prolonged courses of antibiotics do not improve the outcome of post-Lyme syndrome, are potentially associated with adverse events, and are therefore not recommended (Level A recommendation)" [32]. Since clinical practice guidelines are intended for typical patients, clinicians may interpret this statement as: "Although the use of antibiotics is not recommended in this situation, as long as I tell this to my patient who is demanding the antibiotics, it is probably ok to treat."

Alternatively, GRADE recommends using a standardized way to express strong and weak recommendations for or against an intervention, such as: "We recommend to use ..." or "we recommend against the use of ..." or "we suggest to use ..." or "we suggest against the use of ..." the intervention in question. Potentially, a different interpretation may be achieved when the above example is phrased as: "We recommend against the use of antibiotics in post-Lyme syndrome."

Applications of GRADE: A Summary

Figure 3.3 illustrates the GRADE rating process. GRADE can be applied to a wide range of evidence, whether systematic reviews or health technology assessments (top half) or presentations that can be more easily utilized by health care providers, such as clinical practice guidelines, care paths, or decision support systems (lower half). The GRADE system has been adopted by a wide range of specialties and health care settings, suggesting that it has successfully struck a welcome balance between simplicity and methodological rigor.

References

1. Warlow C. The Willis Lecture 2003: evaluating treatments for stroke patients too slowly: time to get out of second gear. Stroke. 2004;35(9):2211–9.
2. Coull BM, Williams LS, Goldstein LB, Meschia JF, Heitzman D, Chaurvedi S, et al. Anticoagulants and antiplatelet agents in acute ischaemic stroke. Report of the Joint Stroke Guideline Development Committee of the American Academy of Neurology and the American Stroke Association (a Division of the American Heart Association). Neurology. 2002;59: 13–22.
3. West S, King V, Carey TS, Lohr KN, McKoy N, Sutton SF, et al. Systems to rate the strength of scientific evidence [Evidence report/technology assessment no 47]. Rockville (MD): Agency for Healthcare Research and Quality; 2002 Mar. AHRQ Publication No 02-E016.
4. Evaluation tools for COMPUS. The Canadian Agency for Drugs and Technologies in Health (Dec 2005). http://www.cadth.ca/media/compus/pdf/COMPUS_Evaluation_Methodology_final_e.pdf. Accessed 28 Feb 2009.
5. Bonow RO, Carabello BA, Chatterjee K, de Leon AC Jr, Faxon DP, Freed MD, Gaasch WH, Lytle BW, Nishimura RA, O'Gara PT, O'Rourke RA, Otto CM, Shah PM, Shanewise JS; 2006 Writing Committee Members; American College of Cardiology/American Heart Association Task Force. 2008 Focused update incorporated into the ACC/AHA 2006 guidelines for the management of patients with valvular heart disease: a report of the American College of Cardiology/American Heart Association Task Force on Practice Guidelines (Writing Committee to Revise the 1998 Guidelines for the Management of Patients With Valvular Heart Disease): endorsed by the Society of Cardiovascular Anesthesiologists, Society for Cardiovascular Angiography and Interventions, and Society of Thoracic Surgeons. Circulation. 2008;118(15):e523–661. Epub 2008 Sep 26.
6. Scottish Intercollegiate Guidelines Network Guideline Number 36, Mar 1999, ISBN 1899893768.

7. Salem DN, O'Gara PT, Madias C, Pauker SG. Valvular and structural heart disease. Antithrombotic and thrombolytic therapy: American College of Chest Physicians Evidence-Based Clinical Practice Guidelines (8th Edition). Chest 2008;133(6 Suppl):593S–629S.
8. Atkins D, Eccles M, Flottorp S, Guyatt GH, Henry D, Hill S, et al. Systems for grading the quality of evidence and the strength of recommendations I: critical appraisal of existing approaches The GRADE Working Group. BMC Health Serv Res. 2004;4(1):38.
9. Schünemann HJ, Woodhead M, Anzueto A, Buist S, Macnee W, Rabe KF, et al. A vision statement on guideline development for respiratory disease: the example of COPD. Lancet. 2008;373:774–9.
10. Guyatt GH, Oxman AD, Vist G, Kunz R, Falck-Ytter Y, Alonso-Coello P, et al. Rating quality of evidence and strength of recommendations GRADE: an emerging consensus on rating quality of evidence and strength of recommendations. BMJ. 2008;336:924–6.
11. Guyatt GH, Oxman AD, Kunz R, Vist GE, Falck-Ytter Y, GRADE Working Group. Rating quality of evidence and strength of recommendations: What is "quality of evidence" and why is it important to clinicians? BMJ. 2008;336(7651):995–8.
12. Schünemann HJ, Oxman AD, Brozek J, Glasziou P, Jaeschke R, Vist GE, et al. Grading quality of evidence and strength of recommendations for diagnostic tests and strategies. BMJ. 2008;336(7653):1106–10.
13. Guyatt GH, Oxman AD, Kunz R, Falck-Ytter Y, Vist GE, Liberati A, et al. Rating quality of evidence and strength of recommendations: Going from evidence to recommendations. BMJ. 2008;336(7652):1049–51.
14. Chaturvedi S, Bruno A, Feasby T, Holloway R, Benavente O, Cohen SN, et al. Therapeutics and Technology Assessment Subcommittee of the American Academy of Neurology. Carotid endarterectomy–an evidence-based review: report of the Therapeutics and Technology Assessment Subcommittee of the American Academy of Neurology. Neurology. 2005;65(6):794–801.
15. The Homocysteine Studies Collaboration. Homocysteine and risk of ischemic heart disease and stroke. JAMA. 2002;288(16):2015–22.
16. Wald NJ, Law MR. A strategy to reduce cardiovascular disease by more than 80%. BMJ. 2003;326(7404):1419–24.
17. Toole JF, Malinow MR, Chambless LE, Spence JD, Pettigrew LC, Howard VJ, et al. Lowering homocysteine in patients with ischemic stroke to prevent recurrent stroke, myocardial infarction, and death: the Vitamin Intervention for Stroke Prevention (VISP) randomized controlled trial. JAMA. 2004;291(5):565–75.
18. Bønaa KH, Njølstad I, Ueland PM, Schirmer H, Tverdal A, Steigen T, Wang H, Nordrehaug JE, Arnesen E, Rasmussen K, NORVIT Trial Investigators. Homocysteine lowering and cardiovascular events after acute myocardial infarction. N Engl J Med 2006;354(15):1578–88.
19. Ebbing M, Bleie Ø, Ueland PM, Nordrehaug JE, Nilsen DW, Vollset SE, et al. Mortality and cardiovascular events in patients treated with homocysteine-lowering B vitamins after coronary angiography: a randomized controlled trial. JAMA. 2008;300(7):795–804.
20. Albert CM, Cook NR, Gaziano JM, et al. Effect of folic acid and B vitamins on risk of cardiovascular events and total mortality among women at high risk for cardiovascular disease: a randomized trial. JAMA. 2008;299(17):2027–36.
21. Cole BF, Baron JA, Sandler RS, et al. Folic acid for the prevention of colorectal adenomas: a randomized clinical trial. JAMA. 2007;297(21):2351–9.
22. Noseworthy JH, Ebers GC, Vandervoort MK, Farquhar RE, Yetisir E, Roberts R. The impact of blinding on the results of a randomized, placebo-controlled multiple sclerosis clinical trial. Neurology. 1994;44(1):16–20.
23. Ederle J, Featherstone RL, Brown MM. Percutaneous transluminal angioplasty and stenting for carotid artery stenosis. A Cochrane review. J Neurol Neurosurg Psychiatry. 2010;81:477–8.
24. De Bruijn S, Stam J. Randomized, placebo-controlled trial of anticoagulant treatment with low-molecular-weight heparin for cerebral sinus thrombosis. Stroke. 1999;30:484–8.
25. Thompson DC, Rivara FP, Thompson R. Helmets for preventing head and facial injuries in bicyclists. Cochrane Database Syst Rev. 2000(2):CD001855.

26. Cannegieter SC, Rosendaal FR, Briet E. Platelets/thromboembolism: thromboembolic and bleeding complications in patients with mechanical heart valve prostheses. Circulation. 1994;89:635–41.
27. Devereaux PJ, Choi PT, Lacchetti C, Weaver B, Schünemann HJ, Haines T, et al. A systematic review and meta-analysis of studies comparing mortality rates of private for-profit and private not-for-profit hospitals. CMAJ. 2002;166(11):1399–406.
28. Levine MN, Raskob G, Beyth RJ, Kearon C, Schulman S. Hemorrhagic complications of anticoagulant treatment: the seventh ACCP conference on antithrombotic and thrombolytic therapy. Chest. 2004;126(3 Suppl):287S–310.
29. Goodin DS, Cohen BA, O'Connor P, Kappos L. Therapeutics and Technology Assessment Subcommittee of the American Academy of Neurology. Assessment: the use of natalizumab (Tysabri) for the treatment of multiple sclerosis (an evidence-based review): report of the Therapeutics and Technology Assessment Subcommittee of the American Academy of Neurology. Neurology. 2008;71(10):766–73.
30. Devereaux PJ, Anderson DR, Gardner MJ, Putnam W, Flowerdew GJ, Brownell BF, et al. Differences between perspectives of physicians and patients on anticoagulation in patients with atrial fibrillation: observational study. BMJ. 2001;323(7323):1218–22.
31. Guyatt GH, Oxman AD, Kunz R, Jaeschke R, Helfand M, Liberati A, et al. Rating quality of evidence and strength of recommendations: incorporating considerations of resources use into grading recommendations. BMJ. 2008;336(7654):1170–3.
32. Halperin JJ, Shapiro ED, Logigian E, Belman AL, Dotevall L, Wormser GP, et al. Quality Standards Subcommittee of the American Academy of Neurology. Practice parameter: treatment of nervous system Lyme disease (an evidence-based review): report of the Quality Standards Subcommittee of the American Academy of Neurology. Neurology. 2007;69(1):91–102.
33. Aguilar MI, Hart R. Oral anticoagulants for preventing stroke in patients with non-valvular atrial fibrillation and no previous history of stroke or transient ischemic attacks. Cochrane Database Syst Rev. 2005(3):CD001927.
34. van Walraven C, Hart RG, Singer DE, Laupacis A, Connolly S, Petersen P, et al. Oral anticoagulants vs aspirin in nonvalvular atrial fibrillation: an individual patient meta-analysis. JAMA. 2002;288(19):2441–8.

Part II
Neurological Diseases

Chapter 4
Stroke

Maria I. Aguilar and Bart M. Demaerschalk

Keywords Stroke • Evidence-based medicine • Critically appraised topics • Transient ischemic attack • Carotid stenosis • Lacunar stroke • Acute ischemic stroke • Cardioembolism • Epidemiology • Diagnosis • Treatment • Prognosis

Transient Ischemic Attack

Introduction

Transient ischemic attack (TIA) is a sudden, focal neurological deficit that lasts less than 24 h, resolves completely, is presumed to be of vascular origin, and is confined to an area of the brain or eye perfused by a specific artery [1]. However, it is known that most TIAs usually last less than 60 min, most resolving within 30 min. The vascular neurology community has then proposed new criteria, where by definition the clinical symptoms would be transient (without a specific time frame defined) and most importantly there would be no evidence of infarction. By using "tissue" rather than "time," this revised definition recognized TIA as a pathophysiological entity. The American Heart Association (AHA) endorsed revised definition as follows: "Transient ischemic attack (TIA): a transient episode of neurological dysfunction caused by focal brain, spinal cord, or retinal ischemia, without acute infarction" [2]. The "old" definition included a time frame of 24 h, although it is known that most TIAs usually last less than 60 min, most resolving within 30 min [3–5].

M.I. Aguilar (✉)
Neurology Department, Mayo Clinic, 5777 East Mayo Blvd., Phoenix, AZ 85054, USA
e-mail: aguilar.maria@mayo.edu

J.G. Burneo et al. (eds.), *Neurology: An Evidence-Based Approach*,
DOI 10.1007/978-0-387-88555-1_4, © Springer Science+Business Media, LLC 2012

TIAs are caused by different clinical situations, i.e., ipsilateral carotid artery stenosis, cardiac embolism, intracranial atherosclerosis, small vessel cerebrovascular disease, among others. The causes of TIA are identical to those of stroke, so secondary prevention strategies are similar for both entities.

Epidemiology

The estimated annual incidence of TIA in the USA is 200,000–500,000. Many episodes never come to medical attention and the above is probably an underestimate. It is presumed that about five million Americans have been given the diagnosis of TIA [1, 6].

Diagnosis

The 2006 guidelines make strong emphasis on prompt evaluation within 24–48 h [7]. The diagnostic evaluation is divided into four groups: general evaluation, brain imaging, carotid imaging, and cardiac evaluation.

General Evaluation

General evaluation should include electrocardiogram (EKG), full blood count, serum electrolytes and creatinine, fasting blood sugar, and lipids.

Brain Imaging

Although the diagnosis of TIA is clinical, brain imaging may reveal infarcts or other pathologies that can mimic TIA. Computed tomography (CT) or magnetic resonance imaging (MRI) of the head should be included in the initial diagnostic evaluation.

Carotid Imaging

Conventional angiography (CA) of the cerebral vessels remains the gold standard diagnostic modality to assess the presence and quantify the location and degree of carotid stenosis. CA is invasive, expensive, and not free of risk (contrast exposure, risk of arterial vasospasm, plaque embolization). Doppler ultrasonography (DUS) is a useful screening tool that provides accurate information [8]. It is noninvasive and inexpensive when compared to other imaging modalities, like magnetic resonance angiography (MRA) or computed tomographic angiography (CTA). MRA has better discriminatory power than DUS recognizing 70–99% stenosis and its sensitivity and specificity is comparable to CA [9, 10]. CTA has high sensitivity and high negative predictive value for carotid disease [11]; however, it is unable to reliably distinguish between moderate (50–69%) and severe (70–99%) stenosis [12] and tends to underestimate clinically relevant grades of stenosis [13]. The 2006 guidelines [7] recommend DUS for screening, MRA or CTA if DUS does not yield reliable results or endarterectomy is seriously considered. CA is recommended for cases, where DUS and MRA/CTA yield discordant results.

The recent AHA 2009 guidelines [2] emphasize again the importance of prompt evaluation (as soon as possible after an event) and recommend the following imaging studies (class I recommendations):

1. Neuroimaging within 24 h of symptom onset, MRI with DWI preferred. CT is an alternative (Level of Evidence B).
2. Routine noninvasive imaging of cervicocephalic vessels (Level A).
3. Noninvasive testing of the intracranial vasculature, when knowledge of intracranial steno-occlusive disease alters management (Level A).

Cardiac Imaging

If a cardioembolic mechanism is suspected, transthoracic echocardiography (TTE) is indicated. Transesophageal echocardiography (TEE) is recommended for patients younger than 45 years, when brain, carotid, and general evaluation provide no clue to the cause of TIA.

Need for admission to the hospital is a topic of great debate, especially in this era of financial grief.

Clinical Case Example

A 58-year-old woman present to the emergency department after a 15-min episode of numbness involving the left side of her face and her left arm. She has no vascular risk factors and is currently on no prescription medications. On clinical examination, her blood pressure (BP) is elevated (150/95) and her neurological examination reveals no focal abnormalities.

Clinical Questions

PICO Question One: Should this woman be admitted to the hospital for observation, management, and further evaluation?

P: Subjects suffering TIA
I: Admission to the hospital
C: Discharge to home from the emergency department
O: Stroke, TIA recurrence, death

PICO Question Two: What is this woman's risk of suffering a stroke in the near future?

P: Subjects suffering TIA
I: Follow-up
C: Subjects without TIA
O: Stroke

Search Strategy

Ovid MEDLINE database was searched from 1996 to February, Week 1, 2009. The Medical Subject Heading (MeSH) terms "ischemic attack, transient" and TIA as a text word were combined using the Boolean operator "OR." Another set was created using the Boolean "OR" of the MeSH terms "survival analysis," "prognosis," "risk," and "risk factors" as a text word. MeSH terms "hospitalization" or "emergency service, hospital" comprised the third set. The three sets were combined using Boolean "AND" and limited to English and humans yielding a final set of 99 citations. From this set, eight articles were reviewed [14–21]. No randomized-controlled trials were identified. One represented a cost–utility analysis [22], and the remaining seven articles were cohort studies describing prognosis [14, 17], risk stratification [20, 21], disposition [15, 18, 19], and the concept of a "TIA clinic" [16].

The Evidence

When deciding if a patient who has just suffered a TIA needs to be institutionalized for work-up and management, the first step is to determine the patient's risk of stroke. From Johnston's cohort study [14], it is well-known that TIAs carry short-term risk of stroke and other adverse events. A significant proportion of strokes (~50%) preceded by a TIA take place in the first 48 h after the TIA. Multiple prediction models have been proposed to help clinicians risk stratify these patients, and the unified ABCD^2 score [23] has been shown to be the most predictive of short-term recurrence [14, 23, 24]. This score takes into account the patient's age, BP during evaluation, clinical features (motor deficit and speech, carry higher risk, respectively, than sensory symptoms), and history of diabetes (Table 4.1).

Based on the ABCD^2 score, the risk of stroke or an adverse event in the subsequent 90 days can be estimated (Table 4.2).

Back to the clinical case, this woman's ABCD^2 score is 2 due to symptom duration 10–59 min and elevated BP. She then belongs in the low-risk group and she probably does not require inpatient evaluation. She should expeditiously, though, undergo general evaluation, brain and carotid imaging, and cardiac evaluation. The higher the score on the ABCD^2 risk stratification model, the higher the risk of an adverse event. Also the higher the score, the higher the likelihood that the episode was indeed a TIA [17].

Table 4.1 ABCD^2 risk stratification score [23]

	Score	Feature
Age	1	≥60
BP	1	SBP >140 or DBP >90
Clinical features	2	Unilateral weakness
	1	Speech impairment
Duration	2	>60 min
	1	10–59 min
	0	<10 min
DM	1	

Table 4.2 Risk of stroke after TIA based on ABCD^2 score [23]

ABCD^2 score	2-Day risk (%)	7-Day risk (%)	90-Day risk (%)
0–3 (low risk)	1.0	1.2	3.1
4–5 (moderate risk)	4.2	5.9	9.8
6–7 (high risk)	8.1	11.7	17.8

The AHA guidelines [2] consider hospitalization reasonable for TIA victims who present within 72 h of the event and meet any of the following criteria (class II recommendations):

1. ABCD^2 score of ≥3 (Level of Evidence C).
2. ABCD^2 score 0–2, and uncertainty that diagnostic work-up can be completed within 48 h in the outpatient setting (Level C).
3. ABCD^2 score 0–2, and other evidence indicating that the event was caused by focal ischemia (Level C).

Treatment

Introduction

Treatment after a TIA is directed toward stroke and cardiovascular disease prevention. The specific treatment depends on the etiology, but overall every effort should be made to modify the individual's vascular risk factors (i.e., HTN, DM, dyslipidemia, atrial fibrillation (AF), smoking cessation, etc.).

Noncardioembolic TIA

Daily long-term antiplatelet therapy should be prescribed immediately [7]. The 2006 guidelines recommend aspirin plus extended-release dypiridamole as the first-line agent. The evidence to support this comes mainly for the ESPIRIT trial [25].

Clopidogrel is indicated when aspirin alone or in combination with dypiridamole is not tolerated. The recent PRoFESS trial though [26], published 2 years after the guidelines, has shown that clopidogrel is somewhat better than previous evidence suggests, and probably aspirin plus extended-release dypiridamole is somewhat worse than previous evidence suggests [27].

Cardioembolic TIA

For patient with paroxysmal or sustained atrial fibrillation (valvular or nonvalvular) who have had a cardioembolic TIA, long-term anticoagulation with warfarin is indicated to a goal INR of 2.5 (2.0–3.0). Risk stratification schemes are available when considering the use of anticoagulation vs. antiplatelet therapy in this patient populations (see section "Cardioembolic Stroke") [7, 28].

Clinical Case Example

While undergoing evaluation at the emergency department, the above mentioned 58-year-old woman goes into atrial fibrillation and has a second TIA, this time with left-sided hemiparesis and dysarthria. Symptoms resolved within 10 min.

Her ABCD^2 score is now a 5, 2 points added for unilateral weakness and 1 for speech impairment. She is now in the "moderate risk" group and the decision is made to admit her to the hospital. CT of the brain is unremarkable; CTA shows no significant stenosis at either carotid bifurcation or intracranial vasculature. TTE shows normal ejection fraction and severe left atrial enlargement. AF is documented on EKG.

Clinical Questions

PICO Question One: Should she be treated with intravenous (IV) heparin while warfarin therapy is initiated and her INR becomes therapeutic?

P: Subjects with atrial fibrillation suffering cardioembolic TIA
I: IV heparin
C: No IV heparin
O: Stroke, recurrent TIA, death

Search Strategy

Ovid MEDLINE database was searched from 1996 to February, Week 1, 2009. The MeSH terms "ischemic attack, transient" and TIA as a text word were combined using the Boolean operator "OR." The "heparin" MeSH term comprised the second set.

The MeSH terms "injections, intravenous" were combined with the text word "iv" using the Boolean "OR." The three sets were combined using the Boolean "AND" and limited to English and human yielding a final result of eight citations [29–36]. No randomized trials addressed our clinical question.

The Evidence

One randomized single-blinded trial addressed the use of a heparin bolus vs. no bolus [32] and found no difference in outcome. In the absence of evidence, information is extrapolated from trials regarding the use of IV heparin after a cardioembolic stroke (not TIA). A meta-analysis of seven trials involving almost 5,000 patients [37] showed that early anticoagulation in this clinical scenario is associated with a nonsignificant reduction in the recurrence of ischemic stroke, no substantial reduction in death and disability, and an increased risk of intracranial bleeding. We then recommend against the use of IV heparin after cardioembolic stroke or TIA as either acute therapy or as bridging therapy to long-term anticoagulation.

Summary Bottom Lines

TIA is a neurological emergency, and as such mandates prompt evaluation with the goal to identify the etiologic cause of the event and implement early therapy to prevent TIA recurrence, stroke, cardiovascular events, and death.

Cardioembolic Stroke

Introduction

Cardioembolic stroke accounts for 20% of all ischemic strokes [38] and its frequency has increased over time, likely reflecting improvement in cardiac imaging [39].

Cardioembolic stroke is typically sudden in onset and involves a large intracranial artery territory (e.g., 3-mm arterial diameter middle cerebral artery (MCA) M1 segment) with corresponding major clinical deficits. Neuroimaging data typically shows a cortical or cortical–subcortical pattern of ischemia corresponding with the arterial territory (MCA M1, M2, or even M3 branch disease).

Occasionally, hemorrhagic infarctions occur from transient large intracranial artery occlusion with subsequent spontaneous recanalization. Embolism has a predilection for the posterior circulation [40], accounting for up to 25% of posterior circulation ischemic infarcts in some registries [41–44]. Posterior inferior cerebellar artery (PICA) and posterior cerebral artery (PCA) territories are particularly prone to cardiac emboli [45, 46]. Cardioembolic stroke can be caused by different cardiac disorders, each with different implications in clinical presentation, management, and prognosis. It occurs most commonly from atrial fibrillation in adults (50%) [39, 47, 48], but other important causes include ventricular thrombus (20%), structural heart defects or tumors (15%), and valvular heart disease (15%) [49–51].

Although the aortic arch (AoA) is not per se a cardiac structure, it is usually considered under sources of cardiac embolism and as such is briefly reviewed in this chapter.

Epidemiology

Atrial fibrillation is the most common cause of cardiac embolism to the central nervous system (CNS). It is also the most common cardiac arrhythmia, affecting almost 1% of the general population of the USA. Its prevalence increases with age, being present in about 5% of persons at age 65 years and in 10% at age 80 years. AF is equally distributed among men and women, and the mean age of individuals affected is about 75 years [52].

The overall incidence of ischemic stroke among people with AF is about 5% per year. The rate of stroke varies widely, however, ranging from 0.5% per year in young patients with "lone AF" to 12% per year in those with prior TIA or stroke. This variation depends on coexisting cardiovascular disorders [53–55]. Identification of subgroups of patients with AF with relatively high vs. low absolute rates of stroke is important for selecting prophylactic antithrombotic therapy [56, 57].

Diagnosis

If a cardioembolic stroke mechanism is suspected based on the history, neurological and general physical examinations or neuroimaging study and evaluation with a 12-lead electrocardiogram (EKG) and echocardiography are recommended as part of the standard [58] diagnostic evaluation. Chest radiography (CXR) was previously recommended as part of the standard acute ischemic stroke diagnostic work-up by the AHA [58], but was recently made optional due to a low yield of information leading to actual changes in clinical management.

TEE is superior to TTE to detect cardioembolic sources of emboli [59]. TEE visualized the left-sided cardiac chambers in more detail and also evaluated the AoA. However, echocardiography sometimes fails to disclose the cardioembolic source despite a suggestive history (e.g., palpitations or valsalva prior to stroke).

We endorse the diagnostic approach recommended in the AHA ischemic stroke guidelines [58].

Overall, the diagnosis of cardiac embolism as the etiology for stroke is made in the absence of arterial stenosis or occlusion in vascular territory involved, absence of a clinical syndrome or radiographic appearance of a lacunar stroke, and absence of unusual causes of stroke (e.g., arterial dissection, vasculitis, drug abuse).

Treatment

Introduction

The treatment of cardioembolic stroke is divided into "acute management" and "secondary prevention of cardioembolic stroke recurrence." The acute management does not differ from the management of acute stroke from an etiology other than cardiac embolism (see section "Acute Ischemic Stroke").

An area of debate is whether or not IV heparin should be used acutely.

Clinical Case Example

A 79-year-old male with history of paroxysmal atrial fibrillation (PAF) on chronic anticoagulation with warfarin presents to the emergency department with aphasia and right-sided weakness. Initially, his NIHSS was 22, but due to abnormal coagulation studies (INR 1.8) he could not receive thrombolytic therapy. After 2 days, his NIHSS was 7 and the brain MRI showed a moderate-sized area of diffusion restriction involving the left MCA territory. The initially occluded left MCA on CTA was recanalized during follow-up vascular imaging (MRA). This patient was managed with rectal aspirin and subcutaneous heparin for deep vein thrombosis (DVT) prophylaxis among others.

Clinical Questions

The clinical question is whether or not IV heparin should be used until his INR become therapeutic.

PICO Question One:

P: Subjects with atrial fibrillation suffering cardioembolic stroke
I: IV heparin
C: No IV heparin
O: Stroke, TIA, systemic embolization, death

Search Strategy

Ovid MEDLINE database was searched from 1996 to February, Week 1, 2009. The text words "cardioembolic" OR "cardioembolism" were combined with the MeSH term "stroke" using the Boolean operator "AND." Another set was created using the Boolean "OR" of the MeSH terms "heparin" and "anticoagulants." The resulting two sets were combined using the Boolean "AND" and limited to English and humans. An evidence-based medicine (EBM) therapy filter that emphasized relevance was applied. A final set of ten citations was obtained [37, 60–68]. A meta-analysis of seven randomized trials, including almost 50,000 patients, addressed our clinical question [37].

The Evidence

This efficacy and safety analysis showed that early anticoagulation in this clinical scenario is associated with nonsignificant reduction in the recurrence of ischemic stroke (3% vs. 4.9%, Odds ratio [OR] 0.68, 95% confidence interval [CI] 0.44–1.06, $P=0.09$, number needed to treat [NNT] 53), no substantial reduction in death and disability (73.5% vs. 73.8%, OR 1.01, 95% CI 0.82–1.24, $P=0.9$), and a significantly increased risk of intracranial bleeding (2.5% vs. 0.7%, OR 2.89, 95% CI 1.19–7.01, $P=0.02$, number needed to harm [NNH] 55). We then recommend against the use of IV heparin after cardioembolic stroke or TIA as either acute therapy or as bridging therapy to long-term anticoagulation.

Treatment: Antiplatelet Therapy Versus Anticoagulation for Stroke Prevention in Atrial Fibrillation

Clinical Question

A 60-year-old woman with history of hypertension, diabetes, and dyslipidemia is diagnosed with PAF. She has history (and radiologic evidence) of a small cerebellar cortical ischemic stroke 2 years ago. At the time, she was prescribed aspirin. She is referred to the neurology clinic to address 2 questions: (1) What is her risk of having a future cardioembolic stroke? (2) Does she need to be anticoagulated or is aspirin therapy optimal for secondary stroke prevention?

Regarding the future risk of stroke, not every patient who has AF must be anticoagulated. The risk of stroke should be addressed and balanced against the benefit and the risk inherent to long-term anticoagulation. Multiple risk stratification schemes exist. The atrial fibrillation investigators (AFIs) systematically pooled data from five AF randomized trials in stroke prevention (BAATAF [69], SPINAF [70], AFASAK [71], CAFA [72], and SPAF [73]), identifying the following independent risk factors for embolism in AF: age, history of stroke or TIA, diabetes mellitus (DM), history of HTN.

In 2000, Pearce and colleagues [74] compared three stroke risk stratification schemes (AFI [75], ACCPC [76], and SPAF [77]) in NVAF. The CHADS^2 score was then implemented [47] taking into consideration risk factors identified by the AFI [76] and SPAF [77]. The acronym stands for

- C = Congestive heart failure (1 point)
- H = Hypertension (1 point)

Table 4.3 CHADS^2 score [47] and annual risk of stroke

CHADS^2	Stroke rate per year (%)	95% Confidence interval
0	1.9	1.2–3.0
1	2.8	2.0–3.8
2	4.0	3.1–5.1
3	5.9	4.6–7.3
4	8.5	6.3–11.1
5	12.5	8.2–7.5
6	18.2	10.5–27.4

- A = Age older than 75 (1 point)
- D = DM (1 point)
- S^2 = History of stroke or TIA (2 points)

The estimated annual risk of stroke based on the CHADS^2 score is shown in Table 4.3.

This woman has then a CHADS^2 score of 4, 2 for previous stroke, 1 for HTN, and 1 for DM. Her estimated risk of stroke per year is around 8.5%.

The next question is how to best decrease her risk of future stroke, antiplatelet therapy vs. anticoagulation.

P: Subjects with atrial fibrillation and history of stroke or TIA
I: Antiplatelet therapy
C: Anticoagulant therapy
O: Stroke, TIA, systemic embolization, intracranial hemorrhage (ICH), death

Search Strategy

Ovid MEDLINE database was searched from 1996 to May, Week 2, 2009. The MeSH term "stroke" and text word stroke were combined using the Boolean operator "OR." "Atrial fibrillation" was searched as a MeSH term and also as a text word. The resulting sets were combined with the Boolean "AND." The MeSH terms "warfarin," "aspirin," "dipyridamole," "platelet aggregation inhibitors," "ticlopidine," and "anticoagulants" and text words warfarin, Aggrenox®, Plavix®, clopidogrel, Coumadin®, anticoagulants, antithrombotics, and antiplatelets were combined with the Boolean operator "OR." The resulting two sets were combined with "AND" and limited to English and humans. After further limiting the results to randomized controlled trials and meta-analysis, the final yield was 85 citations. The Cochrane Database of Systematic Reviews was also searched utilizing the terms above.

The Evidence

The meta-analysis by Hart and colleagues [78] seemed to best address this clinical question. Twenty-nine trials, including 28,044 participants, showed that compared with control, adjusted-dose warfarin and antiplatelet agents reduced stroke by 64% and 24%, respectively, in patients with atrial fibrillation. Warfarin was substantially more efficacious (by approximately 40%) than antiplatelet therapy. Increased risk of major hemorrhage by antithrombotic therapies did not offset the benefit for selected patients.

Applying this information to the previous case scenario, this patient's estimated risk of stroke per year of 8.5% would be reduced to 3.4% by using adjusted-dose warfarin and to 6.8% by using antiplatelet agents.

Warfarin-related intracerebral hemorrhage (W-ICH) is the most feared complication of anticoagulant therapy. Optimal patient selection for warfarin therapy remains crucial to prevent elderly patients from unnecessary warfarin anticoagulation. Aggressive management of HTN and rigorous anticoagulation control are the key to decrease the risk of W-ICH.

Treatment: Patent Foramen Ovale

Patent foramen ovale (PFO) is a flap-like defect in the interatrial septum and a common finding (25%) in the general population. PFO closes in the majority of infants at birth. The relationship of PFO and ischemic stroke remains an area of considerable *debate* [49–51]. The mechanism by which PFO causes ischemic stroke remains speculative; available theories include paradoxical embolism from the venous circulation, in situ thrombosis at the PFO, and availability of vasoactive substances (e.g., serotonin) in the systemic circulation, which would normally be deactivated in the pulmonary circulation [79]. Regardless of hypothetical mechanism, prospective studies provide evidence that PFO is found more commonly in patients with a cryptogenic stroke mechanism in both younger and older adults [49–51]. Others suggest that the size of the PFO defect is important, with a large PFO (≥2 mm) more likely to be associated with an embolic stroke than a small PFO (<2 mm) [80]. Studies investigating medical therapy for PFO are largely retrospective and do not show any advantage of warfarin over aspirin. Most of these studies, however, have been limited by insufficient power to compare aspirin to warfarin, nonrandomized treatment allocation or nonmasked treatment or allocation, crossover, or unblinded ascertainment of end points [51]. Regarding PFO closure, because of the lack of randomized trial data comparing closure to standard medical therapy, the American Academy of Neurology issued practice parameters concluding insufficient evidence to recommend routine percutaneous closure of PFOs in patients with cryptogenic stroke [81].

Treatment: Aortic Arch Atherosclerosis

Proximal AoA atherosclerosis is an overlooked but potentially serious source of embolic stroke [82]. Patients with ascending aorta or proximal arch plaques of

≥4 mm thickness are up to seven times more likely to have cerebral infarction than controls (14.4% vs. 2%, $P<0.001$) [82, 83]. For nonmobile aortic plaque, statin therapy appears protective in preventing stroke while uncertainty remains about the optimal antithrombotic regimen, aspirin, or warfarin [84]. However, mobile aortic plaques seem best treated with adjusted-dose warfarin (target INR 2–3), 5% vs. 45% incidence of vascular events, $P=0.006$ (stroke 0 vs. 27%) [85]. The dimensions of the mobile atheroma are not predictive of stroke risk; only the presence or absence of the mobile component predicts such risk.

Summary Bottom Lines

Cardioembolic stroke is a syndrome with diverse causes and not a single disease entity.

A systematic approach, including detail history, general, cardiac, and neurological examination, review of neuroimaging studies, ECG, and echocardiographic data, may disclose the cause of embolism and guide subsequent stroke prevention strategies.

Acute Ischemic Stroke

Introduction

A stroke is the rapidly developing loss of brain function(s) due to disturbance in the blood supply to the brain. This can be due to ischemia caused by blockage (thrombosis or arterial embolism) or due to a hemorrhage. A stroke is a medical emergency and can cause permanent neurological damage, complications, and death. It is the leading cause of adult disability in the USA and Europe and it is the number two cause of death worldwide. Risk factors for stroke include advanced age, hypertension, previous stroke or TIA, diabetes, high cholesterol, cigarette smoking, and atrial fibrillation.

Epidemiology

Introduction

On average, every 40 s, someone in the USA has a stroke.

Clinical Case Example

A 79-year-old man who sustained the witnessed acute onset of aphasia and right-sided hemiparesis at 11:00 a.m. presented by ambulance to the emergency department of a community hospital at 11:27 a.m.

Clinical Questions

What is the incidence of stroke in the USA?
What is the prevalence of stroke in the USA?

Incidence

Each year, about 795,000 people in the USA experience a new or recurrent stroke. Approximately 610,000 of these are first attacks, and 185,000 are recurrent attacks. Of all strokes, 87% are ischemic.

Prevalence

Among adults aged 20 and older, the estimated prevalence of stroke is approximately 6,400,000. Of all strokes, 87% are ischemic.

Clinical Bottom Lines

Incidence of ischemic stroke in the USA is approximately 692,000 per year.
Prevalence of ischemic stroke in the USA is approximately 5,568,000.

Diagnosis

Introduction

There exists, in acute stroke management, a distinct rural–urban disparity due to a shortage of vascular neurologists and few primary stroke centers in rural settings. Two-way audio–video communication through telemedicine is a reliable tool for assessment of stroke-related neurological deficits and may have greater diagnostic utility than the telephone for determination of thrombolytic eligibility.

Diffusion-weighted imaging (DWI) is the principle method for reliably detecting acute ischemic stroke. Radiology departments are now equipped with new 3.0 Tesla (T) MRI units. Early reports suggest a potential advantage of 3.0 T DWI.

Clinical Case Example

Refer to the case example above. The rural hospital participates in a regional stroke network. The treating emergency physician can communicate by telephone and telemedicine with an available on-call vascular neurologist at a regional primary stroke center 200 miles away.

Clinical Questions

1. Do stroke telemedicine consultations have superior diagnostic utility over telephone-only consultations for determination of a thrombolysis-eligible acute ischemic stroke patient?
2. Does 3.0 T MRI improve accuracy for imaging acute ischemic stroke compared with 1.5 T?

Search Strategy

Ovid MEDLINE database was searched from 1996 to November, Week 2, 2008. The MeSH term "Stroke/di,th" (diagnosis and therapy subheadings) was exploded and yielded 9,510 citations. The exploded MeSH terms of "Remote Consultation," "Telemedicine," "Telephone," and "Videoconferencing" as well as the text words "teleconsultation," "telephonic guidance," and "teleneurology" were combined by the Boolean "OR" yielding 14,472 citations. The two resulting sets were combined with the Boolean "AND" with a result of 67 citations. The text words "telestroke," "stroke telehealth," and "stroke telemedicine" were searched with the Boolean "OR" and combined with the previous set resulting in 73 citations. Limits of English, human, and randomized controlled trial as a publication type were applied with a final result of two citations. Meyers et al. [86] was chosen as this was the only true randomized controlled study that focused on stroke neurology. Campangan et al. [87] provided a critical appraisal of the Meyers publication.

The Evidence

A single randomized, blinded, prospective trial comparing telephone-only consultations to telemedicine consultations for stroke emergencies was appraised. Correct acute stroke treatment decisions were made more frequently in the telemedicine group vs. the telephone-only group [98% vs. 82%, (number needed to assess (NNA)=6)]. Stroke telemedicine when compared to telephone-only consultations was more sensitive (100% vs. 58%), more specific (98% vs. 92%), had a more favorable positive likelihood ratio (LR 41 vs. 7) and negative likelihood ratio (0 vs. 0.5), and had higher predictive values (positive predictive value 94% vs. 76%, and negative predictive value 100% vs. 84%) for the determination of thrombolysis eligibility.

Table 4.4 Diagnostic utility parameters of telemedicine and telephone consultative modalities for determination of thrombolysis eligibility

	Telemedicine (95% CI)	Telephone (95% CI)
Sensitivity (%)	100 (NC)	58 (41–74)
Specificity (%)	98 (94–100)	92 (86–98)
Positive likelihood ratio	41 (11–156)	7 (3–16)
Negative likelihood ratio	0 (NC)	0.5 (0.3–0.6)
Positive predictive value (%)	94 (85–100)	76 (59–93)
Negative predictive value (%)	100 (NC)	84 (76–92)
Overall accuracy (%)	98 (96–100)	82 (75–89)

Table adapted from data presented in ref. [87]
NC not calculated

Rosso et al. [88] blindly reviewed the DWI of 135 acute stroke patients and 34 controls performed at 1.5 T ($n = 108$) or 3.0 T ($n = 61$). All stroke patients had anterior territory ischemic stroke and were imaged within the first 6 h after onset. Four readers (neuroradiologists and vascular neurologists) blinded to clinical data and MRI field strength recorded the presence of ischemic lesions on DWI. Diagnostic utility was assessed. The accuracy of DWI was superior at 1.5 T (98.8%) than at 3.0 T (90.9%, $P = 0.03$). The sensitivity decreased from 99.1% at 1.5 T to 92.5% at 3.0 T ($P = 0.06$) and the specificity from 97.8% to 84.1% ($P = 0.002$). False negative rate was 0.6% at 1.5 T and 6.1% at 3.0 T.

Clinical Bottom Lines

Both consultative modalities, telemedicine and telephone-only, achieved similar rates of thrombolysis use in acute stroke patients (overall rate 25%).

Telemedicine consultations took longer to initiate (11 min) and to conduct (32 min) than telephone-only consults (2 min, 23 min, respectively).

Correct acute stroke treatment decisions were made more often in the telemedicine group vs. the telephone-only group [98% vs. 82% (NNA = 6)].

Stroke telemedicine when compared to telephone-only consultations was more sensitive (100% vs. 58%), more specific (98% vs. 92%), had a more favorable positive likelihood ratio (41 vs. 7) and negative likelihood ratio (0 vs. 0.5), and had higher predictive values (positive predictive value 94% vs. 76%, and negative predictive value 100% vs. 84%) for the determination of thrombolysis eligibility.

Technical complications were noted in 19% of telemedicine consultations.

1.5 T DWI MRI is better than 3.0 T for the imaging of acute ischemic stroke during the first 6 h.

Table 4.4.

Treatment

Clinical Questions

1. What is the expected benefit and anticipated harm for intravenous tPA for acute ischemic stroke patients treated in <3 h?
2. What visual aids are available for thrombolysis decision making in acute ischemic stroke?
3. What is the expected benefit and anticipated harm for intravenous tPA for acute ischemic stroke patients treated in the 3–4.5-h window?
4. What is the expected benefit and anticipated harm for intraarterial tPA for acute ischemic stroke patients treated in the 3–6-h window?
5. Does a combined IV–IA therapy offer advantages over traditional IV tPA therapy?

Treatment: Intravenous Thrombolysis <3-h Window

Saver developed a method for estimating NNT for nonbinary outcomes from parallel design clinical trials and illustrated its application to outcomes of thrombolytic stroke therapy across the full range of stroke-related disability [89]. The result was an average estimated NNT of 3.1 (95% CI 2.6–3.6) to have a better outcome by ≥1 grade on Modified Rankin Scale (mRS). The estimated NNH was 30.1 (95% CI 25.1–36.0). For every 100 acute stroke patients treated with intravenous tPA, approximately 32 would be predicted to experience a better outcome, and 3 a worse outcome, as a result of the treatment.

Saver also undertook a study to derive NNH values for the impact of symptomatic intracerebral hemorrhage (SICH) upon the 3-month poststroke disability score, the mRS [90]. Saver's study was well-conceived and methodologically sound. The study compared the observed 3-month mRS outcomes among the patients experiencing SICH after tPA and the predicted outcomes had they been treated with placebo. The NNH for one more patient to have a final disabled or death outcome (mRS≥3) attributable to tPA-related SICH was 707; for severely disabled or death outcome (mRS≥4), NNH was 126; for fatal outcome, NNH was 36.5; and for worsened outcome by any degree (≥1 mRS grade), NNH was between 29.7 and 40.1. The average estimated NNT for one additional patient to have a better outcome by ≥1 mRS grade as a result of tPA treatment is approximately 3 and the average NNH for one more patient to have a worsened outcome by ≥1 mRS grade attributable to tPA-related SICH is approximately 30. Therefore, the likelihood of being helped vs. harmed (LHH) is expressed as 30/3 = 10. It is evident that tPA is ten times more likely to help than to harm eligible patients with acute ischemic stroke.

Table 4.5 Number of patients benefited (by ≥1 mRS grade) and harmed (by ≥1 mRS grade) per 100 patients treated with tPA by different routes and in different time windows at 3-month post-stroke follow-up

	IV tPA 0–3 h (NINDS tPA trials)	IV tPA 3–4.5 h (ECASS 3 trial)	IA tPA 3–6 h (PROACT 2 trial)
Benefit per 100	32.3	16.4	20.8
NNT	3.1 (95% CI, 2.6–3.6)	6.1 (95% CI, 5.6–6.7)	5
Harm per 100	3.3	2.7	3.5
NNH	30.1 (95% CI, 25.1–36.0)	37.5 (95% CI, 34.6–40.5)	100/3.5 = 29
LHH (approximate)	30/3 = 10	37/6 = 6	29/5 = 6

NNT Number needed to treat, *NNH* Number needed to harm, *LHH* Likelihood of being helped vs. harmed

Treatment: Thrombolysis Treatment Decision Making in Acute Ischemic Stroke

The decision of whether or not to use intravenous thrombolysis for a patient with an acute ischemic stroke within 3 h of onset requires collaborative discussion among patients, family members, and health care providers. Sometimes, visual displays help individuals to more rapidly comprehend the expected response patterns to treatment. Gadhia et al. evaluated, refined, and improved existing visual aids for stroke thrombolysis decision making [91]. Ultimately, a new decision matrix visual aid with the highest possible quality score was developed to efficiently and informatively convey the health benefits and risks of thrombolysis for stroke to patients and family.

Treatment: Intravenous Thrombolysis 3–4.5-h Window

The ECASS 3 trial demonstrated a statistically significant benefit of intravenous tPA for acute ischemic stroke in the 3–4.5-h window. Saver et al., using the joint outcome table specification, derived NNT and NNH values summarizing treatment impact over the entire outcome range on the mRS of global disability [92]. Refer to Table 4.5.

Treatment: Intraarterial Thrombolysis 3–6-h Window

Refer to Table 4.5.

Treatment: Combined Intravenous Thrombolysis – Intraarterial Thrombolysis/Thrombectomy Approaches

Algorithms for current-era treatment of acute ischemic stroke emphasize the importance of successful recanalization and subsequent reperfusion to preserve brain tissue at risk and diminish disability. IV thrombolysis has the advantage of speed but the disadvantage of lower rates of recanalization of larger artery occlusions as compared to IA treatment methods. Conversely, IA treatments report higher recanalization rates, but are impeded by limited availability, procedural delays, and increased risks. Higher rates of recanalization in IA trials using mechanical thrombectomy devices have not always translated into improved patient outcomes. Combined IV–IA treatments offer advantages of both routes, speed, and enhanced recanalization. Equipoise among recanalization approaches still exists.

Lacunar Stroke

Introduction

Lacunar strokes are small subcortical infarctions that result from occlusion of a single penetrating artery and account for approximately 25% of all ischemic strokes. The prognosis after a lacunar stroke may not be as benign as previously thought. There is a recognized risk of recurrence, vascular cognitive impairment and dementia, and death in the long term. Acute treatment may include thrombolysis for eligible patients, and secondary prevention should include antiplatelet medications, rigorous management of hypertension, hyperlipidemia, and hyperglycemia and promotion of a healthy vascular lifestyle [93].

Epidemiology

Clinical Case Example

A 58-year-old female hypertensive diabetic cattle rancher was riding her horse when she noted acute onset of right arm and leg weakness and clumsiness, causing her to fall. Her examination in urgent clinic revealed a right ataxic hemiparesis syndrome. Her MRI brain displayed an acute small 9-mm left subcortical corona radiata infarction. Neurovascular imaging excluded intra- and extracranial arterial stenosis, and cardiovascular testing did not identify any obvious cardiac source for embolism. The rancher's presenting neurological syndrome was determined to be due to lacunar stroke.

Clinical Question

1. What is the incidence rate of lacunar stroke?
2. What is the prevalence of vascular risk factors in lacunar and nonlacunar strokes?
3. How common are ataxic hemiparesis lacunar stroke syndromes and what are their relative frequencies compared with other lacunar stroke syndromes?

Incidence

Bejot et al. evaluated the incidence of symptomatic lacunar stroke in patients included from 1989 to 2006 in a prospective population-based stroke registry, which complies with rigorous epidemiological criteria for incidence studies [94]. In the whole study period, standardized incidence rates according to world populations were 18.3 per 100,000 per year in men and 10.3 per 100,000 per year in women. There was a progressive increase in the incidence of lacunar stroke with each decade of life.

Prevalence of Vascular Risk Factors in Lacunar Stroke

Bejot et al. determined the distribution of vascular risk factors in patients with lacunar and nonlacunar stroke [94]. A history of atrial fibrillation was significantly more frequent in patients with nonlacunar ischemic stroke (31%; 95% CI, 0.29–0.33) than in lacunar stroke (15%; 95% CI, 0.13–0.18). There were no other significant differences in the distribution of other vascular risk factors.

Benavente et al. reported the frequency of common clinical lacunar stroke syndrome presentations in the ongoing SPS3 trial cohort of lacunar stroke patients: pure motor 33%, sensorimotor 29%, ataxic hemiparesis 11%, pure sensory 10%, and other miscellaneous 16% [95]. Anatomic location of lacunar stroke in the SPS3 cohort was 52% in basal ganglia, internal capsule, corona radiate, and centrum semiovale, 27% in pons, medulla, and midbrain, and 22% in the thalamus.

Clinical Bottom Lines

Incidence rates of lacunar stroke were 18.3 per 100,000 per year in men and 10.3 per 100,000 per year in women.

A history of atrial fibrillation was significantly more frequent in patients with nonlacunar ischemic stroke (31%; 95% CI, 0.29–0.33) than in lacunar stroke (15%; 95% CI, 0.13–0.18).

Ataxic hemiparesis syndromes represent approximately 11% of all lacunar stroke syndromes.

Diagnosis

Clinical Questions

1. What is the utility of MRI in diagnosing a lacunar stroke?
2. What is the utility of the clinical examination determination of a lacunar syndrome in diagnosing a lacunar stroke?

The Evidence

MRI is the imaging technique of choice for the demonstration of lacunar strokes. The overall sensitivity of DWI for acute subcortical infarction was 94.9%, specificity was 94.1%, positive predictive value was 97.4%, negative predictive value was 88.9%, and accuracy was 94.6% [96, 97].

A lacunar syndrome is not highly specific for a lacunar infarction. Causes other than penetrating small vessel disease are present in up to one-third of cases [93, 97]. These findings emphasize the importance of conducting a comprehensive diagnostic work-up for patients with lacunar stroke.

Clinical Bottom Lines

MRI is the diagnostic test of choice for lacunar stroke.
Do not rely exclusively on the discovery of a clinical lacunar syndrome as proof that a patient's stroke was caused by a lacunar stroke.

Treatment

Clinical Questions

1. What is the most effective antiplatelet(s) for prevention of recurrent lacunar stroke?
2. Is intravenous thrombolysis an effective and safe treatment for an acute lacunar stroke?

The Evidence

To date, there have been no prevention trials in antiplatelet therapy focused on lacunar stroke. The SPS3 is the first trial of secondary stroke prevention focusing specifically on patients with strokes secondary to small vessel disease. Its aims are to define the optimal interventions (antiplatelet therapy of either aspirin 325 mg/day or aspirin plus clopidogrel 75 mg/day, and two targets of systolic blood pressures, intensive <130 mm Hg or usual 130–149 mm Hg) to prevent stroke recurrence and cognitive decline [98].

In the acute phase, patients with lacunar infarctions respond to IV tPA similarly to those patients with other ischemic stroke subtypes [97]. Postthrombolysis intracerebral hemorrhages (all/symptomatic) were similar in lacunar stroke (12.3%/4.6%) and non-lacunar stroke (13.4%/5.3%; $P > 0.8$). Lacunar stroke patients reached independence more often than nonlacunar stroke patients (75.4% vs. 58.9%; $P = 0.001$), but this association became insignificant after adjustment for age, gender, and stroke severity [99].

Clinical Bottom Lines

Tailored antiplatelet combinations are under investigation for prevention of recurrent lacunar stroke.

Intravenous thrombolysis in eligible acute lacunar stroke patients is as effective and safe as in ischemic stroke caused by other common mechanisms.

Prognosis

Clinical Question

1. What is the prognosis of lacunar stroke?

The Evidence

Bejot et al. described survival rates in patients with lacunar stroke as 96% at 1 month (95% CI, 0.94–0.97), 86% at 1 year (95% CI, 0.83–0.89), and 78% (95% CI, 0.75–0.81) after 2 years of follow-up [94]. In comparison, survival rates of non-lacunar stroke patients were 82% (95% CI, 0.80–0.84), 68% (95% CI, 0.66–0.71), and 62% (95% CI, 0.59–0.64). The survival rate after lacunar stroke was significantly higher than that after nonlacunar stroke (hazard ratio, 2.05; 95% CI, 1.70–2.47; $P < 0.001$). Jackson et al. performed a systematic review of cohort studies with ischemic stroke subtype-specific short- and long-term follow-up data on death and recurrent stroke [100]. One month odds of death and recurrent stroke were significantly greater following nonlacunar than lacunar stroke, but the difference decreased thereafter. 1–5-year mortality: OR 1.77, 95% CI, 1.28–2.45 and 1–5-year stroke recurrence: OR 1.61, 95% CI, 0.96–2.70.

Sacco et al. reported, also, that in the short term patients with nonlacunar stroke had more vascular events, but that in the long term the risk of death and stroke recurrence was similar [101].

In prospective studies, approximately 11% of patients with first-ever lacunar strokes developed vascular dementia over the following 3 years, approximately 3–5% per year [95].

Clinical Bottom Lines

Although early mortality and stroke recurrence risks are higher among nonlacunar than lacunar stroke patients, the risks appear not to differ in the long term.

Summary

1. Lacunar infarction accounts for one quarter of all cerebral infarctions.
2. Not all lacunar syndromes are secondary to a lacunar infarction.
3. DWI MRI is the most sensitive and specific imaging method to detect lacunes.
4. Fifty percent of all patients with first-ever lacunar stroke present with mild neuropsychological abnormalities.
5. Lacunar strokes are not benign; there is high risk of recurrence and vascular dementia.
6. Response to IV tPA appears similar to other subtypes of ischemic stroke.

Carotid Stenosis

Clinical Case

A 65-year-old train photographer, scheduled to embark on a major assignment, sustained a minor right hemispheric ischemic stroke caused by symptomatic high-grade (80%) right internal carotid stenosis. Two days later, a carotid revascularization by endarterectomy (CEA) or angioplasty and stenting (CAS) was recommended by his vascular surgeon. He, his family members, and his health care providers gathered at his bedside and wrestled with the advantages and disadvantages of the two approaches.

Treatment

For patients with recent TIA or ischemic stroke within the last 6 months and ipsilateral severe (70–99%) carotid artery stenosis, carotid revascularization via CEA or CAS is recommended. See below for the question of selecting CEA vs. CAS.

For patients with recent TIA or ischemic stroke and ipsilateral moderate (50–69%) carotid stenosis, carotid revascularization is also recommended depending on patient-specific factors, such as age, gender, comorbidities, and severity of initial symptoms. When the degree of stenosis is <50%, there is no indication for carotid revascularization. Medical management is sufficient. When a revascularization is indicated for patients with symptomatic carotid stenosis, performing the procedure within 2 weeks is suggested rather than delaying. Among patients with symptomatic moderate or severe stenosis (>50%) being considered for revascularization, high surgical risk categorization includes instances when stenosis is difficult to access surgically; medical conditions are present that greatly increase the risk for surgery; or other specific circumstances exist, such as radiation-induced stenosis or restenosis after CEA. In these high surgical risk cases, CAS is not inferior to CEA and is the preferred revascularization modality. Among patients with symptomatic carotid occlusion, EC/IC bypass surgery is not routinely recommended.

Question: For standard (or conventional) risk symptomatic carotid stenosis patient candidates for carotid artery revascularization, how does CAS compare to the gold standard CEA in terms of periprocedural complications and ipsilateral stroke long term?

The Evidence

CREST reported on 2,502 carotid stenosis patients (53% symptomatic) who were randomly assigned to undergo CAS or CEA. There was no significant difference in the estimated 4-year rates of the primary end point (stroke, myocardial infarction, or death during periprocedural period or any ipsilateral stroke during follow-up) between CAS and CEA (7.2% and 6.8%, respectively). There was no difference in treatment effect to primary outcome according to symptomatic status. Periprocedural rates of some individual components of the end points differed between the CAS and CEA groups: for death (0.7% vs 0.3%, $P=0.18$), for stroke (4.1% vs 2.3%, $P=0.01$), and for MI (1.1% vs 2.3%, $P=0.03$). After periprocedural period, the incidences of ipsilateral stroke with CAS and CEA were similarly low (2.0% vs 2.4%, $P=0.85$). Prespecified analysis demonstrated an interaction between age and treatment efficacy ($P=0.02$), with a crossover at an age of approximately 70 years; CAS demonstrated greater efficacy at younger ages and CEA at older ages. Post-hoc analyses demonstrated that minor and major periprocedural stroke had a greater effect on quality of life status than did periprocedural MI. The likelihood of the primary end point was not significantly affected by the specialty of the interventionalist performing the CAS procedure.

Clinical Bottom Lines

Carotid revascularization performed by highly qualified surgeons and interventionalists is effective and safe.
Periprocedural stroke is more likely after CAS.

Periprocedural MI is more likely after CEA, but its effect on quality of life is less than the effect of periprocedural stroke.

Younger patients have fewer periprocedural complications after CAS than after CEA.

Older patients have fewer periprocedural complications after CEA than after CAS.

Both CAS and CEA are clinically durable interventions.

Carotid revascularization, in combination with medical therapy, results in very low absolute risk of recurrent stroke.

References

1. Johnston SC. Clinical practice. Transient ischemic attack. N Engl J Med. 2002;347:1687–92.
2. Easton JD, Saver JL, Albers GW, et al. Definition and evaluation of transient ischemic attack: a scientific statement for healthcare professionals from the American Heart Association/American Stroke Association Stroke Council; Council on Cardiovascular Surgery and Anesthesia; Council on Cardiovascular Radiology and Intervention; Council on Cardiovascular Nursing; and the Interdisciplinary Council on Peripheral Vascular Disease: The American Academy of Neurology affirms the value of this statement as an educational tool for neurologists. Stroke. 2009;40:2276–93.
3. Levy DE. How transient are transient ischemic attacks? Neurology. 1988;38:674–7.
4. Pessin MS, Duncan GW, Mohr JP, Poskanzer DC. Clinical and angiographic features of carotid transient ischemic attacks. New Engl J Med. 1977;296:358–62.
5. Weisberg LA. Clinical characteristics of transient ischemic attacks in black patients. Neurology. 1991;41:1410–4.
6. Bots ML, van der Wilk EC, Koudstaal PJ, Hofman A, Grobbee DE. Transient neurological attacks in the general population. Prevalence, risk factors, and clinical relevance. Stroke. 1997;28:768–73.
7. Johnston SC, Nguyen-Huynh MN, Schwarz ME, et al. National Stroke Association guidelines for the management of transient ischemic attacks. Ann Neurol. 2006;60:301–13.
8. Furst G, Saleh A, Wenserski F, et al. Reliability and validity of noninvasive imaging of internal carotid artery pseudo-occlusion. Stroke. 1999;30:1444–9.
9. Forsting M, Wanke I. Funeral for a friend [comment]. Stroke. 2003;34:1324–32.
10. Nederkoorn PJ, van der Graaf Y, Hunink MG. Duplex ultrasound and magnetic resonance angiography compared with digital subtraction angiography in carotid artery stenosis: a systematic review. Stroke. 2003;34:1324–32.
11. Josephson SA, Bryant SO, Mak HK, Johnston SC, Dillon WP, Smith WS. Evaluation of carotid stenosis using CT angiography in the initial evaluation of stroke and TIA. Neurology. 2004;63:457–60.
12. Anderson GB, Ashforth R, Steinke DE, Ferdinandy R, Findlay JM. CT angiography for the detection and characterization of carotid artery bifurcation disease. Stroke. 2000;31:2168–74.
13. Silvennoinen HM, Ikonen S, Soinne L, Railo M, Valanne L. CT angiographic analysis of carotid artery stenosis: comparison of manual assessment, semiautomatic vessel analysis, and digital subtraction angiography. Am J Neuroradiol. 2007;28:97–103.
14. Johnston SC, Gress DR, Browner WS, Sidney S. Short-term prognosis after emergency department diagnosis of TIA. JAMA. 2000;284:2901–6.
15. Nguyen-Huynh MN, Johnston SC. Is hospitalization after TIA cost-effective on the basis of treatment with tPA? Neurology. 2005;65:1799–801.
16. Fallon C, Noone I, Ryan J, O'Shea D, O'Laoide R, Crowe M. Assessment and management of transient ischaemic attack–the role of the TIA clinic. Irish J Med Sci. 2006;175:24–7.

17. Josephson SA, Sidney S, Pham TN, Bernstein AL, Johnston SC. Higher ABCD2 score predicts patients most likely to have true transient ischemic attack. Stroke. 2008;39:3096–8.
18. Josephson SA, Sidney S, Pham TN, Bernstein AL, Johnston SC. Factors associated with the decision to hospitalize patients after transient ischemic attack before publication of prediction rules. Stroke. 2008;39:411–3.
19. Coben JH, Owens PL, Steiner CA, Crocco TJ. Hospital and demographic influences on the disposition of transient ischemic attack. Acad Emerg Med. 2008;15:171–6.
20. Byrne A, Daly C, Rocke L, Gray J. Can risk stratification of transient ischaemic attacks improve patient care in the emergency department? Emerg Med J. 2007;24:637–40.
21. Bray JE, Coughlan K, Bladin C. Can the ABCD Score be dichotomised to identify high-risk patients with transient ischaemic attack in the emergency department? Emerg Med J. 2007;24:92–5.
22. Nguyen-Huynh MN, Johnston SC. Transient ischemic attack: a neurologic emergency. Curr Neurol Neurosci Rep. 2005;5:13–20.
23. Rothwell PM, Giles MF, Flossmann E, et al. A simple score (ABCD) to identify individuals at high early risk of stroke after transient ischaemic attack. Lancet. 2005;366:29–36.
24. Johnston SC, Rothwell PM, Nguyen-Huynh MN, et al. Validation and refinement of scores to predict very early stroke risk after transient ischaemic attack. Lancet. 2007;369:283–92.
25. Group ES, Halkes PH, van Gijn J, Kappelle LJ, Koudstaal PJ, Algra A. Aspirin plus dipyridamole versus aspirin alone after cerebral ischaemia of arterial origin (ESPRIT): randomised controlled trial. Lancet. 2006;367:1665–73.
26. Sacco RL, Diener HC, Yusuf S, et al. Aspirin and extended-release dipyridamole versus clopidogrel for recurrent stroke. New Engl J Med. 2008;359:1238–51.
27. Kent DM, Thaler DE. Stroke prevention–insights from incoherence. New Engl J Med. 2008;359:1287–9.
28. Sacco RL, Adams R, Albers G, et al. Guidelines for prevention of stroke in patients with ischemic stroke or transient ischemic attack: a statement for healthcare professionals from the American Heart Association/American Stroke Association Council on Stroke: co-sponsored by the Council on Cardiovascular Radiology and Intervention: the American Academy of Neurology affirms the value of this guideline. Stroke. 2006;37:577–617.
29. Albers GW, Amarenco P, Easton JD, Sacco RL, Teal P, American College of Chest. Antithrombotic and thrombolytic therapy for ischemic stroke: American College of Chest Physicians Evidence-Based Clinical Practice Guidelines (8th Edition). Chest 2008;133:630S–69.
30. Singer DE, Albers GW, Dalen JE, et al. Antithrombotic therapy in atrial fibrillation: American College of Chest Physicians Evidence-Based Clinical Practice Guidelines (8th Edition). Chest. 2008;133:546S–92.
31. Albers GW, Amarenco P, Easton JD, Sacco RL, Teal P. Antithrombotic and thrombolytic therapy for ischemic stroke: the Seventh ACCP Conference on Antithrombotic and Thrombolytic Therapy. Chest. 2004;126:483S–512.
32. Toth C. The use of a bolus of intravenous heparin while initiating heparin therapy in anticoagulation following transient ischemic attack or stroke does not lead to increased morbidity or mortality. Blood Coagul Fibrinolysis. 2003;14:463–8.
33. Lengyel M, Vandor L. The role of thrombolysis in the management of left-sided prosthetic valve thrombosis: a study of 85 cases diagnosed by transesophageal echocardiography. J Heart Valve Dis. 2001;10:636–49.
34. Levine MN, Raskob G, Landefeld S, Kearon C. Hemorrhagic complications of anticoagulant treatment. Chest. 2001;119:108S–21.
35. Morgan MK, Sekhon LH, Finfer S, Grinnell V. Delayed neurological deterioration following resection of arteriovenous malformations of the brain. J Neurosurg. 1999;90:695–701.
36. del Zoppo GJ, Higashida RT, Furlan AJ, Pessin MS, Rowley HA, Gent M. PROACT: a phase II randomized trial of recombinant pro-urokinase by direct arterial delivery in acute middle cerebral artery stroke. PROACT Investigators. Prolyse in Acute Cerebral Thromboembolism. Stroke. 1998;29:4–11.

37. Paciaroni M, Agnelli G, Micheli S, Caso V. Efficacy and safety of anticoagulant treatment in acute cardioembolic stroke: a meta-analysis of randomized controlled trials. Stroke. 2007;38:423–30.
38. Asinger RW, Dyken ML, Fisher M, Hart RG, Sherman DG. Cardiogenic brain embolism: the second report of Cerebral Embolism Task Force. Arch Neurol. 1989;46:723–43.
39. Bogousslavsky J, Cachin C, Regli F, Despland PA, Van Melle G, Kappenberger L. Cardiac sources of embolism and cerebral infarction–clinical consequences and vascular concomitants: the Lausanne Stroke Registry. Neurology. 1991;41:855–9.
40. Caplan L. Posterior circulation ischemia: then, now, and tomorrow. The Thomas Willis Lecture-2000. Stroke. 2000;31:2011–23.
41. Caplan LR, Wityk RJ, Glass TA, et al. New England Medical Center Posterior Circulation registry. Ann Neurol. 2004;56:389–98.
42. Bogousslavsky J, Regli F, Maeder P, Meuli R, Nader J. The etiology of posterior circulation infarcts: a prospective study using magnetic resonance imaging and magnetic resonance angiography. Neurology. 1993;43:1528–33.
43. Glass TA, Hennessey PM, Pazdera L, et al. Outcome at 30 days in the New England Medical Center Posterior Circulation Registry [see comment]. Arch Neurol. 2002;59:369–76.
44. Schonewille WJ, Wijman CA, Michel P, Algra A, Kappelle LJ. The Basilar Artery International Cooperative Study (BASICS). Int J Stroke. 2007;2:220.
45. Pessin MS, Lathi ES, Cohen MB, Kwan ES, Hedges 3rd TR, Caplan LR. Clinical features and mechanism of occipital infarction. Ann Neurol. 1987;21:290–9.
46. Yamamoto Y, Georgiadis AL, Chang HM, Caplan LR. Posterior cerebral artery territory infarcts in the New England Medical Center Posterior Circulation Registry. Arch Neurol. 1999;56:824–32.
47. Gage BF, Waterman AD, Shannon W, Boechler M, Rich MW, Radford MJ. Validation of clinical classification schemes for predicting stroke: results from the National Registry of Atrial Fibrillation. JAMA. 2001;285:2864–70.
48. Sila CA. Cardioembolic Stroke. In: Noseworthy JH, editor. Neurological Therapeutics: Principles and Practice, vol. 1. London: Martin Dunitz; 2003. p. 450–7.
49. Handke M, Harloff A, Olschewski M, Hetzel A, Geibel A. Patent foramen ovale and cryptogenic stroke in older patients. New Engl J Med. 2007;357:2262–8.
50. Mas JL, Arquizan C, Lamy C, et al. Recurrent cerebrovascular events associated with patent foramen ovale, atrial septal aneurysm, or both. New Engl J Med. 2001;345:1740–6.
51. Kizer JR, Devereux RB. Clinical practice. Patent foramen ovale in young adults with unexplained stroke [see comment][erratum appears in N Engl J Med. 2006 Jun 1;354(22):2401]. New Engl J Med. 2005;353:2361–72.
52. Feinberg WM, Blackshear JL, Laupacis A, Kronmal R, Hart RG. Prevalence, age distribution, and gender of patients with atrial fibrillation. Analysis and implications. Arch Intern Med. 1995;155:469–73.
53. Hart RG, Halperin JL. Atrial fibrillation and thromboembolism: a decade of progress in stroke prevention. Ann Intern Med. 1999;131:688–95.
54. Hart RG, Halperin JL. Atrial fibrillation and stroke: concepts and controversies. Stroke. 2001;32:803–8.
55. Albers GW, Dalen JE, Laupacis A, Manning WJ, Petersen P, Singer DE. Antithrombotic therapy in atrial fibrillation. Chest. 2001;119:194S–206.
56. Flaker GC, Blackshear JL, McBride R, Kronmal RA, Halperin JL, Hart RG. Antiarrhythmic drug therapy and cardiac mortality in atrial fibrillation. The Stroke Prevention in Atrial Fibrillation Investigators. J Am Coll Cardiol. 1992;20:527–32.
57. Flaker GC, Fletcher KA, Rothbart RM, Halperin JL, Hart RG. Clinical and echocardiographic features of intermittent atrial fibrillation that predict recurrent atrial fibrillation. Stroke Prevention in Atrial Fibrillation (SPAF) Investigators. Am J Cardiol. 1995;76:355–8.
58. Adams Jr HP, del Zoppo G, Alberts MJ, et al. Guidelines for the early management of adults with ischemic stroke: a guideline from the American Heart Association/American Stroke

Association Stroke Council, Clinical Cardiology Council, Cardiovascular Radiology and Intervention Council, and the Atherosclerotic Peripheral Vascular Disease and Quality of Care Outcomes in Research Interdisciplinary Working Groups: The American Academy of Neurology affirms the value of this guideline as an educational tool for neurologists. Circulation. 2007;115:e478–534.

59. Douglas PS, Khandheria B, Stainback RF, et al. ACCF/ASE/ACEP/ASNC/SCAI/SCCT/ SCMR 2007 appropriateness criteria for transthoracic and transesophageal echocardiography: a report of the American College of Cardiology Foundation Quality Strategic Directions Committee Appropriateness Criteria Working Group, American Society of Echocardiography, American College of Emergency Physicians, American Society of Nuclear Cardiology, Society for Cardiovascular Angiography and Interventions, Society of Cardiovascular Computed Tomography, and the Society for Cardiovascular Magnetic Resonance endorsed by the American College of Chest Physicians and the Society of Critical Care Medicine. J Am Coll Cardiol. 2007;50:187–204.

60. Bath PM, Lindenstrom E, Boysen G, et al. Tinzaparin in acute ischaemic stroke (TAIST): a randomised aspirin-controlled trial.[see comment][erratum appears in Lancet 2001 Oct 13;358(9289):1276]. Lancet. 2001;358:702–10.

61. Bruno A, Biller J, Adams Jr HP, et al. Acute blood glucose level and outcome from ischemic stroke. Trial of ORG 10172 in Acute Stroke Treatment (TOAST) Investigators. Neurology. 1999;52:280–4.

62. Dalal PM, Mishra NK, Bhattacharjee M, Bhat P. Antithrombotic agents in cerebral ischaemia. J Assoc Physicians India. 2006;54:555–61.

63. Graham SP. To anticoagulate or not to anticoagulate patients with cardiomyopathy. Cardiol Clin. 2001;19:605–15.

64. Hart RG, Pearce LA, Miller VT, et al. Cardioembolic vs. noncardioembolic strokes in atrial fibrillation: frequency and effect of antithrombotic agents in the stroke prevention in atrial fibrillation studies. Cerebrovasc Dis. 2000;10:39–43.

65. Homma S, Sacco RL, Di Tullio MR, Sciacca RR, Mohr JP. Atrial anatomy in non-cardioembolic stroke patients: effect of medical therapy [see comment]. J Am Coll Cardiol. 2003;42: 1066–72.

66. Sandercock P. Full heparin anticoagulation should not be used in acute ischemic stroke. Stroke. 2003;34:231–2.

67. Teitelbaum JS, von Kummer R, Gjesdal K, et al. Effect of ximelagatran and warfarin on stroke subtypes in atrial fibrillation. Can J Neurol Sci. 2008;35:160–5.

68. Yasaka M, Yamaguchi T. Secondary prevention of stroke in patients with nonvalvular atrial fibrillation: optimal intensity of anticoagulation. CNS Drugs. 2001;15:623–31.

69. Anonymous. The effect of low-dose warfarin on the risk of stroke in patients with nonrheumatic atrial fibrillation. The Boston Area Anticoagulation Trial for Atrial Fibrillation Investigators [see comment]. New Engl J Med. 1990;323:1505–11.

70. Ezekowitz MD, Levine JA. Preventing stroke in patients with atrial fibrillation. JAMA. 1999;281:1830–5.

71. Petersen P, Boysen G, Godtfredsen J, Andersen ED, Andersen B. Placebo-controlled, randomised trial of warfarin and aspirin for prevention of thromboembolic complications in chronic atrial fibrillation. The Copenhagen AFASAK study. Lancet. 1989;1:175–9.

72. Connolly SJ, Laupacis A, Gent M, Roberts RS, Cairns JA, Joyner C. Canadian Atrial Fibrillation Anticoagulation (CAFA) Study. J Am Coll Cardiol. 1991;18:349–55.

73. Anonymous. Stroke Prevention in Atrial Fibrillation Study. Final results [see comment]. Circulation 1991;84:527–39.

74. Pearce LA, Hart RG, Halperin JL. Assessment of three schemes for stratifying stroke risk in patients with nonvalvular atrial fibrillation. Am J Med. 2000;109:45–51.

75. Anonymous. Risk factors for stroke and efficacy of antithrombotic therapy in atrial fibrillation. Analysis of pooled data from five randomized controlled trials [erratum appears in Arch Intern Med 1994 Oct 10;154(19):2254]. Arch Intern Med. 1994;154:1449–57.

76. Laupacis A, Albers G, Dalen J, Dunn MI, Jacobson AK, Singer DE. Antithrombotic therapy in atrial fibrillation. Chest. 1998;114:579S–89.
77. Anonymous. Patients with nonvalvular atrial fibrillation at low risk of stroke during treatment with aspirin: Stroke Prevention in Atrial Fibrillation III Study. The SPAF III Writing Committee for the Stroke Prevention in Atrial Fibrillation Investigators [see comment]. JAMA 1998;279:1273–7.
78. Hart RG, Pearce LA, Aguilar MI. Meta-analysis: antithrombotic therapy to prevent stroke in patients who have nonvalvular atrial fibrillation. Ann Intern Med. 2007;146:857–67.
79. Wilmshurst PT, Nightingale S, Walsh KP, Morrison WL. Effect on migraine of closure of cardiac right-to-left shunts to prevent recurrence of decompression illness or stroke or for haemodynamic reasons. Lancet. 2000;356:1648–51.
80. Maisel WH, Laskey WK. Patent foramen ovale closure devices: moving beyond equipoise. JAMA. 2005;294:366–9.
81. Messe SR, Silverman IE, Kizer JR, et al. Practice parameter: recurrent stroke with patent foramen ovale and atrial septal aneurysm: report of the Quality Standards Subcommittee of the American Academy of Neurology [see comment]. Neurology. 2004;62:1042–50.
82. Amarenco P, Cohen A, Tzourio C, et al. Atherosclerotic disease of the aortic arch and the risk of ischemic stroke [see comment]. New Engl J Med. 1994;331:1474–9.
83. Fujimoto S, Yasaka M, Otsubo R, Oe H, Nagatsuka K, Minematsu K. Aortic arch atherosclerotic lesions and the recurrence of ischemic stroke. Stroke. 2004;35:1426–9.
84. Tunick PA, Nayar AC, Goodkin GM, et al. Effect of treatment on the incidence of stroke and other emboli in 519 patients with severe thoracic aortic plaque [see comment]. Am J Cardiol. 2002;90:1320–5.
85. Dressler FA, Craig WR, Castello R, Labovitz AJ. Mobile aortic atheroma and systemic emboli: efficacy of anticoagulation and influence of plaque morphology on recurrent stroke [see comment]. J Am Coll Cardiol. 1998;31:134–8.
86. Meyer BC, Raman R, Hemmen T, Obler R, Zivin JA, Rao R, et al. Efficacy of site-independent telemedicine in the STRokE DOC trial: a randomised, blinded, prospective study. Lancet Neurol. 2008;7(9):787–95.
87. Capampangan DJ et al. Telemedicine versus telephone for remote emergency stroke consultations. A critically appraised topic. Neurologist. 2009;15:163–6.
88. Rosso C et al. Diffusion-weighted MRI in acute stroke within the first 6 hours: 1.5 or 3.0 Tesla. Neurology. 2010;74:1946–53.
89. Saver JL. Number needed to treat estimates incorporating effects over the entire range of clinical outcomes. Novel derivation method and application to thrombolytic therapy for acute stroke. Arch Neurol. 2004;61:1066–70.
90. Saver JL. Hemorrhage after thrombolytic therapy for stroke: the clinically relevant number needed to harm. Stroke. 2007;38:2279–83.
91. Gadhia J et al. Assessment and improvement of figures to visually convey benefit and risk of stroke thrombolysis. Stroke. 2010;41:300–6.
92. Saver JL et al. Number needed to treat to benefit and to harm for intravenous tissue plasminogen activator therapy in the 3- to 4.5-hour window. Joint outcome table analysis of the ECASS trial. Stroke. 2009;40:2433–7.
93. Norrving B. Lacunar infarcts: no black holes in the brain are benign. Pract Neurol. 2008;8:222–8.
94. Bejot Y, Catteau A, Caillier M, Rouaud O, Durier J, et al. Trends in incidence, risk factors, and survival in symptomatic lacunar stroke in Dijon, France, from 1989 to 2006: a population based study. Stroke. 2008;39:1945–51.
95. Benavente O et al. Small vessel strokes. Curr Cardiol Rep. 2005;7:23–8.
96. Schonewille WJ, Tuhrim S, Singer MB, Atlas SW. Diffusion-weighted MRI in acute lacunar syndromes. A clinical-radiological correlation study. Stroke. 1999;30(10):2066–9.
97. Arboix A, Marti-Vilalta JL. Lacunar stroke. Expert Rev Neurother. 2009;9(2):179–96.

98. Benavente OR et al. and for the SPS3 Investigators. The secondary prevention of small subcortical strokes (SPS3) study. International journal of stroke. 2011;6:164–75. doi: 10.1111/j.1747-4949.2010.00573.x.
99. Fluri F et al. Intravenous thrombolysis in patients with stroke attributable to small artery occlusion. Eur J Neurol. 2010;17:1054–60.
100. Jackson C et al. Comparing risks of death and recurrent vascular events between lacunar and non-lacunar infarction. Brain. 2005;128:2507–17.
101. Sacco S et al. A population based study of the incidence and prognosis of lacunar stroke. Neurology. 2006;66:1335–8.

Chapter 5
Headache

Esma Dilli and David W. Dodick

Keywords Migraine • Headache • Trigeminal autonomic cephalalgia • Cluster headache • Treatment • Evidence based

Migraine

Introduction

Migraine is a neurological disorder characterized by recurrent disabling attacks of moderate or severe headache associated with gastrointestinal (e.g., nausea, emesis) and autonomic (pallor, flushing, increased urination) symptoms, and heightened sensitivity to environmental stimuli (e.g., light, sound). Reversible focal neurological symptoms may precede the onset of headache by 20–60 min (migraine with aura). Migraine with aura affects about 30% of patients with migraine and usually consists of visual symptoms including spots of light, zigzag lines, or regions of visual loss (scotomas); nonvisual symptoms include somatosensory symptoms (tingling and numbness) and/or language impairment.

D.W. Dodick (✉)
Neurology Department, Mayo Clinic, 5777 East Mayo Boulevard 5E, Phoenix, AZ 85054, USA
e-mail: dodick.david@mayo.edu

J.G. Burneo et al. (eds.), *Neurology: An Evidence-Based Approach*,
DOI 10.1007/978-0-387-88555-1_5, © Springer Science+Business Media, LLC 2012

Epidemiology

Incidence

The incidence of migraine with and without aura in females has been shown to peak between ages 12 and 13 (14.1/1,000 person-years) and 14 and 17 (18.9/1,000 person-years), respectively [1, 2]. In males, migraine with and without aura peaks in incidence several years earlier, around 5 years of age at 6.6/1,000 person-years and 10–11 years at 10/1,000 person-years, respectively. The median age of onset of migraine is approximately 19–23 for males and 20–25 for females, while the cumulative lifetime incidence is 7.4% for males and 21% for females [3, 4]. The cumulative incidence of migraine by age 85 is 18.5% in males and 44.3% in females [4]. These findings suggest that migraine is associated with high rates of onset and remission.

Prevalence

The prevalence of migraine in the United States has been studied and replicated in three large population-based studies over the past two decades. The prevalence of migraine in all three studies has remained stable at approximately 18% in women and 6% in men [5]. In general, migraine prevalence is higher in boys than in girls before puberty, but as adolescence approaches, incidence and prevalence increases significantly in girls more than in boys. The prevalence increases throughout childhood and early adult life until approximately age 40, after which it declines. Overall, prevalence is highest from 25 to 55.

Clinical Case Example

A 38-year-old attorney, and mother of two children, experienced her first migraine attack without aura at the age of 13 years. During adolescence, attacks occurred monthly, usually 2 days prior to the onset of menstrual flow. However, after the birth of her second child 5 years ago, her attacks increased in frequency and severity. Currently, she experiences two attacks per week, each lasting up to 16 h untreated. If treated with sumatriptan 100 mg oral tablets, the pain and associated symptoms resolve in approximately 2–4 h, but she is left with symptoms of fatigue, poor concentration, and photophobia. Symptoms during attacks invariably consist of a bilateral squeezing/pressure headache that is severe, worsened with routine physical activity, and associated with photophobia and nausea. The patient's past medical history is noteworthy for obesity (BMI 33.4), glucose intolerance, and asthmatic bronchitis.

1. What are the criteria for making a diagnosis of migraine?
2. What are the indications for initiating treatment with preventive medication?
3. What is the evidence for the use of preventive medications in migraine?

Table 5.1 Migraine without aura

A. At least five attacks fulfilling criteria B–D
B. Headache attacks lasting 4–72 h (untreated or unsuccessfully treated)
C. Headache has *at least two* of the following characteristics:
1. Unilateral location
2. Pulsating quality
3. Moderate or severe pain intensity
4. Aggravation by or causing avoidance of routine physical activity (for example, walking or climbing stairs)
D. During headache *at least one* of the following:
1. Nausea and/or vomiting
2. Photophobia and phonophobia
E. Not attributed to another disorder

Table 5.2 Migraine with aura

A. At least 2 attacks fulfilling B–E
B. Fully reversible visual and/or sensory and/or speech symptoms but no motor weakness
C. At least *two* of the following:
1. *Unilateral* symptoms including positive and/or negative features
2. At least one symptom develops gradually over >5 min and/or different symptoms occur in succession (e.g., visual symptoms followed by sensory symptoms or language dysfunction)
3. Each symptom lasts >5 min and <60 min
D. Headache meets criteria for migraine without aura and begins during the aura or follows aura within 60 min
E. Not attributable to another disorder

Adapted from ref. [6]

Diagnosis

Operational diagnostic criteria for migraine have been established by the International Classification of Headache Disorders (ICHD-II) [6]. The diagnostic criteria for migraine with and without aura are outlined in Tables 5.1 and 5.2. The diagnostic criteria are highly sensitive, but not specific. The classification criteria therefore always has a minimum threshold number of attacks required for the diagnosis and a criterion that stipulates that secondary causes have been excluded ("not attributed to another disorder").

Treatment Section Search Strategy

Studies were identified through computerized searches of the MEDLINE, PsychINFO, and CINAHL databases. The search strategy used the MeSH term "headache" (exploded) and a published search strategy for identifying randomized controlled trials published between June 1999 and May 2010. A total of 284 articles were identified. Clinical studies reviewed were limited to those assessing efficacy of pharmacologic treatments for prevention of episodic migraine in adults. Studies were excluded if they assessed the efficacy of therapeutic agents for prevention or treatment of chronic migraine, intractable migraine, tension-type headache, or headache in adolescents or children. Studies were also excluded if they assessed acute treatment for migraine, treatment or prevention of migraine aura, or nonpharmacological treatments (e.g., behavioral approaches). Studies using quality of life measures, disability assessment, or nonstandardized outcomes as primary efficacy endpoints were not included. Drugs not available in the United States were not reviewed. The following classification of recommendations was used.

Level A. Established as effective, ineffective, or harmful (or established as useful/predictive or not useful/predictive) for the given condition in the specified population. (Level A rating requires at least two consistent Class I studies).

Level B. probably effective, ineffective, or harmful (or probably useful/predictive or not useful/predictive) for the given condition in the specified population. (Level B rating requires at least one Class I study or two consistent Class II studies – see Appendix).

Migraine Preventive Drug Treatment

Preventive therapy is used in an attempt to reduce the frequency, duration, or severity of attacks [7]. Additional benefits include enhancing the response to acute treatments, improving a patient's ability to function, and reducing disability. Preventive treatment may also result in health care cost reductions [8]. Recent US and European Guidelines [9, 10] have established the circumstances that might warrant preventive treatment (1) recurring migraine that significantly interferes with quality of life and patient's daily routine despite acute treatment; (2) frequency of attacks per month is two or higher; (3) failure of, contraindication to, or troublesome side effects from acute medications; and (4) frequent, very long, or uncomfortable auras. A migraine preventive drug is considered successful if the frequency of migraine attacks is reduced by at least 50% within 3 months. For treatment evaluation, a migraine diary is highly recommended.

The major medication groups for preventive migraine treatment include certain β-adrenergic blockers and anticonvulsants, flunarizine and amitriptyline. If preventive medication is indicated, the agent should be chosen from one of these first-line categories, based on the drug's relative efficacy in double-blind, placebo-controlled trials, its side effect profile, and the patient's preference, as well as coexistent and comorbid conditions.

Divalproex sodium, sodium valproate, topiramate, metoprolol, propranolol, and timolol, are effective for migraine prevention and should be offered to patients with migraine to reduce the frequency and severity of migraine attacks (Level A) [7]. The following medications are probably effective and should be considered for migraine prevention; amitriptyline, fluoxetine, venlafaxine, gabapentin, atenolol, nadolol, nimodipine, verapamil, and for short-term prevention of menstrually related migraine – naratriptan and zolmitriptan (Level B) [7].

Treatment Section Clinical Bottom Lines

1. Preventive treatment should be offered to patients whose attack frequency exceeds one attack per week.
2. Medications with the highest level of evidence should be considered first when selecting a preventive medication for migraine.
3. Comorbid and coexisting conditions should influence the selection of preventive medication.

In the particular case example, topiramate is a reasonable first choice for prevention based on the level of supporting evidence and Level A recommendation. Topiramate is associated with weight loss, which could improve her glucose intolerance, however word finding difficulties may occur with topiramate. Tricyclic antidepressants and divalproex sodium would be less desirable choices based on the potential for weight gain in a patient with obesity and glucose intolerance, and beta-blockers are relatively contraindicated in this woman due to her history of asthmatic bronchitis.

Cluster Headache and Other Trigeminal Autonomic Cephalalgias

Introduction

The trigeminal autonomic cephalalgias (TACs) are a group of primary headaches characterized by excruciating unilateral, side-locked pain, which occur in paroxysms lasting minutes to hours. The term comes from the trigeminal (often first division) distribution of the pain, and the accompanying cranial autonomic features including Horner's syndrome, lacrimation, conjunctival injection, and nasal congestion. The attacks may "cluster" daily for a period of weeks to months, and intervening periods of complete remission. Chronic forms of each disorder may occur, where patients do not have sustained respite from attacks for periods of longer than 4 weeks. These disorders are distinguished from each other by the frequency of attacks that occur within a 24 h period, the duration of each attack, and the response to medication. The TACs are listed in the ICHD-II under their own section, and include Cluster headache (CH), Paroxysmal hemicrania (PH), and Short unilateral neuralgiform headache with conjunctival injection and tearing/cranial autonomic symptoms (SUNCT/SUNA).

Epidemiology

Incidence

Unlike other primary headache disorders such as migraine and tension-type headache, the incidence and prevalence of CH is substantially lower. Incidence and prevalence figures for other, even rarer TACs, such as PH and SUNCT are not available.

In a population-based study conducted in Olmstead County, Minnesota involving 6,400 patients screened between 1979 and 1981, the age-adjusted incidence was determined to be 9.8 per 100,000 (15.6 per 100,000 person-years for men and 4.0 per 100,000 person-years for women) [11]. The incidence fell to 2.07 per 100,000 person-years in a follow up study that evaluated a similar population in the same region from 1989 to 1990 [12]. While the reasons are not clear, the authors speculated that this decline correlated with a decline in the prevalence of cigarette smoking, a feature that is highly prevalent in CH patients (>90%). This data, however, was similar to the findings from another population-based study in Italy, which demonstrated an incidence of 2.5 per 100,000 person-years [13].

Prevalence

A recent meta-analysis of population-based studies that have evaluated the prevalence of CH demonstrated lifetime prevalence of 124 per 100,000 and a 1-year prevalence of 53 per 100,000 [14]. The overall sex ratio was 4.3 (male to female), but the ratio was higher in chronic CH (15.0) compared with episodic CH (3.8). The ratio of episodic vs. chronic CH was 6.0. The lifetime prevalence was relatively stable and suggested that about one in 1,000 people suffer from CH, the prevalence being independent of the region of the population study.

Clinical Case Example

A 32-year-old man presents with a 6 year history of recurrent, severe, right periorbital headaches. He has had six bouts of headache over this time, each bout lasting about 3 months. Attacks usually occur during the fall season. He experiences three attacks per day, at least one of which occurs about 2 h after falling asleep each night. The pain is the worst pain he has ever experienced, even worse than the pain he had with two prior kidney stones. Each attack lasts about 90 min, the pain peaks within 5 min, and it's impossible for him to sit or lie still during the pain. Each attack is associated with bilateral lacrimation (worse on the right) nasal stuffiness and rhinorrhea on the right, ipsilateral photophobia in the right eye, and conjunctival injection bilateral (worse on the right). Attacks can be triggered by minimal amounts of alcohol, but only when he is in a cycle of attacks. He has 12-year history of tobacco use (one pack per day), but no other significant past medical history. There is no family history of a similar headache disorder.

1. What is the diagnosis, and how does one distinguish between CH and other TACs?
2. What is the evidence to support the acute and preventive treatment of this disorder?
3. What is the prognosis for this patient?

Treatment Section Search Strategy

A comprehensive systematic review and meta-analysis was recently published on the treatment of CH [15]. In this meta-analysis, the search strategy employed was a search of MEDLINE (1950 to June 2009) and EMBASE (1980 to June 2009) databases for double-blind randomized controlled clinical trials. Studies were rated "Class I" if all of the following criteria are met (a) allocation concealment, (b) primary outcome(s) clearly defined, (c) inclusion/exclusion criteria clearly defined, (d) adequate accounting for drop outs and crossovers with numbers sufficient to have minimal potential for bias, and (e) relevant baseline characteristics are presented and substantially equivalent among treatment groups or there is appropriate adjustment for differences. A "Class II" study, is a prospective matched group cohort study, in a representative population with masked outcome assessment that meets (a)–(e) above, or an RCT in a representative population that lacks one criteria (a)–(d). A "Class III" study is a controlled trial, including well-defined natural history controls or patients serving as own controls – in a representative population, where outcome is independently assessed, or independently derived by objective outcome measurement, or an RCT that lacks two criteria (a)–(d). "Class IV" studies include uncontrolled studies, case series, case reports, or expert opinion.

This group of authors employed American Academy of Neurology Classification of Recommendations: A = Established as effective, ineffective, or harmful (or established as useful/predictive or not useful/predictive) for the given condition in the specified population. (Level A rating requires at least two consistent Class I studies.) B = Probably effective, ineffective, or harmful (or probably useful/predictive or not useful/predictive) for the given condition in the specified population. (Level B rating requires at least one Class I study or at least two consistent Class II studies.) C = Possibly effective, ineffective, or harmful (or possibly useful/predictive or not useful/predictive) for the given condition in the specified population. (Level C rating requires at least one Class II study or two consistent Class III studies.) U = Data inadequate or conflicting; given current knowledge, treatment (test, predictor) is unproven (Studies not meeting criteria for Class I–Class III). In addition, a systematic search of MedLine (1950–June 2009), Science Citation Index and the Cochrane Library databases was performed, using keywords "cluster," "headache," "PH," "SUNCT," "treatment," and "trial" (last search in January 2006). All papers published in English were considered if they described a controlled trial or a case series (in PH or SUNCT syndrome).

Table 5.3 Trigeminal autonomic cephalalgias

Feature	PH	SUNCT	Cluster
Sex F:M	2:1	1:2	1:3
Attack duration	~15 min	~1 min	60 min
Attack frequency	11	~30	1

The trigeminal autonomic cephalalgias may be distinguished by the sex ratio, but more importantly, the frequency of attacks in a 24 h period and the duration of individual attacks

PH Paroxysmal hemicrania, *SUNCT* Short lasting unilateral neuralgiform pain with conjunctival injection and tearing

Diagnosis

The diagnosis of CH is made according to the ICHD-II. However, there is considerable phenotypic overlap amongst the TACs. These disorders are distinguished primarily on the basis of the duration and frequency of individual discrete attacks (Table 5.3). The TACs are distinguished from migraine by their circannual and circadian periodicity, the side-locked nature of the attacks, robust cranial autonomic features, agitation and restlessness during attacks, and the presence of ipsilateral photophobia and phonophobia. In addition, each paroxysm of pain, regardless of the diagnosis, lasts between 30 s–3 h, while the pain of migraine, by definition, lasts more than 4 h. The importance of distinguishing between the individual TACs cannot be overemphasized because of the different response to treatment. The preventive treatment of choice for CH, PH, and SUNCT syndrome are verapamil, indomethacin, and lamotrigine, respectively.

Treatment

The treatment of CH invariably requires both acute treatment to minimize the severity of duration of individual attacks, and preventive therapy to reduce the frequency of attacks. In general, preventive treatment is initiated at the onset of a cluster cycle and continued at least for the usual duration of a cluster attack, or 2–4 weeks beyond the expected duration of a cluster cycle.

There is robust (Level A) evidence to support the use of subcutaneous sumatriptan 6 mg, intranasal zolmitriptan 5 and 10 mg, and 100% oxygen for the acute treatment of CH attacks [15]. Intranasal sumatriptan 20 mg and oral zolmitriptan 5 and 10 mg have a level of evidence (B) to support their use for acute treatment, while lower levels of evidence (Level C) exists for the use of intranasal 10% cocaine, intranasal 10% lidocaine, and subcutaneous octreotide 100 μg for the acute treatment of CH.

Currently, there is no preventive treatment for CH with sufficient evidence to support a Level A recommendation. However, intranasal civamide 100 μL and occipital nerve blockade with corticosteroids and lidocaine have evidence to support a Level B recommendation, while Level C advice can be given for melatonin 10 mg, verapamil 360 mg, and lithium 900 mg.

The evidence for the preventive treatment of patients with chronic CH (absence of remission periods less than 4 weeks) is scant. While open-label pilot studies have demonstrated promising results for the use of anticonvulsants [16, 17], as well as peripheral (suboccipital nerve) and central (hypothalamic) deep brain stimulation in patients with medically intractable CH, the implementation of these treatment modalities will depend on the results of randomized controlled studies [18–22].

Because of the rare nature of other TACs such as PH and SUNCT/SUNA, there is insufficient evidence to support a Level A recommendation for any preventive treatment. Moreover, because of the brief duration and high diurnal frequency of individual attacks, acute therapy for patients with PH and SUNCT/SUNA is not feasible or advisable. Nevertheless, indomethacin is widely considered by the academic and clinical headache community to be the treatment of choice for patients with PH, while the ICHD-II considers a complete response to indomethacin an obligatory criterion for the diagnosis of PH [6]. Open-label case series suggest that lamotrigine, topiramate, intravenous lidocaine, and gabapentin may be effective treatments for patients with SUNCT syndrome [23, 24].

Prognosis

The available evidence on the natural history of CH, while scarce, suggests that it is a lifelong disorder in the majority of patients. In one study, about one-tenth of patients with episodic CH (ECH) evolved into chronic CH (CCH), whereas one-third of patients with CCH transformed into ECH [25]. Another study did reveal encouraging evidence in that a substantial proportion of CH sufferers may develop longer remission periods with age [26].

There is a paucity of literature on the natural history and long-term prognosis of PH. The available evidence suggests that it is a life-long condition, although pediatric cases have not been followed for more than 1 year, so the natural history in childhood onset is uncertain. Patients with PH can expect sustained efficacy of indomethacin treatment without developing tachyphylaxis, though about one-quarter develop gastrointestinal side effects [27]. Indomethacin does not appear to alter the long-term course, though a significant proportion of patients can decrease the dose of indomethacin required to maintain a pain-free state [27].

The natural history of SUNCT, the rarest of the TACs, is poorly understood. The average duration of symptoms in one study was 7 years [24]. The longest reported duration of SUNCT is 48 years [28]. SUNCT appears to be a life-long disorder, though more prospective data is needed.

Clinical Bottom Lines

1. The TACs are uncommon, incapacitating primary headache disorders characterized by first division trigeminal pain and robust cranial autonomic symptoms and signs.
2. While there is significant phenotypic overlap, the TACs can be distinguished based on the duration and frequency of individual attacks, and importantly, the response to different medications.
3. Preventive therapy is absolutely necessary for all TACs, mainly because of the high attack frequency, the daily occurrence, and the brevity of attacks that renders treating individual attacks not feasible. The preventive treatments of choice based on evidence for cluster, PH, and SUNCT syndrome are, respectively, verapamil, indomethacin, and topiramate or lamotrigine.
4. The acute treatments of choice for CH, based on evidence, are subcutaneous sumatriptan 6 mg, intranasal zolmitriptan 5 and 10 mg, and 100% oxygen.

The patient presented has CH, based on the frequency of three attacks per 24 h period and a duration of 90 min attacks.

Appendix: Definition of Class I and Class II Studies

Class I: A randomized, controlled clinical trial of the intervention of interest with masked or objective outcome assessment, in a representative population. Relevant baseline characteristics are presented and substantially equivalent among treatment groups or there is appropriate statistical adjustment for differences.

The following are also required:

a. Concealed allocation
b. Primary outcome(s) clearly defined
c. Exclusion/inclusion criteria clearly defined
d. Adequate accounting for drop outs (with at least 80% of enrolled subjects completing the study) and crossovers with numbers sufficiently low to have minimal potential for bias.
e. For noninferiority or equivalence trials claiming to prove efficacy for one or both drugs, the following are also required:

   1. The authors explicitly state the clinically meaningful difference to be excluded by defining the threshold for equivalence or noninferiority.
   2. The standard treatment used in the study is substantially similar to that used in previous studies establishing efficacy of the standard treatment. (e.g., for a drug, the mode of administration, dose, and dosage adjustments are similar to those previously shown to be effective).
   3. The inclusion and exclusion criteria for patient selection and the outcomes of patients on the standard treatment are comparable to those of previous studies establishing efficacy of the standard treatment.

4. The interpretation of the results of the study is based upon a per protocol analysis that takes into account dropouts or crossovers.

Class II: A randomized controlled clinical trial of the intervention of interest in a representative population with masked or objective outcome assessment that lacks one criteria a–e above or a prospective matched cohort study with masked or objective outcome assessment in a representative population that meets b–e above. Relevant baseline characteristics are presented and substantially equivalent among treatment groups or there is appropriate statistical adjustment for differences.

References

1. Lipton RB, Bigal ME, Diamond M, Freitag F, Reed ML, Stewart WF. Migraine prevalence, disease burden, and the need for preventative therapy. Neurology. 2007;68:343–9.
2. Stovner LJ, Hagen K, Jensen R, et al. The global burden of headache: a documentation of headache prevalence and disability worldwide. Cephalalgia. 2007;27:193–210.
3. Stewart WF, Linet MS, Celentano DD, et al. Age- and sex-specific incidence rates of migraine with and without visual aura. Am J Epidemiol. 1991;134(10):1111–20.
4. Stewart WF, Bigal ME, Lipton RB, et al. Lifetime migraine incidence. Results from the American Migraine Prevalence and Prevention study. Headache. 2005;46:52–60.
5. Lipton RB, Bigal ME, Diamond M, et al. Migraine prevalence, disease burden, and the need for preventive therapy. Neurology. 2007;68:343–9.
6. Headache Classification Subcommittee of the International Headache Society. The international classification of headache disorders: 2nd edition. Cephalalgia. 2004;24:9–160.
7. Dodick DW, Silberstein SD. Migraine prevention. Prac Neurol. 2007;7:383–93.
8. Silberstein SD, Winner PK, Chmiel JJ. Migraine preventive medication reduces resource utilization. Headache. 2003;43:171–8.
9. Silberstein SD. Practice parameter: evidence-based guidelines for migraine headache (an evidence-based review) report of the Quality Standards Subcommitte of the American Academy of Neurology. Neurology. 2000;55:754–62.
10. Evers S, Afra J, Frese A, Goadsby PJ, et al. EFNS guideline on the drug treatment of migraine-report of an EFNS task force. Eur J Neurol. 2006;13:560–72.
11. Swanson JW, Yanagihara T, Stang PE, et al. Incidence of cluster headaches: a population-based study in Olmsted County, Minnesota. Neurology. 1994;44:433–7.
12. Black DF, Swanson JW, Stang PE. Decreasing incidence of cluster headache: a population-based study in Olmsted County, Minnesota. Headache. 2005;45:220–3.
13. Tonon C, Guttmann S, Volpini M, et al. Prevalence and incidence of cluster headache in the Republic of San Marino. Neurology. 2002;58:1407.
14. Fischera M, Marziniak M, Gralow I, et al. The incidence and prevalence of cluster headache: a meta-analysis of population-based studies. Cephalalgia. 2008;28:614–8.
15. Francis GJ, Becker WJ, Pringsheim TM. Acute and preventive pharmacologic treatment of cluster headache. Neurology. 2010;75:463–73.
16. Wheeler SD, Carrazana EJ. Topiramate-treated cluster headache. Neurology. 1999;53:234–6.
17. Schuh-Hofer S, Israel H, Neeb L, Reuter U, Arnold G. The use of gabapentin in chronic cluster headache patients refractory to first-line therapy. Eur J Neurol. 2007;14:694–6.
18. Schoenen J, Di Clemente L, Vandenheede M, et al. Hypothalamic stimulation in chronic cluster headache: a pilot study of efficacy and mode of action. Brain. 2005;128:940–7.
19. Leone M, Franzini A, Broggi G, Bussone G. Hypothalamic stimulation for intractable cluster headache: long-term experience. Neurology. 2006;67:150–2.
20. Leone M, Proiette Cecchini A, Franzini A, et al. Lessons from 8 years experience of hypothalamic stimulation in cluster headache. Cephalalgia. 2008;28:789–97.

21. Burns B, Watkins L, Goadsby PJ. Treatment of intractable cluster headache by occipital nerve stimulation in 14 patients. Neurology. 2009;72:341–5.
22. May A, Leone M, Afra J, Linde M, Sandor PS, Evers S, et al. EFNS guidelines on the treatment of cluster headache and other trigeminal autonomic cephalalgias. Eur J Neurol. 2006;13:1066–77.
23. Cohen AS, Goadsby PJ. Paroxysmal hemicrania responding to topiramate. JNNP. 2007;78:96–7.
24. Cohen AS, Matharu MS, Goadsby PJ. Shortlasting unilateral neuralgiform headache attacks with conjunctival injection and tearing (SUNCT) or cranial autonomic features (SUNA)-a prospective clinical study of SUNCT and SUNA. Brain. 2006;129:2746–60.
25. Manzoni GC, Micieli G, Granella F, et al. Cluster headache-course over ten years in 189 patients. Cephalalgia. 1991;11:169–74.
26. Igarashi H, Sakai F. Natural history of cluster headache. Cephalalgia. 1996;16:390–1.
27. Pareja JA, Caminero AB, Franco E, et al. Dose, efficacy and tolerability of long-term indomethacin treatment of chronic paroxysmal hemicrania and hemicrania continua. Cephalagia. 2001;21:869–938.
28. Pareja JA, Sjaastad O. SUNCT syndrome. A clinical review. Headache. 1997;37:195–202.

Chapter 6
Epilepsy

Jorge G. Burneo and Robert C. Knowlton

Keywords Epilepsy • Seizures • Antiepileptics • Status epilepticus • Epilepsy surgery

Introduction

Epileptic seizures are defined as transient clinical events that result from the abnormal, excessive activity of a more or less extensive population of cerebral neurons. The clinical events that constitute epileptic seizures can be extremely diverse. Epilepsy can be defined as a condition characterized by a tendency for recurrent epileptic seizures (2 or 3 or more) unprovoked by any known proximate insult.

New Onset Seizures

Introduction

As defined by the International League Against Epilepsy (ILAE), an unprovoked seizure is a seizure without an identified proximate precipitant or multiple such seizures within a 24-h period. These diagnoses exclude individuals with only febrile seizures, neonatal seizures, or acute symptomatic seizures.

J.G. Burneo (✉)
Neurology, Biostatistics and Epidemiology, Clinical Neurological Sciences,
The University of Western Ontario, 339 Windermere Road B10-118, London,
ON, Canada N6A 5A5
e-mail: jorge.burneo@lhsc.on.ca

J.G. Burneo et al. (eds.), *Neurology: An Evidence-Based Approach*,
DOI 10.1007/978-0-387-88555-1_6, © Springer Science+Business Media, LLC 2012

Epidemiology

Clinical Case Scenario

A 25-year-old, right-handed male presented to the emergency department after having a witnessed, generalized, tonic–clonic seizure at home while watching TV around 10 a.m., 3 h after he woke up. He is not on any medications. His physical/ neurological exam was unremarkable. His basic blood work, including electrolytes and complete blood count, was within normal limits. He had a CT scan of the head while in ER that was normal. Once stable, the neurology service was consulted, he was diagnosed with having a seizure, but was not placed on any medication. He wants to know how often we see patients like him.

Clinical Questions

What is the incidence of a first unprovoked seizure?

Search Strategy

Ovid MEDLINE database was searched since its inception to February 26, 2010. Medical Subject Heading (MeSH) terms "incidence or prevalence" and "seizures" were searched and combined using the Boolean "AND."[1] After limiting the retrieval to English and human and excluding letters and editorials, a final set of 464 citations were obtained. From this set, a systematic review and a population-based study were selected, as they represented the latest publications on the topic [1, 2]. EMBASE, PubMed, LILACS, and the Cochrane Library databases were also searched implementing the same strategy of MeSH terms and keywords. No additional relevant articles were detected.

Incidence of Unprovoked First Seizure

The populational-based study was performed in the northern part of Manhattan and in the Bronx as well as in hospitals and nursing homes in the Northern Manhattan communities. The authors were able to identify incident unprovoked seizures between June 1, 2003 and June 1, 2005. Out of more than 270,000 people, the authors

---

[1]("Seizures"[Mesh] AND "incidence"[Mesh]) OR ("seizures"[Mesh] AND "prevalence"[Mesh]) OR ("Seizures/epidemiology"[Mesh] AND ("humans"[MeSH Terms] AND English[lang] AND (Clinical Trial[ptyp] OR Meta-Analysis[ptyp] OR Randomized Controlled Trial[ptyp]))).

identified 123 cases of a single unprovoked incident seizure, making a crude incidence of 38.6 cases per 100,000 person-years (95% CI: 33.4–43.8). The authors also found that the age- and sex-adjusted incidence was 41.1 (35.4–46.8). The age- and sex-adjusted incidence was 23.9 (19.6–28.2) for single unprovoked seizure and 16.4 (12.8–20.0) for epilepsy. Incidence was highest in the first year of life and among those 75 years and older. This pattern was seen for males and females. Incidence for children less than 1-year-old was 134.4/100,000 (51.1–217.7), decreasing to 50.4/100,000 (24.9–75.9) for children 1–4 years old, and continuing to decrease across age categories until the fourth decade of life. The highest incidence rate among females occurred in the 85 years and older age group (235.5; 95% CI 123.6–347.5), although in the male population the highest incidence rate was found among the 75–84-year olds. Incidence was lowest among 25–34-year olds, and this was true for both sexes.

In the systematic review, the authors based their analysis on 161 English publications, eight French, one German, and one Dutch; but only 13 studies met their inclusion criteria. There was considerable heterogeneity in study methodology. The median incidence rate of unprovoked seizures was 56 per 100,000 people. The age-specific incidence showed a U-shaped pattern with higher rates for children and the elderly than for adults. Overall, the distribution of the age-specific incidence rates of epilepsy differed significantly ($p = 0.008$). In particular, children differed significantly from the other age categories ($p = 0.002$). Furthermore, the incidence was slightly higher for males than for females. However, this difference was not significant. Finally, the results showed that median seizure-specific incidence rates were higher for partial than for generalized seizures, but this difference was not significant. The median incidence rate of partial seizures was higher in children than in adults. Correspondingly, the median incidence rate of generalized seizures was 45.2 in children and decreased to 21 in adults.

Clinical Bottom Lines

The incidence of unprovoked seizures falls between 40 and 56 per 100,000 people. This rate follows a bimodal distribution, being higher in children and in the elderly. It appears to be higher in developing than in developed countries.

Summary

There are many methodological limitations, as studies on unprovoked seizures lack a standard definition, despite the current definition given by the ILAE. There is a lack of incidence studies in developing countries and there appears to be remarkable heterogeneity between studies.

Diagnosis

Introduction

After an adult who presents with a first seizure is stabilized and returns to baseline function, a physician must determine if the event was a seizure and, if so, whether this was the first such event. A history of prior seizures supports a diagnosis of epilepsy. Diagnosing the first unprovoked seizure is not easy. The diagnosis is usually made in clinical grounds, and an electroencephalogram (EEG) or any neuroimaging study after the seizure may aid in the diagnosis but is usually helpful in prognosis and treatment.

Case Scenario

Assuming that our previous 25-year-old patient was not investigated, you are called to see him. His general physical and neurological examinations are performed.

Clinical Question

What is the added value or yield of investigations, including laboratory tests, EEG, CT, and magnetic resonance imaging (MRI), to determine seizure etiology?

Search Strategy

Ovid MEDLINE database was searched since its inception to February 26, 2010. MeSH terms "seizures," "CT," "MRI," "Electroencephalography," and "cerebrospinal fluid" were searched and combined using the Boolean "AND/OR."[2] After limiting the retrieval to English and human and excluding letters and editorials, a final set of 464 citations were obtained. EMBASE, PubMed, LILACS, and the Cochrane Library databases were also searched implementing the same strategy of MeSH terms and keywords. Electronic search of practice parameters from the American Academy of Neurology revealed a practice parameter on the issue [3]. No additional relevant articles were detected.

---

[2]"Seizure" AND (("cerebrospinal fluid"[Mesh]) OR ("CT"[Mesh]) OR ("MRI"[Mesh]) OR ("Electroencephalography"[Mesh])) AND ((Humans[Mesh]) AND (English[lang]) AND (Clinical Trial[ptyp] OR Meta-Analysis[ptyp] OR Practice Guideline[ptyp] OR Randomized Controlled Trial[ptyp])).

The Evidence

The practice parameter represents a systematic review of the literature on the topic. The search was conducted using MEDLINE, 1966 to November 2004, and also included CINAHL and The Cochrane Trials Register. To be included in the review, studies had to report results of any diagnostic or monitoring intervention pertinent to a first or new seizure in adults or adolescents (>18 years of age) with at least ten patients as total sample size. Studies with mixed age populations were reviewed for data pertaining to patients >18 years of age when possible. Of an initial number of 793 articles, 157 articles were considered based on a number of inclusion and exclusion criteria [3].

EEG

EEGs were reported as abnormal in 12–73% (average yield 51%) and reported as significantly abnormal in 8–50% (average 29%). The abnormality considered as significant by the authors was the presence of epileptiform activity in the form of spikes or sharp waves as interpreted by the local or reading electroencephalographer in patients clinically judged to present with a new onset seizure. However, it was also clear from the evidence that a normal EEG does not exclude the presence of a seizure disorder. Indeed, on average, about 50% of individuals clinically diagnosed with a seizure have a normal EEG.

Neuroimaging

Seven studies were considered. The panel assessed the yield and value (with or without contrast agents) of the CT or MRI in adults initially presenting with a seizure (1,092 patients). The neuroimaging study was reported as abnormal in 1 to 57% (average yield 15%) and was significantly abnormal in 1 to 47% (average 10%). These significant abnormalities affected patient management and included previously unrecognized brain tumors, vascular lesions, and cerebral cysticercosis.

Interestingly, almost all of the studies were reported on CT rather than MRI. One reason for this is that some of the studies were older, but another is that many of these studies were of patients seen acutely in emergency departments, where the CT is the procedure of choice because of the relative speed and ease of obtaining the study and its effectiveness in excluding catastrophic problems that may require immediate attention. However, one MRI study of new onset seizures indicated that the yield of MRI was at least as high and likely higher than CT, but it included patients with provoked seizures and those presenting after multiple seizures or with preexisting epilepsy.

CSF Analysis

Two studies were considered for review, as they evaluated the value of a lumbar puncture in patients with a first seizure; both were from emergency departments and reported significant lumbar puncture abnormalities in up to 8% of patients. A substantial number of patients had acute symptomatic seizures. In these studies, the lumbar punctures were performed selectively, as they were performed in only 68% of the patients in one study and 24% of the other, and this depended on such presenting clinical features as fever or at the discretion of the staff. The practice parameter did not find convincing studies to support a lumbar puncture in patients who are alert, oriented, afebrile, and not immunocompromised.

Blood Work

Six studies assessed the yield and value of blood counts, blood glucose, and electrolyte panels [4–9]. The authors reported abnormalities in 0–15% for each of these tests, but no clinically significant by the authors. All these studies were based in emergency departments, and the patients were obviously ill with other comorbidities. A large proportion was patients with acute symptomatic or provoked rather than apparent unprovoked seizures. Among the reported acute symptomatic causes for the seizures were alcohol withdrawal, acute stroke, tumor, sepsis, or trauma. The authors of the systematic review concluded that despite the limitations and acknowledgment that yield is very low, the studies were consistent in proposing some value to routine screening of blood glucose for hypoglycemia and serum electrolytes for hyponatremia because unanticipated and clinically relevant hypoglycemia and hyponatremia were found in about 1% of these patients.

Bottom Lines

Based on the current evidence, EEG and CT or MRI of the brain should be considered part of the routine evaluation in patients after the first unprovoked seizure. Other testing, including CSF analysis, may be performed as there is no data supporting or refuting their use.

Summary

Despite the existence of evidence that supports the use of certain tools for the assessment of patients with a first unprovoked seizure, there is no data to support the use of a test to diagnose seizure, other than clinical history and physical examination.

Treatment

Introduction

Antiepileptic drugs (AEDs) are successful in preventing the recurrence of seizures in 50–70% of newly diagnosed patients with epilepsy. There is broad agreement that treatment should begin after the occurrence of the second seizure, even though AEDs frequently cause adverse reactions. The best approach to adopt after a first unprovoked seizure is more controversial.

Case Scenario

Continuing with our previous 25-year-old patient; his neurological examination was normal. He was investigated and had a normal EEG and CT scan. He wants to know whether he should take an antiepileptic drug.

Clinical Question

Should we treat patients with a single unprovoked tonic–clonic generalized seizure?
Is treatment of a first unprovoked seizure effective?

Search Strategy

Ovid MEDLINE database was searched since its inception to February 26, 2010. MeSH terms "seizures" and "treatment" were searched and combined using the Boolean "AND." We searched Pubmed using the terms "first seizure" AND "treatment." We also limited the retrieval to English and human, and we excluded letters and editorials. EMBASE, PubMed, LILACS, and the Cochrane Library databases were also searched implementing the same strategy of MeSH terms and keywords. The search allowed us to obtain eight articles [10–17]. Electronic search of practice parameters from the American Academy of Neurology revealed a practice parameter on the issue [18]. No additional relevant articles were detected.

The Evidence

All studies selected were randomized clinical trials, with the exception of the practice parameter which is a systematic review of the evidence. In this latter one, the authors had multiple questions regarding first unprovoked seizures, but the one of interest was: *How effective is treatment after a first seizure in prevention of recurrences?*

The authors included four randomized clinical trials (four of the ones we selected based on our search), including children and adolescents that have examined the efficacy of treatment after a first seizure [10–12, 17]. Only one of these studies consisted solely of children randomized to treatment versus no treatment after a first nonfebrile seizure [10]. In this study, with a total of 31 children, 2 of 14 children (14%) treated with carbamazepine experienced a recurrence compared with 9 of 17 (53%) who were not treated. Follow-up was for 1 year, and compliance was monitored. Although the recurrence rate up to 1 year was significantly lower in the treated group, only 6 of 14 (43%) patients randomized to carbamazepine completed the year with no significant side effects or seizure recurrence and 7 of 17 (41%) assigned to no medication had no seizure recurrence.

The other studies involved both children and adults and the outcome was not provided based on age. The results of these studies as well as the ones we selected are presented in Table 6.1.

The presence of side effects has been an important reason for discontinuation of the antiepileptic medication, once this was initiated after a first seizure. In the FIRST study [15], adverse events were reasons for drug discontinuation in 7% of cases (14 out of 204). In Marson et al. study [16], patients under treatment were more likely to report at least one adverse event than those without immediate treatment (8.6%, 95% CI: 3.6–13.6).

Bottom Lines

Treatment of the first unprovoked seizure does not influence the long-term prognosis of epilepsy.

Summary

The results of this review indicate that none of the drugs evaluated can prevent the establishment of a chronic seizure disorder. The American Academy of Neurology based on their review [18] has recommended that treatment can be considered in circumstances, where the benefits of reducing the risk of a second seizure outweigh the risk of pharmacological and psychosocial side effects.

Prognosis

Introduction

Approximately 10% of the population have at least one seizure at some point in their life [19]. Some go on to have further seizures. The following section touches on to this issue.

Table 6.1 Studies included in the systematic review

Author	Setting	Population	Medication used (number of patients)	Recurrence at 12 months	2 years	10 years
Chandra [11]	University and private hospitals	228 adults	VPA (115) vs. placebo (113)	VPA (56) vs placebo (4)	–	–
Gilad [14]	ER	91 adults	CBZ (46) vs. no treatment (45)	Treated (13) vs. untreated (59)	–	–
Das [17]	Outpatient neurology service	76 children and adults	Any AED (36) vs. no treatment (40)	Treated (11) vs. untreated (45)	–	–
Marson [16]	Multicenter	812 children and adults	Treatment (697) vs. no treatment (115)	Information not clear	Treatment (602) vs. untreated (19)	–
Musicco [12]	Multicenter	419 adults and children	Treatment (215) vs. no treatment (204)	–	Treated (52) vs. untreated (85)	–
Leone [13]	Multicenter	264 adults and children	Treatment (136) vs. no treatment (128)	–	–	Treated (50) vs. untreated (46)
FIRST [15]	Multicenter	419 adults and children	Treatment (17) vs. no treatment (28)	–	–	–

Case Scenario

Our 25-year-old patient would like to know what his risk of having another seizure is.

Clinical Question

In an otherwise healthy individual with a first, unprovoked, generalized, tonic–clonic seizure and normal neurological examination, what is the risk of seizure recurrence?

Search Strategy

We combined free text and MeSH terms in PubMed, MEDLINE, Cochrane, and EMBASE: "seizure recurrence," "unprovoked seizure," "first seizure," "single seizure," and "prognosis." The search provided us with 209 references of which 32 seemed relevant [4, 7, 12–15, 18–43].

The Evidence

The most important (in hierarchy) is a meta-analysis of 13 studies involving 1,930 patients [19]. In this study, the recurrence of seizures happened in 36% and 47% of patients in prospective and retrospective studies, respectively. Abnormalities on neurologic examination as well as on EEG predicted a second seizure. The authors of this study calculated a pooled, overall risk of recurrence of 46% (95% CI = 44–49%) at 2–5 years. The risk of recurrence was quite similar in children and adults (43%, 95% CI = 38–47%, in both).

Some clinical features may determine the recurrence of seizures [25]. Most patients with a single unprovoked seizure were found to be between 16 and 60 years of age [4, 12, 41]. This may increase the suspicion that higher risk of recurrent seizures probably occur in the elderly and the childhood population. Presence of febrile seizures, positive family history, and two or more seizures are markers of recurrence [44–46]. Furthermore, an initial abnormal neurological exam and the presence of a brain lesion are associated with seizure recurrence [44]. But, some studies have actually not found any risk factors for recurrence [33, 47].

A prediction rule was created in 2006 to identify patients with various probabilities for seizure recurrence [43]. This was based on a large, randomized trial in which the authors compared immediate versus deferred antiepileptic treatment for early epilepsy and single seizures [16]. The index takes into account the past history of seizures (one seizure = 0 points, 2–3 seizures = 1 point, 4 or more = 2 points), the presence of neurological deficit, learning disability, or developmental delay (1 point for each) and abnormalities in the EEG (1 point). The final score may range from 0 to 4: 0 points = low risk of recurrence, 1 points = medium risk, and 2–4 points = high risk. No validation has been performed though.

Bottom Lines

For patients who have a single unprovoked, generalized, tonic–clonic seizure, there is a 46% chance of seizure recurrence.

Risk factors for seizure recurrence are: abnormal neurological exam, abnormal EEG, developmental delay, and learning disability.

Temporal Lobe Epilepsy

Introduction

The ILAE groups temporal lobe epilepsy (TLE) within a broad category of "localization-related symptomatic epilepsies characterized by seizures with specific modes of precipitation" [48] and offers a tentative description based on strongly clinical and electrographic (EEG) features. Furthermore, epileptologists allow two subcategories: mesial (or amygdalohippocampal) and lateral (or neocortical) TLE. But, the ILAE classification does not take into account MRI findings, and for that reason fails to include mesial temporal sclerosis, perhaps the commonest pathological substrate of TLE.

Epidemiology

Case Scenario

A 42-year-old female presents to clinic with frequent complex partial seizures for the last 10 years. She has a history of two febrile seizures at the age of 4. She was investigated before and was found to have right temporal spikes and evidence of right hippocampal sclerosis (mesial temporal sclerosis) on MRI. She has been given the diagnosis of TLE and has tried three antiepileptic medications in the past. She is wondering how common her condition is.

Clinical Question

What is the prevalence of TLE?

Search Strategy

Ovid MEDLINE database was searched since its inception to June 30, 2010. MeSH terms "prevalence" and "temporal lobe epilepsy" were searched and combined using the Boolean "AND."[3] After limiting the retrieval to English and humans and excluding letters and editorials, a final set of 1,137 citations were obtained. EMBASE, PubMed, LILACS, and the Cochrane Library databases were also searched implementing the same strategy of MeSH terms and keywords. No additional relevant articles were detected.

The Evidence

There is a lack of studies in this regard. A nonsystematic review that included literature on the topic was identified [49]. In this review, the author identified a chapter in a book [50] that provided the results of a worldwide census of 107 epilepsy surgery centers. In this census, it was found that TLE is by far the most common type of localization-related epilepsy. Of 8,234 operations performed between 1985 and 1990, 66% involved the temporal lobe. But, as the author of this review mentioned, series from specialty units are biased toward patients who are surgical candidates, have more severe epilepsy, and are more intensely investigated.

On the same page, most patients with TLE, as in our patient, are referred for surgical treatment after they had received treatment with multiple medications, as they would be considered medically-intractable or therapy-resistant.

Despite difficulties defining intractability, there are systematic studies on its epidemiology. Two studies have been found [51, 52] in children. In one of those studies, 15% of children with incidence epilepsy met criteria for intractability of at least one seizure per month for a 2-year period [51] while in the other one, the frequency was 7% of all incidence cases, excluding children with minor motor seizures and infantile spasms [52]. In adults, the studies are lacking, but Kwan and Brodie [53] found that close to 30% of adults with epilepsy become refractory. No specific studies in TLE have been done, but perhaps the percentage of patients developing intractability is higher in those with hippocampal sclerosis.

Bottom Lines

Two-thirds of patients seen in epilepsy programs across the globe have TLE.

---

[3]("temporal lobe epilepsy") OR ("temporal lobe epilepsy" AND "prevalence"[Mesh]) OR ("temporal lobe epilepsy" AND "epidemiology" AND ("humans"[MeSH Terms] AND English[lang] AND (Clinical Trial[ptyp] OR Meta-Analysis[ptyp] OR Randomized Controlled Trial[ptyp]))).

Summary

There is a need for studies assessing the epidemiology of TLE.

Diagnosis

Clinical Question

1. What clinical features are useful in diagnosing TLE?
2. What investigational tests are useful in diagnosing TLE?

Search Strategy

MEDLINE database was searched since its inception to June of 2010. MeSH terms and text words *Epilepsy, Temporal Lobe,* and *diagnosis* were searched and combined using the Boolean "AND." After limiting the retrieval to "English," "human," "clinical trial," "meta-analysis," "randomized-controlled trial," and "practice guidelines," a final set of 262 citations were obtained. From this search, all citations and abstracts were searched for relevance to the clinical question revealing nine articles. All nine articles were reviewed and included if they met the following criteria: address a focused clinical question, contain a thorough search of the literature, and assess the validity of the studies.

A second search was conducted using the MeSH terms and text words *Epilepsy, Temporal Lobe,* and *diagnosis (sensitivity OR specificity) (physical examination OR magnetic resonance imaging OR positron emission tomography OR EEG OR video-EEG OR magnetoencephalography OR SPECT OR magnetic resonance spectroscopy OR physical examination OR diagnostic tests)* and combined using the Boolean "AND." After limiting the retrieval to "English," "human," "clinical trial," "meta-analysis," "randomized-controlled trial," and "practice guidelines," a final set of 56 citations were obtained. All 56 articles were reviewed and included if they contributed new information not reported in the meta-analysis or systematic practice guidelines and if they met the following criteria: appropriate spectrum of patients included, presence of a defined gold standard, diagnostic test was compared to the gold standard in a blinded fashion, and greater than ten participants in the each cohort.

Cochrane Database was searched from inception to June 2010 for the terms *temporal lobe epilepsy* and *diagnosis* revealing no additional reviews.

The Evidence

Clinical Features

All the information available comes from retrospective and prospective cohort studies. The ictal clinical manifestations can be in the form of auras and objective observations from video-EEG monitoring. They are further classified as mesial or neocortical.

The mesial temporal auras can consist of a visceral sensation usually in the abdomen and often with a raising component [54–57]. Less common phenomenology would include: fear, déjá vu, jamais vu, olfactory hallucinations, and depersonalization [55]. The inability to describe the aura has also been reported in many case series, but some authors have attributed this to the phenomenon of amnesia that occurs during a complex partial seizure [58]. Objective manifestations include motor arrest, staring, and automatisms; this latter one can be oroalimentary (lip smacking, chewing, licking, and tooth-grinding type of movements) or manual [59]. Unilateral dystonic posture of an arm as a localizing feature (to the contralateral temporal lobe) has been described and is highly accurate when associated with unilateral automatisms of the contralateral hand [60–63]. Other less common manifestations include spitting, postictal nose rubbing or wiping, vomiting, and unilateral eye blinking [64–67]. Postictal aphasia, always thought to be a lateralizing sign, has been the debate of controversy due to contradictory findings in the literature, most likely related to the methodology used in the studies. Aphasia can be easily confused with postictal confusion [68].

Electroencephalography

There are multiple manuscripts on the use of EEG for the diagnosis of epilepsy. But there are no specific controlled trials on the use of EEG in TLE, despite being accepted as part of the standard care when evaluating patients with epilepsy. Most of the existent information comes from retrospective, descriptive case series and cohort studies [69].

The characteristic interictal (in-between seizures) EEG abnormality is anterior temporal sharp waves, spikes, and slow waves. Ictal recordings are characterized by unilateral 5–7 Hz rhythmic discharges, seen in temporal scalp electrodes and appearing within 30 s of the first ictal EEG abnormality [70]. Specific ictal patterns can help the clinician differentiate lateral or neocortical from mesial TLE [71].

EEG recording with intracranial electrodes has been also used for a long time, even though there have not been any randomized, controlled trials supporting its use. Intracranial electrodes can be in the form of depth electrodes or lines or strips usually placed subdurally.

Neuroimaging

Computed tomography (CT) of the head and MRI of the brain are standard tools for the evaluation of patients with epilepsy. They are considered structural imaging techniques. MRI, preferably of high resolution, can demonstrate atrophy of the hippocampal structures (a marker of mesial temporal lobe sclerosis) [69, 72] and can visualize other abnormalities in the temporal lobe that can be the epilepsy's culprit.

In regards with functional imaging, positron emission tomography with ^{18}F-fluorodeoxyglucose (FDG-PET) is a very sensitive interictal imaging technique [73].

Interictal single photon emission computed tomography (SPECT) is also capable of showing unilateral temporal hypoperfusion, but with a much lower specificity than PET. Ictal SPECT, on the contrary, may reveal hyperperfusion of the area involved during a seizure [74, 75]. Other studies used in the evaluation of patients with TLE are: magnetic resonance spectroscopy (MRS), which has demonstrated a decrease in N-acetylaspartate in the area involved in the generation of seizures [76], and magnetic source imaging (MSI) with magnetoencephalography (MEG), which can localize interictal epileptiform discharges to the area involved in the seizure generation [77].

In a recent study, with a large number of subjects (160 patients), different neuroimaging techniques were compared to what is considered the "gold standard" tool for the localization of focal epilepsy [78]. Even though the study was not focused to TLE, the results are of importance. Seventy-two patients underwent implantation of intracranial electrodes and had seizures recorded. Sensitivity ranged from 58 to 64% for MSI, 22 to 40% for PET, and 39 to 48% for ictal SPECT. Specificity ranged from 58 to 64% for MSI, 53 to 63% for PET, and 44 to 50% for ictal SPECT. Gains in diagnostic yield were seen only with the combination of MSI and PET or MSI and ictal SPECT. Localization concordance with intracranial recordings was greatest with MSI, but a significant difference was demonstrated only between MSI and PET. Moderate redundancy was seen between PET and ictal SPECT (kappa$=0.452$; $p=0.011$) [78]. The same group of investigators enrolled the same patients in a study to predict seizure-free outcome following epilepsy surgery [79]. Sixty-two patients completed intracranial EEG recording and subsequent surgical resection. MSI sensitivity for a conclusively localized study was 55% with a positive predictive value of 78%. Eliminating nondiagnostic MSI cases (no spikes captured during recording) yielded a corrected negative predictive value of 64%. With available comparison subgroups, FDG-PET and ictal SPECT values were similar to MSI. The odds ratio (adjusted for epilepsy and MRI findings) for MSI prediction of seizure-free outcome was 4.4 ($p=0.01$). In cases with both PET and MSI, the adjusted OR for PET was 7.1 ($p<0.01$) and for MSI 6.4 ($p=0.01$). In the cases with all three tests ($n=27$), ictal SPECT had the highest OR of 9.1 ($p=0.05$). Finally, a systematic review was done to analyze how useful was MSI/MEG in the presurgical evaluation of patients with focal epilepsy (not only temporal lobe) [80]. The authors selected 17 studies based on rigorous criteria and found that when compared with seizure outcome (seizure freedom as the expected goal), the sensitivity of this technique ranged from 0.2 to 1.0, the specificity from 0.6 to 1.0, and the positive and negative likelihood ratios were 0.67–2 and 0.4–2.13, respectively. The authors concluded that there was insufficient evidence in the literature to support the relationship between the use of MEG and seizure-free outcome after epilepsy surgery [80].

Bottom Lines and Summary

The information regarding the usefulness and utility of clinical signs and symptoms during the peri-ictal and ictal period comes from small retrospective and prospective cohort studies. Larger studies, including a stricter methodology, are needed.

There are no strong studies (Class I) on the use of EEG and video-EEG, but despite that, they are considered standard clinical care.

Even though MRI is widely used for the diagnosis and management of patients with epilepsy, the evidence lacks randomized, controlled trials. Functional neuroimaging studies look promising, but there is a need of randomized, controlled trials.

Treatment

Case Scenario

Our patient has been diagnosed with TLE.

Clinical Question

What are the best options or treatment?

Search Strategy

Ovid MEDLINE database was searched since its inception to June 26, 2010. MeSH terms "epilepsy" and "temporal lobe" were searched and combined using the Boolean "AND." We searched Pubmed using the terms "epilepsy" AND "temporal lobe" AND "treatment." We also limited the retrieval to English and human, and we excluded letters, case reports, and editorials. EMBASE, PubMed, LILACS, and the Cochrane Library databases were also searched implementing the same strategy of MeSH terms and keywords. The search allowed us to obtain 396 abstracts. Electronic search of practice parameters from the American Academy of Neurology revealed a practice parameter on the issue [81]. Review of abstracts to recent epilepsy and neurology meetings allowed us to identify two abstracts on surgery for epilepsy [82, 83]. They were included as well.

The Evidence

Medical Treatment

There is a lack of evidence in regards of medical treatment for TLE. Existent studies have not made a distinction between the different types of epilepsy, as they mainly focused on types of seizures.

Surgical Treatment

Resective Surgery

The short-term efficacy and safety of epilepsy surgery for TLE have been established through a large number of cohort studies and one randomized controlled trial (RCT) [84]. This RCT was a 1:1 RCT of 80 patients with TLE that were felt to be difficult to treat with medications. The trial assessed the safety and efficacy of temporal lobe surgery as compared to the best medical treatment. Optimal medical therapy and primary outcomes were assessed by blinded epileptologists. The primary outcome was freedom from seizures that impair awareness of self and surroundings. Secondary outcomes were the frequency and severity of seizures, the quality of life, disability, and death.

In the RCT, the NNT to render patients free from all seizures at 1 year was 3 (95% CI: 2–5) while it was 2 (95% CI: 1.5–3) to render patients free from seizures impairing awareness. The proportion of patients that remained seizure-free of seizures impairing awareness at 1 year was 58% in the surgical group and 8% in the medical group ($p < 0.001$). The proportion of patients that remained seizure-free of all seizures was 38% for the surgical group and 3% for the medical group ($p < 0.001$). The quality of life was better among the patients in the surgical group than among those in the medical group ($p < 0.001$) and improved over time in both groups ($p < 0.003$). Surgery was safe in patients with TLE (NNH: 9); however, this study was limited to outcomes at 1 year, and there was no clear definition of medical intractability.

Following this RCT, three rigorous meta-analysis or systematic reviews have been published [81, 85, 86]. These studies grouped temporal and extratemporal epilepsy surgery. In the practice parameter [81], the authors included 32 studies with 2,250 patients. Overall, 65% of patients were seizure-free, 21% improved, and 14% did not improve after anteromesial temporal resections (standard TLE surgery). In the second study [86], 126 studies of TLE surgery were included. Seizure-free rates varied widely (33–93%) with a median of 70% (Fig. 6.1). Number of patients was not specified. The last published systematic review [85] included 83 studies, with a total of 3,895 patients with TLE. Sixty-six percent was the median proportion of long-term seizure-free patients. This study even revealed a trend toward better seizure outcome in patients operated after 1980, in children, and in younger patients.

A recent systematic review [83] done by the Canadian Appropriateness and Necessity Study of Epilepsy Surgery (CASES), in order to make recommendations about referral for epilepsy surgery evaluation [82], has been presented (Table 6.2). The systematic review focused on all epilepsy surgeries (temporal and extratemporal). A total of 75 articles after 2003 (the last systematic review published in 2005 included studies conducted up to 2003) were considered, including a total of 7,784 patients. Seventeen studies focused on TLE surgery, including 1,577 patients. The follow-up ranged from 6 months to 29.9 years (±4.9 years). Most of the studies had a follow-up of 1–2 years. Seizure freedom rates varied significantly among studies,

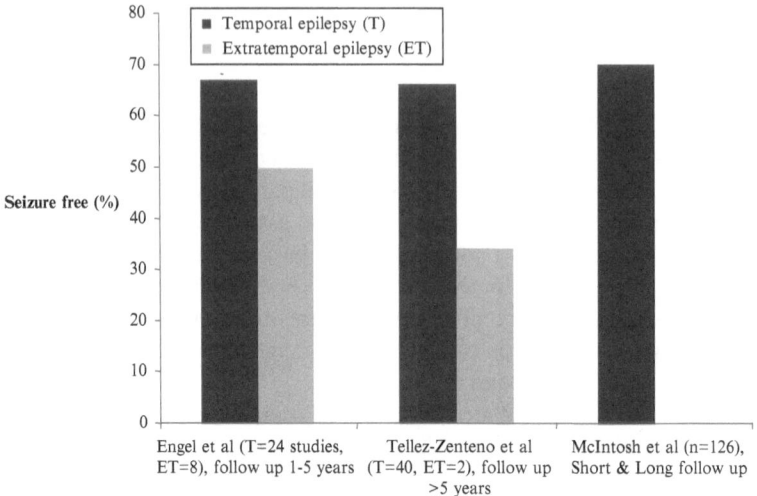

Fig. 6.1 Seizure outcome in three meta-analyses-RAND study. In this graph, we display the results of three rigorous systematic reviews involving short-term, intermediate, and long-term outcomes' report results that are similar for temporal lobe surgery, but less favorable in the long term for extratemporal surgery. From ref. [87] http://www.epilepsycases.com/. With permission from Nathalie Jette

with 33–95.5% of patients being seizure-free at the time of last follow-up. One study focused on long-term follow-up (29.9 ± 4.9 years) and found 50% of patients being seizure-free [88]. Twenty-two studies focused on mesial TLE surgery, including 2,351 patients. The most common etiology was hippocampal sclerosis. Overall seizure freedom ranged between 40.7 and 76%.

Other Surgeries

There were three studies found on the use of electrical hippocampal stimulation in patients with TLE [89–91]. The first article by Boon et al. [90] was an open pilot study, and 2 of the 12 consecutive patients with refractory MTL seizures underwent resective surgery. The other study by Tellez-Zenteno et al. [89], even though it used an individual patient RCT design, included only four patients. The study by Velasco et al. [91] had the largest published study using a double-blinded protocol. They evaluated the safety, efficacy of hippocampal electrical stimulation, and long-term follow-up in nine nonconsecutive patients with medically refractory mesial TLE. All patients had complex, partial seizures with 7/9 also having secondary, generalized tonic–clonic seizures. Patients were selected from a larger group of patients who underwent bilateral hippocampal electrode implantation for diagnostic purposes. The study group consisted of nine patients (six male, three female) between the ages 14 and 43. Average number of seizures per month was 28 (15–70) measured within a 3-month period. Five had normal MRIs and remaining four had mesial temporal

Table 6.2 Temporal lobe surgery: Seizure-free rates by prognostic variable (40 studies involving 3,895 patients)

Group of studies	Patients (n)	Pooled (%)	95% CI	RR[a]	95% CI
Studies with patients operated after 1980 (n=35)	3,512	64	61, 67	1.1	0.9, 1.5
Studies with patients operated before 1980 (n=5)	383	54	48, 60		
Studies with 5–10 years of follow-up (n=35)	3,407	61	59, 63	1.3	1.0, 1.7
Studies with more than 10 years of follow-up (n=5)	488	45	41, 49		
Studies in adults (n=30)[b]	2,947	63	61, 65	1.0	0.7, 1.3
Studies in children (n=9)[b]	444	62	57, 67		
Studies using Engel's outcome classification (n=19)	1,803	66	64, 69	1.0	0.8, 1.4
Studies using other classification systems (n=21)	2,092	61	59, 64		
Other groups					
Studies including patients older than 50 years (n=2)[c]	50	41	29, 53	0.6	0.4, 0.8
Studies including patients with tumors (n=3)[c]	269	76	73, 79	1.1	0.9, 1.4

From ref. [85]. Reprinted with kind permission from Oxford University Press
Risk ratio ([a]RR): Ratio of probability of being seizure-free in one group relative to its comparison. <1 denotes lower and >1 higher chance of being seizure-free
[b]One of forty studies did not specify the age group
[c]Ratio of probability of being seizure-free in these studies relative to all other studies of temporal lobe epilepsy

sclerosis. Three patients had bilateral foci and six had a unilateral focus of MTL seizure activity. Patients were randomized to a double-blind stimulation protocol: five of the patients had an initial 1-month "off" period and the remaining four initiated stimulation immediately after implantation. Patients were evaluated at baseline (3 months prior to electrode implantation) and subsequently every 3 months up to 84 months (mean 37 months). Every 3 months up to 18 months, patients were evaluated with EEG, neuropsychological testing, neurophysiological testing, seizure frequency, and complications. No changes were made to antiepileptic therapy. For the purpose of the study, all participants were evaluated up to month 18 for main outcome measures (seizure frequency and neuropsychological performance) in addition to 3 months of baseline. Complications were reported regardless of duration of follow-up. A seizure reduction of 79% ($p < 0.0005$) occurred in all patients with electrical stimulation of the hippocampus. In patients without mesial temporal sclerosis (MTS) compared to those with MTS, seizure reduction appeared earlier (at 1 month vs. 8 months) and to a greater extent (95%, $p < 0.0005$ vs. 69%, $p < 0.05$ at 18 months). There was a significant rate of complication consisting of skin erosion resulting in infection requiring the removal of the stimulation device in three out of nine participants (33%). The limitations of the study included the following: patients were aware of allocation, selection was nonconsecutive, inclusion and exclusion criteria were not clearly defined, and the characteristics of the patients in the two groups were not specified; 1 month follow-up was not sufficient to see the effect of hippocampal stimulation in the MTS group; statistical comparisons could not be made for the efficacy of hippocampal stimulation within the various subgroups (bilateral vs. left vs. right implantation) or on neuropsychological changes over time by group because of the small sample size of the study; no confidence intervals or effect sizes were calculated; it is unclear what the neuropsychological cutoffs (i.e., standard deviation on tests) were used for degree of memory impairment; a complete follow-up in all patients of 18 months (18–84) was short; and limited information was given on patient's antiepileptic medications and whether they were changed during the base-line period. There are ongoing trials on the use of the hippocampal stimulator in Canada and Europe. They are currently in the process of recruiting patients.

Bottom Lines and Summary

There is a lack of studies evaluating the use of antiepileptic drugs in the treatment of TLE.
The surgical treatment for TLE (medically refractory) appeared to be safe. Short-term studies reported that approximately 60–65% of patients are seizure-free after surgery.
The evidence is not strong for the use of hippocampal electrical stimulation. There is a need for a large study.

Status Epilepticus

Convulsive status epilepticus has been defined as a continuous seizure lasting at least 30 min or cluster of seizures without recovery of awareness or consciousness for at least 30 min as well. Studies on the topic have been done in medical centers and not in the community; hence, the epidemiology of this condition is not clear.

Diagnosis and Assessment of Status Epilepticus

The search of the evidence allowed us to find one practice parameter from the American Academy of Neurology, which was based on a systematic review [92]. This review applies only to the diagnostic assessment of status in children. The authors performed a literature search from 1970 to 2005 and found 20 studies (including 2,093 children).

They found that laboratory studies were abnormal in 6% while cultures (blood and spinal fluid) were abnormal in 2.5%. CNS infection was found in 12.8% of patients. AED levels were low in 32%. Inborn errors of metabolism were found in 4.2%. EEG was helpful in 43% of cases, and abnormalities on neuroimaging studies were found in 8% of children. The authors concluded that the evidence was insufficient for blood work, blood, and CSF cultures. But if the child is taking AEDs, measurement of blood levels was recommended, as well as performance of EEG and neuroimaging studies [92].

Treatment

Introduction

Because status epilepticus is a medical emergency due to its association with significant mortality and morbidity, treatment is recommended. The ethics of RCT in this group of patients have limited their performance. Nonetheless, there is evidence in the literature about it.

Case Scenario

A 30-year-old man was brought to the emergency room seizing for longer than 30 min. The seizure was a generalized tonic–clonic. The ABC rule was applied (airway was protected, breathing was confirmed, and he was started on an IV line). The physician is about to start treatment.

Clinical Question

What is the adequate treatment for status epilepticus?

Search Strategy

MEDLINE and EMBASE were interrogated using the MeSH word "status epilepticus," limited to human, clinical trials, meta-analysis, reviews, and English. We found 162 abstracts. Thirteen were finally selected, as they were focused on treatment. Search of the Cochrane Database of Systematic Reviews allowed us to identify two reviews.

The Evidence

The systematic reviews from the Cochrane library focused their search up to July of 2007 [93, 94]. We found four other studies [95–98].

The first systematic review [94] included 11 studies with 2,017 participants. The authors included RCT of participants with status epilepticus using random or quasi-random allocation of treatments. They found:

– Diazepam vs. placebo:

- Risk of noncessation of seizures → RR = 0.73, 95% CI: 0.57–0.92
- Requirement for ventilator support → RR = 0.39, 95% CI: 0.16–0.94
- Continuation of SE requiring a different drug → RR = 0.73, 95% CI: 0.57–0.92

– Lorazepam vs. placebo:

- Noncessation of seizures → RR = 0.52, 95% CI: 0.38–0.71
- Continuation of SE requiring a different drug → RR = 0.52, 95% CI: 0.38–0.71

– Lorazepam vs. diazepam:

- Noncessation of seizures → RR = 0.64, 95% CI: 0.45–0.9
- Continuation of SE requiring a different drug → RR; 0.63, 95% CI: 0.45–0.88

– Lorazepam vs. phenytoin:

- Noncessation of seizures → RR = 0.62, 95% CI: 0.45–0.86

– Intrarectal gel of diazepam 30 mg vs. 20 mg

- Risk of seizure continuation → RR = 0.39, 95% CI: 0.18–0.86

The second review included the same studies, but also obtained information on the management of tonic–clonic convulsions, not the topic of this section [93].

One recent study was not included in any of the systematic reviews [97]. In this study, the authors randomly allocated 178 children with status epilepticus to receive either IV lorazepam (0.1 mg/kg) or the combination of diazepam (0.2 mg/kg) and phenytoin (18 mg/kg). The children were followed for 18 h. Ninety were enrolled in the lorazepam group and 88 in the diazepam–phenytoin one. The results did not show any significant difference. Six patients (6.7%) in the lorazepam group required more than one dose while 14 in the combination group (15.9%) did so (adjusted RR = 0.38, 95% CI: 0.34–1.05). The number of patients affected by respiratory depression was similar in each group (4.4% in the lorazepam group vs. 5.6% in the combination group).

Another recent study [95] evaluated the use of IV valproate and phenytoin in a group of patients who were refractory to benzodiazepine use. The authors allocated 50 patients in each group (phenytoin versus valproate) in a randomized fashion. A successful outcome was quantified as cessation of motor or EEG activity within 20 min after administration of the drug and no return of seizure activity during the following 12 h. The authors found that 88% of patients responded to IV valproate while 84% to phenytoin ($p < 0.05$), but there was no difference with regards to recurrence after 12 h.

Bottom Lines

- Lorazepam appeared to be better than diazepam or phenytoin alone based on a systematic review [94], but had similar effect than a combined phenytoin–diazepam protocol in an RCT [97].
- Valproate appeared to be an option for the management of benzodiazepine-related status epilepticus [95].

Summary

The literature is still scarce in regards to the optimal treatment of status epilepticus, even though the drugs being used currently in clinical settings are fairly effective. More trials are needed.

References

1. Kotsopoulos IA, van Merode T, Kessels FG, de Krom MC, Knottnerus JA. Systematic review and meta-analysis of incidence studies of epilepsy and unprovoked seizures. Epilepsia. 2002;43:1402–9.
2. Benn EK, Hauser WA, Shih T, et al. Estimating the incidence of first unprovoked seizure and newly diagnosed epilepsy in the low-income urban community of Northern Manhattan, New York City. Epilepsia. 2008;49:1431–9.
3. Krumholz A, Wiebe S, Gronseth G, et al. Practice Parameter: evaluating an apparent unprovoked first seizure in adults (an evidence-based review): report of the Quality Standards Subcommittee of the American Academy of Neurology and the American Epilepsy Society. Neurology. 2007;69:1996–2007.
4. Hopkins A, Garman A, Clarke C. The first seizure in adult life. Value of clinical features, electroencephalography, and computerised tomographic scanning in prediction of seizure recurrence. Lancet. 1988;1:721–6.
5. Edmondstone WM. How do we manage the first seizure in adults? J R Coll Phys Lond. 1995;29:289–94.
6. Sempere AP, Villaverde FJ, Martinez-Menendez B, Cabeza C, Pena P, Tejerina JA. First seizure in adults: a prospective study from the emergency department. Acta Neurol Scand. 1992;86:134–8.
7. Tardy B, Lafond P, Convers P, et al. Adult first generalized seizure: etiology, biological tests, EEG, CT scan, in an ED. Am J Emerg Med. 1995;13:1–5.
8. Turnbull TL, Vanden Hoek TL, Howes DS, Eisner RF. Utility of laboratory studies in the emergency department patient with a new-onset seizure. Ann Emerg Med. 1990;19:373–7.
9. Henneman PL, DeRoos F, Lewis RJ. Determining the need for admission in patients with new-onset seizures. Ann Emerg Med. 1994;24:1108–14.
10. Camfield P, Camfield C, Dooley J, Smith E, Garner B. A randomized study of carbamazepine versus no medication after a first unprovoked seizure in childhood. Neurology. 1989;39:851–2.
11. Chandra B. First seizure in adults: to treat or not to treat. Clin Neurol Neurosurg. 1992;94(Suppl):S61–3.

12. Musicco M, Beghi E, Solari A, Viani F. Treatment of first tonic-clonic seizure does not improve the prognosis of epilepsy. First Seizure Trial Group (FIRST Group). Neurology. 1997;49:991–8.

13. Leone MA, Solari A, Beghi E. Treatment of the first tonic-clonic seizure does not affect long-term remission of epilepsy. Neurology. 2006;67:2227–9.

14. Gilad R, Lampl Y, Gabbay U, Eshel Y, Sarova-Pinhas I. Early treatment of a single generalized tonic-clonic seizure to prevent recurrence. Arch Neurol. 1996;53:1149–52.

15. Randomized clinical trial on the efficacy of antiepileptic drugs in reducing the risk of relapse after a first unprovoked tonic-clonic seizure. First Seizure Trial Group (FIR.S.T. Group). Neurology 1993;43:478–83.

16. Marson A, Jacoby A, Johnson A, Kim L, Gamble C, Chadwick D. Immediate versus deferred antiepileptic drug treatment for early epilepsy and single seizures: a randomised controlled trial. Lancet. 2005;365:2007–13.

17. Das CP, Sawhney IM, Lal V, Prabhakar S. Risk of recurrence of seizures following single unprovoked idiopathic seizure. Neurol India. 2000;48:357–60.

18. Hirtz D, Berg A, Bettis D, et al. Practice parameter: treatment of the child with a first unprovoked seizure: Report of the Quality Standards Subcommittee of the American Academy of Neurology and the Practice Committee of the Child Neurology Society. Neurology. 2003;60:166–75.

19. Berg AT, Shinnar S. The risk of seizure recurrence following a first unprovoked seizure: a quantitative review. Neurology. 1991;41:965–72.

20. Annegers JF, Shirts SB, Hauser WA, Kurland LT. Risk of recurrence after an initial unprovoked seizure. Epilepsia. 1986;27:43–50.

21. Wiebe S. An evidence based approach to the first unprovoked seizure. Can J Neurol Sci. 2002;29:120–4.

22. Sathasivam S, Nicolson A. First seizure – to treat or not to treat? Int J Clin Practice. 2008;62:1920–5.

23. Haut SR, Shinnar S. Considerations in the treatment of a first unprovoked seizure. Semin Neurol. 2008;28:289–96.

24. Beghi E. Management of a first seizure. General conclusions and recommendations. Epilepsia 2008;49(Suppl 1):58–61.

25. Wiebe S, Tellez-Zenteno JF, Shapiro M. An evidence-based approach to the first seizure. Epilepsia. 2008;49 Suppl 1:50–7.

26. Kho LK, Lawn ND, Dunne JW, Linto J. First seizure presentation: do multiple seizures within 24 hours predict recurrence? Neurology. 2006;67:1047–9.

27. Zupanc ML. The first seizure in childhood: don't just do something, stand there! Neurology 2005;64:774–5.

28. Herman ST. Single unprovoked seizures. Curr Treat Opt Neurol. 2004;6:243–55.

29. Winckler MI, Rotta NT. Clinical and electroencephalographic follow-up after a first unprovoked seizure. Pediatr Neurol. 2004;30:201–6.

30. King M. The new patient with a first seizure. Aust Fam Physician. 2003;32:221–8.

31. Falip-Centellas M, Rovira RM, Gratacos-Vinyola M, Lluis C, Perez-Perez S, Padro-Ubeda L. First tonic clonic generalized seizure: recurrence, and prognosis factors. Revista de neurologia. 2002;34:924–8.

32. Baumhackl U, Billeth R, Graf M. Type-specific diagnostic analysis of first epileptic seizure in adults. Eur Neurol. 1994;34 Suppl 1:71–3.

33. Bora I, Seckin B, Zarifoglu M, Turan F, Sadikoglu S, Ogul E. Risk of recurrence after first unprovoked tonic-clonic seizure in adults. J Neurol. 1995;242:157–63.

34. Elwes RD, Chesterman P, Reynolds EH. Prognosis after a first untreated tonic-clonic seizure. Lancet. 1985;2:752–3.

35. Forsgren L, Bucht G, Eriksson S, Bergmark L. Incidence and clinical characterization of unprovoked seizures in adults: a prospective population-based study. Epilepsia. 1996;37:224–9.

36. Gupta SK, Satishchandra P, Venkatesh A, Subbakrishna DK. Prognosis of single unprovoked seizure. J Assoc Physicians India. 1993;41:709–10.
37. Hart YM, Sander JW, Johnson AL, Shorvon SD. National General Practice Study of Epilepsy: recurrence after a first seizure. Lancet. 1990;336:1271–4.
38. Hauser WA, Anderson VE, Loewenson RB, McRoberts SM. Seizure recurrence after a first unprovoked seizure. New Engl J Med. 1982;307:522–8.
39. Olafsson E, Hauser WA, Gudmundsson G. Long-term survival of people with unprovoked seizures: a population-based study. Epilepsia. 1998;39:89–92.
40. van Donselaar CA, Geerts AT, Schimsheimer RJ. Idiopathic first seizure in adult life: who should be treated? BMJ 1991;302:620–3.
41. van Donselaar CA, Schimsheimer RJ, Geerts AT, Declerck AC. Value of the electroencephalogram in adult patients with untreated idiopathic first seizures. Arch Neurol. 1992;49:231–7.
42. Wolf P. Non-medical treatment of first epileptic seizures in adolescence and adulthood. Seizure. 1995;4:87–94.
43. Kim LG, Johnson TL, Marson AG, Chadwick DW. Prediction of risk of seizure recurrence after a single seizure and early epilepsy: further results from the MESS trial. Lancet Neurol. 2006;5:317–22.
44. Hauser WA, Rich SS, Lee JR, Annegers JF, Anderson VE. Risk of recurrent seizures after two unprovoked seizures. New Engl J Med. 1998;338:429–34.
45. Shinnar S, Berg AT, O'Dell C, Newstein D, Moshe SL, Hauser WA. Predictors of multiple seizures in a cohort of children prospectively followed from the time of their first unprovoked seizure. Ann Neurol. 2000;48:140–7.
46. Hauser WA, Rich SS, Annegers JF, Anderson VE. Seizure recurrence after a 1st unprovoked seizure: an extended follow-up. Neurology. 1990;40:1163–70.
47. Pohlmann-Eden B, Beghi E, Camfield C, Camfield P. The first seizure and its management in adults and children. BMJ 2006;332:339–42.
48. Proposal for revised classification of epilepsies and epileptic syndromes. Commission on Classification and Terminology of the International League Against Epilepsy. Epilepsia. 1989;30:389–99.
49. Wiebe S. Epidemiology of temporal lobe epilepsy. Can J Neurol Sci 2000;27(Suppl 1):S6–10; discussion S20–1.
50. Engel Jr J, Shewmon DA. Overview. Who Should be Considered a Surgical Candidate? In: Engel Jr J, editor. Surgical Treatment of the Epilepsies. 2nd ed. New York: Raven; 1993. p. 23–34.
51. Casetta I, Granieri E, Monetti VC, et al. Early predictors of intractability in childhood epilepsy: a community-based case-control study in Copparo, Italy. Acta Neurol Scand. 1999;99:329–33.
52. Camfield CS, Camfield PR, Gordon K, Wirrell E, Dooley JM. Incidence of epilepsy in childhood and adolescence: a population-based study in Nova Scotia from 1977 to 1985. Epilepsia. 1996;37:19–23.
53. Kwan P, Brodie MJ. Early identification of refractory epilepsy. New Engl J Med. 2000;342:314–9.
54. Duncan JS, Sagar HJ. Seizure characteristics, pathology, and outcome after temporal lobectomy. Neurology. 1987;37:405–9.
55. French JA, Williamson PD, Thadani VM, et al. Characteristics mesial temporal sclerosis temporal lobe epilepsy: I. Results of history and physical examination. Ann Neurol. 1993;34:774–80.
56. Palmini A, Gloor P. The localizing value of auras in partial seizures: a prospective and retrospective study. Neurology. 1992;42:801–8.
57. Van Buren JM. The abdominal aura. A study of abdominal sensations occurring in epilepsy and produced by depth stimulation. Electroencephalogr Clin Neurophysiol. 1963;15:1–19.
58. Engel Jr J. Diagnostic evaluation. In: Engel Jr J, editor. Seizures and epilepsy. Philadelphia: FA Davis; 1989.

59. Manford M, Fish DR, Shorvon SD. An analysis of clinical seizure patterns and their localizing value in frontal and temporal lobe epilepsies. Brain. 1996;119(Pt 1):17–40.

60. Kotagal P, Luders H, Morris HH, et al. Dystonic posturing in complex partial seizures of temporal lobe onset: a new lateralizing sign. Neurology. 1989;39:196–201.

61. Chee MW, Kotagal P, Van Ness PC, Gragg L, Murphy D, Luders HO. Lateralizing signs in intractable partial epilepsy: blinded multiple-observer analysis. Neurology. 1993;43:2519–25.

62. Acharya JN, Wyllie E, Luders HO, Kotagal P, Lancman M, Coelho M. Seizure symptomatology in infants with localization-related epilepsy. Neurology. 1997;48:189–96.

63. Yu HY, Yiu CH, Yen DJ, et al. Lateralizing value of early head turning and ictal dystonia in temporal lobe seizures: a video-EEG study. Seizure. 2001;10:428–32.

64. Hecker A, Andermann F, Rodin EA. Spitting automatism in temporal lobe seizures with a brief review of ethological and phylogenetic aspects of spitting. Epilepsia. 1972;13:767–72.

65. Geyer JD, Payne TA, Faught E, Drury I. Postictal nose-rubbing in the diagnosis, lateralization, and localization of seizures. Neurology. 1999;52:743–5.

66. Kramer RE, Luders H, Goldstick LP, et al. Ictus emeticus: an electroclinical analysis. Neurology. 1988;38:1048–52.

67. Benbadis SR, Kotagal P, Klem GH. Unilateral blinking: a lateralizing sign in partial seizures. Neurology. 1996;46:45–8.

68. Theodore WH, Porter RJ, Penry JK. Complex partial seizures: clinical characteristics and differential diagnosis. Neurology. 1983;33:1115–21.

69. Williamson PD, French JA, Thadani VM, et al. Characteristics of medial temporal lobe epilepsy: II. Interictal and ictal scalp electroencephalography, neuropsychological testing, neuroimaging, surgical results, and pathology. Ann Neurol. 1993;34:781–7.

70. Risinger MW, Engel Jr J, Van Ness PC, Henry TR, Crandall PH. Ictal localization of temporal lobe seizures with scalp/sphenoidal recordings. Neurology. 1989;39:1288–93.

71. Ebersole JS, Pacia SV. Localization of temporal lobe foci by ictal EEG patterns. Epilepsia. 1996;37:386–99.

72. Berkovic SF, Andermann F, Olivier A, et al. Hippocampal sclerosis in temporal lobe epilepsy demonstrated by magnetic resonance imaging. Ann Neurol. 1991;29:175–82.

73. Knowlton RC, Laxer KD, Ende G, et al. Presurgical multimodality neuroimaging in electroencephalographic lateralized temporal lobe epilepsy. Ann Neurol. 1997;42:829–37.

74. Newton MR, Berkovic SF, Austin MC, Rowe CC, McKay WJ, Bladin PF. SPECT in the localisation of extratemporal and temporal seizure foci. J Neurol Neurosurg Psychiatry. 1995;59:26–30.

75. Ho SS, Berkovic SF, Berlangieri SU, et al. Comparison of ictal SPECT and interictal PET in the presurgical evaluation of temporal lobe epilepsy. Ann Neurol. 1995;37:738–45.

76. Hetherington H, Kuzniecky R, Pan J, et al. Proton nuclear magnetic resonance spectroscopic imaging of human temporal lobe epilepsy at 4.1 T. Ann Neurol. 1995;38:396–404.

77. Knowlton RC, Laxer KD, Aminoff MJ, Roberts TP, Wong ST, Rowley HA. Magnetoencephalography in partial epilepsy: clinical yield and localization accuracy. Ann Neurol. 1997;42:622–31.

78. Knowlton RC, Elgavish RA, Limdi N, et al. Functional imaging: I. Relative predictive value of intracranial electroencephalography. Ann Neurol. 2008;64:25–34.

79. Knowlton RC, Elgavish RA, Bartolucci A, et al. Functional imaging: II. Prediction of epilepsy surgery outcome. Ann Neurol. 2008;64:35–41.

80. Lau M, Yam D, Burneo JG. A systematic review on MEG and its use in the presurgical evaluation of localization-related epilepsy. Epilepsy Res. 2008;79:97–104.

81. Engel Jr J, Wiebe S, French J, et al. Practice parameter: temporal lobe and localized neocortical resections for epilepsy: report of the Quality Standards Subcommittee of the American Academy of Neurology, in association with the American Epilepsy Society and the American Association of Neurological Surgeons. Neurology. 2003;60:538–47.

82. Jette N, Tellez-Zenteno J, Hader W, et al. Epilepsy: when to think surgery! Neurology. 2010;74:A108.

83. Burneo JG, Tellez-Zenteno J, Jette N. Seizure outcome after resective epilepsy surgery: a systematic review. Proceedings of the 28th International Epilepsy Congress (International League Against Epilepsy) 2009.
84. Wiebe S, Blume WT, Girvin JP, Eliasziw M. A randomized, controlled trial of surgery for temporal-lobe epilepsy. New Engl J Med. 2001;345:311–8.
85. Tellez-Zenteno JF, Dhar R, Wiebe S. Long-term seizure outcomes following epilepsy surgery: a systematic review and meta-analysis. Brain. 2005;128:1188–98.
86. McIntosh AM, Kalnins RM, Mitchell LA, Fabinyi GC, Briellmann RS, Berkovic SF. Temporal lobectomy: long-term seizure outcome, late recurrence and risks for seizure recurrence. Brain. 2004;127:2018–30.
87. Jette N, CASES-investigators. A literature review of the natural history, epidemiology and surgical outcomes of epilepsy, with focus on localization-related epilepsy. In. Calgary; 2009. http://www.epilepsycases.com/pdf/Literature%20Review%20FINAL.pdf.
88. Kelley K, Theodore WH. Prognosis 30 years after temporal lobectomy. Neurology. 2005;64:1974–6.
89. Tellez-Zenteno JF, McLachlan RS, Parrent A, Kubu CS, Wiebe S. Hippocampal electrical stimulation in mesial temporal lobe epilepsy. Neurology. 2006;66:1490–4.
90. Boon P, Vonck K, De Herdt V, et al. Deep brain stimulation in patients with refractory temporal lobe epilepsy. Epilepsia. 2007;48:1551–60.
91. Velasco AL, Velasco F, Velasco M, Trejo D, Castro G, Carrillo-Ruiz JD. Electrical stimulation of the hippocampal epileptic foci for seizure control: a double-blind, long-term follow-up study. Epilepsia. 2007;48:1895–903.
92. Riviello Jr JJ, Ashwal S, Hirtz D, et al. Practice parameter: diagnostic assessment of the child with status epilepticus (an evidence-based review): report of the Quality Standards Subcommittee of the American Academy of Neurology and the Practice Committee of the Child Neurology Society. Neurology. 2006;67:1542–50.
93. Appleton R, Macleod S, Martland T. Drug management for acute tonic-clonic convulsions including convulsive status epilepticus in children. Cochrane Database Syst Rev. 2008:CD001905.
94. Prasad K, Al-Roomi K, Krishnan PR, Sequeira R. Anticonvulsant therapy for status epilepticus. Cochrane Database Syst Rev. 2005:CD003723.
95. Agarwal P, Kumar N, Chandra R, Gupta G, Antony AR, Garg N. Randomized study of intravenous valproate and phenytoin in status epilepticus. Seizure. 2007;16:527–32.
96. Lewena S, Pennington V, Acworth J, et al. Emergency management of pediatric convulsive status epilepticus: a multicenter study of 542 patients. Pediatr Emerg Care. 2009;25:83–7.
97. Sreenath TG, Gupta P, Sharma KK, Krishnamurthy S. Lorazepam versus diazepam-phenytoin combination in the treatment of convulsive status epilepticus in children: a randomized controlled trial. Eur J Paediatr Neurol. 2010;14:162–8.
98. Rossetti AO, Novy J, Ruffieux C, et al. Management and prognosis of status epilepticus according to hospital setting: a prospective study. Swiss Med Wkly. 2009;139:719–23.

Chapter 7
Movement Disorders

Mary E. Jenkins, Janis M. Miyasaki, and Oksana Suchowersky

Keywords Parkinson's disease • Essential tremor • Dystonia • Epidemiology
• Diagnosis • Treatment

Parkinson's Disease

Introduction

Parkinson's disease (PD) is a common neurodegenerative disorder caused by loss of dopaminergic cells in the substantia nigra pars compacta [1]. The diagnosis is based on clinical criteria and requires the presence of bradykinesia, in association with at least one of rigidity, rest tremor, or postural instability [2]. There is no definitive ancillary test and the diagnosis continues to rest on clinical grounds.

Clinical Scenario

A 60-year-old man presents with symptoms of right-sided rest tremor, micrographia, and slowness of gait. The neurological examination reveals bradykinesia, rigidity, and unilateral rest tremor. He meets the diagnostic criteria of PD. The patient inquires about risk factors, diagnostic tests, and treatment options.

J.M. Miyasaki (✉)
Division of Neurology, Medicine Department, University of Toronto, Toronto, ON, Canada

The Movement Disorders Centre, University Health Network, Toronto Western Hospital,
Toronto, ON, Canada
e-mail: miyasaki@uhnresearch.ca

J.G. Burneo et al. (eds.), *Neurology: An Evidence-Based Approach*,
DOI 10.1007/978-0-387-88555-1_7, © Springer Science+Business Media, LLC 2012

Epidemiology

Clinical Questions

1. What is the incidence and prevalence of Parkinson's disease (PD)?
2. Are there risk factors for the development of PD?

Search Strategy

See Appendix for all search strategies.

Incidence and Prevalence in PD

One well-designed meta-analysis reviewed the incidence and prevalence of PD [3]. The inclusion criteria were published after 1990 (as the rate of disease may change over time), population based, well-defined, and accepted diagnostic criteria, and diagnosis confirmed by an expert diagnostician who applied the criteria to all cases. Two studies evaluated incident rates across all age groups (from England and Finland) and reported a median incidence of 14/100,000 (range 12–15). Six studies evaluated incident rates for individuals over 65 years (one each from the Netherlands, Italy, Spain, and three studies from the United States), and reported a median incidence of 160/100,000 (range 62–332) in this age group. Incidence increased with increasing age to 80 years of age; beyond 80 years the data were insufficient to accurately report rates. Men appeared to be affected more commonly than women [relative risk (RR) 1.8 (range 1.4–2.0)].

The PD prevalence in individuals over 65 years was reported in six class I studies (Germany, Finland, Faroe Islands in Denmark, Inuit population in Greenland, the Netherlands, and Spain) and six class II studies (England, United States, France, Norway, and two from Spain) [3]. The median prevalence was 9.5/1,000 (range 7.0–43.8) for individuals over 65 years of age.

Risk Factors for the Development of PD: Genetics and Environment

Genetics and environmental factors have both been implicated in the development of PD. As illustrated from the incidence studies listed above, increasing age has been established to be a definite risk factor in the development of PD [3].

One meta-analysis of familial aggregation studies examined the familial risk of development of PD [4]. Studies were chosen based on the following criteria: identification of affected relatives, confirmed diagnosis by neurological examination, population based, and specified data analysis. The data from six studies were combined to provide the best estimate of relative risk (RR). For individuals with a first degree relative with PD, the RR was 2.9 (95% CI 2.2–3.8). More specifically, the RR for a child–parent pair was 2.7 (95% CI 2.0–3.7) and for a sibling pair was 4.4 (95% CI 3.1–6.1). When stratified by age, the RR for a first degree relative of an individual with late onset PD was 2.7 (95% CI 1.9–3.9) and for early onset PD was 4.7 (95% CI 3.2–6.8).

Two meta-analyses reviewed the literature regarding environmental factors and risk of PD. In both meta-analyses, the authors evaluated case-control studies and extracted the data to calculate odds ratio (OR) from the original results. The first meta-analysis evaluated the risk of pesticide exposure in the development of PD [5]. From 19 case-control studies, exposure to pesticides was higher in the PD cases than controls (OR 1.94, 95% CI 1.49–2.53). No significant dose-response relationship was found, although there was a trend for an increased PD risk with longer duration of pesticide exposure. The second meta-analysis assessed the risk of rural living (16 studies), well water drinking (18 studies), farming (11 studies), and pesticides (14 studies). The combined ORs revealed an increase risk in the development of PD for rural living (OR 1.56, 95% CI 1.18–2.07), farming (OR 1.42, 95% CI 1.05–1.91), and pesticide exposure (OR 1.85, 95% CI 1.31–2.60). There was a nonsignificant trend for well water drinking. A subsequent case-control study evaluated similar exposures and found only well water drinking to be a significant risk factor [6]. Although head injury has been historically associated with PD, a meta-analysis of case-control studies did not find a clear association [7].

Coffee and cigarette smoking have both been evaluated as protective factors. From one well-designed meta-analysis, which included the pooled data of eight case-controlled and five cohort studies, the relative risk (RR) of developing PD was significantly lower in coffee drinkers (consuming a mean of three cups of coffee daily) than noncoffee drinkers (RR 0.69, 95% CI 0.59–0.80) [8]. The proposed mechanism is felt to be related to caffeine [9]. Caffeine, an inhibitor of the adenosine A2 receptor, has been found to improve motor function is a PD mouse model [9].

Two well-designed meta-analyses evaluated the risk of smoking in the development of PD. Based on review of 44 case-control and four cohort studies, the RR for development of PD was significantly lower for "ever smokers" compared to nonsmokers (RR 0.59, 95% CI 0.54–0.63) [8]. The pooled RR for 10 additional pack years was RR 0.84 (95% CI 0.81–0.88) [8]. The second meta-analysis reviewed the evidence of risk of smoking and development of PD from prospective cohort studies only [10]. Based on review of six prospective studies, the risk of developing PD was significantly lower among "ever smokers" than nonsmokers (OR 0.51, 95% CI 0.43–0.61) and even lower in the current smoking group. The proposed mechanism for the protective factor of cigarette smoking is most likely related to nicotine [9]. Possible pathophysiological mechanisms include nicotine actions as a stimulator of dopamine, as an antioxidant, or as a monoamine oxidase B inhibitor [9].

Clinical Bottom Lines

1. The incidence of PD is 14 (range 12–15) per 100,000 for all age groups and 160/100,000 (range 62–332) over 65 years. PD may occur slightly more frequently in men.
2. The prevalence of PD is 9.5 (range 7.0–43.8) per 1,000 over 65 years.
3. The incidence of PD increases with increasing age up to 80 years. There is insufficient evidence beyond 80 years of age.
4. There is good evidence that the risk of PD is increased in individuals with an affected first degree relative. The risk is higher for relatives of young-onset PD and sibling pairs.
5. Farming, rural living, and pesticide exposure are probably associated with an increased risk of developing PD. Well water may also be a factor, but the evidence is weaker.
6. Coffee drinking and cigarette smoking are associated with a lower risk of developing PD. The evidence is stronger for smoking.
7. Genetic testing for known mutations is not recommended at this time as there is no evidence that it aids in diagnosis or treatment.

Diagnosis

Clinical Questions

1. What clinical features are useful in diagnosing PD and distinguishing PD from other parkinsonian disorders?
2. What investigational tests are useful in diagnosing PD and distinguishing PD from other parkinsonian disorders?

Clinical Features Useful in the Diagnosis of Parkinson's Disease

The diagnosis of PD rests on clinical criteria. From neuropathological studies, 20% of patients initially diagnosed with PD antemortem by community physicians and specialists combined had an alternative diagnosis established by autopsy [2, 11, 12]. The alternative diagnoses included Progressive Supranuclear Palsy (PSP), Multiple Systems Atrophy (MSA), Alzheimer's disease (AD), Cortical Basal Degeneration, or cerebrovascular disease [2, 11, 12]. A retrospective clinicopathological review of 100 patients diagnosed with Parkinson's disease examined the sensitivity of the UK Brain Bank criterion (Table 7.1) compared to the gold standard of pathological diagnosis. The UK Brain Bank criterion had a sensitivity of 90% when administered by neurologists, geriatricians, or internists [13]. A retrospective review using movement disorders specialists' clinical diagnosis had a sensitivity of 91% (95% CI 85–97) and a specificity of 98% (95% CI 95–100) compared with pathologic diagnosis [11].

Table 7.1 UK Parkinson's Disease Society Brain Bank Criteria [2]

Inclusion criteria
- (1) Bradykinesia AND
- At least one of: (2) Rigidity, (3) Rest tremor, (4) Postural instability

Exclusion criteria
- Repeated stroke
- Repeated head injury
- Encephalitis
- Oculogyric crisis
- Neuroleptic treatment
- More than one affected relative
- Sustained remission
- Strictly unilateral feature after 3 years
- Supranuclear gaze palsy
- Cerebellar signs
- Early severe dysautonomia
- Early severe dementia
- Babinski sign
- CNS Tumor or hydrocephalus
- Negative response to levodopa
- MPTP exposure

Supportive prospective criteria
- Unilateral onset
- Rest tremor present
- Progressive disorder
- Persistent asymmetry of symptoms
- Excellent response to levodopa
- Severe levodopa-induced chorea
- Levodopa response for >5 years
- Clinical course of 10 years or more

Table 7.2 Clinical features distinguishing atypical parkinsonism from idiopathic PD

Atypical Parkinsonism: clinical features

- Falls at presentation or within first year
- Poor response to levodopa
- Symmetrical onset of symptoms
- Rapid progression
- Lack of tremor
- Autonomic dysfunction
- Eye movement abnormalities
- Ataxia
- Dementia

Based on a systematic review of three retrospective case-control studies using pathological diagnosis as the gold standard and one retrospective cohort using clinical diagnosis over time as the gold standard, the American Academy of Neurology (AAN) determined a set of physical examination characteristics that are useful in distinguishing atypical parkinsonism from early idiopathic PD (Table 7.2) [12]. The diagnostic certainty increased if more than one characteristic was present. Follow-up with reevaluation over a 2-year period was also helpful in improving diagnostic accuracy.

Levodopa or Apomorphine Challenge

Two studies examined the utility of the levodopa and apomorphine challenge in the diagnosis of PD [12], using clinical diagnosis as the gold standard. Patients received 250/50 mg of levodopa/carbidopa or 1.5–4.5 mg of apomorphine and were assessed for improvement in motor scores on a standardized PD scale. For the levodopa challenge, the sensitivity was 71% and the specificity was 81%. For the apomorphine challenge, the sensitivity was 65% and the specificity was 70–77% [14]. Levodopa or apomorphine challenge was probably useful to differentiate idiopathic PD from other parkinsonian syndromes, but there was no evidence that these tests were more useful than clinical examination [12].

Diagnostic Tests Useful to Distinguish PD from Other Parkinsonian Syndromes

Olfaction Testing

Three well-designed clinical studies (two case-controls and one cohort) of standard-ized olfaction testing in the diagnosis of PD found that patients with PD had moder-ate to severe hyposomnia, while patients with PSP or CBD scored in the normal range and MSA patients scored in the mild to moderate range of impairment [12]. Therefore, olfaction testing may be useful to distinguish PD from PSP and CBD, but not from MSA. There was insufficient evidence to recommend olfaction testing over clinical diagnosis.

In a recent evidence-based critically appraised topic review, olfaction testing was found to be moderately sensitive and specific (sensitivity 77%, 95% CI 70–85 and specificity 85%, 95% CI 74–85) to distinguish idiopathic PD from other parkinsonian disorders [15]. However, olfactory testing is time consuming (taking approximately 30 min to administer) limiting its utility.

Magnetic Resonance Imaging

Numerous well-designed, blinded-rater, prospective, and retrospective studies evaluated the utility of routine MRI, volumetric MRI, and diffusion-weighted MRI in differentiating PD from other parkinsonian syndromes. In all cases, clinical diag-nosis was used as a surrogate gold standard limiting the strength of the evidence.

Three studies evaluated the use of MRI to differentiate MSA from PD. Routine MRI was assessed by consensus of two blinded raters in a retrospective study of 35 patients with MSA and 17 patients with PD [16]. The study reported a sensitivity of 70% and a specificity of 100% for MRI abnormalities in the putamen, pons, middle cerebellar peduncle, and cerebellum to differentiate MSA from PD. Another study prospectively evaluated T2-weighted MRI by two blinded raters in 52 patients with MSA and 88 patients with PD [17]. T2-weighted signal changes in the putamen had a sensitivity of 64–69% and a specificity of 91% to differentiate MSA from PD. A third prospective study evaluated the utility of diffuse-weighted MRI to distinguish 16 subjects each with MSA, PD, and PSP using blinded raters [18]. Diffusion-weighted MRI changes in the middle cerebral peduncles distinguished MSA from PD and MSA from PSP in all cases (sensitivities and specificities 100%).

Two other studies evaluated the use of MRI to distinguish PSP from PD, using clinical diagnosis by a movement disorders specialist as the gold standard. In the first study, two independent blinded raters prospectively evaluated MRI brain scans in 25 patients with PSP and 27 patients with PD and found that midbrain profile changes differentiated PSP from PD with a sensitivity of 68% and a specificity of 77% [19]. In the second study, two independent blinded raters prospectively used MRI brain scans to calculate an "index measurement" from measurements of the pons, midbrain, middle, and superior cerebellar peduncles in 33 patients with PSP, 108 patients with PD, and 19 patients with MSA-P [20]. The index, although not validated in other studies, was 100% sensitive and specific in distinguishing PSP from PD and MSA.

Although the MRI findings presented above may be useful in differentiating PSP or MSA (high specificity), the absence of the MRI findings does not necessarily indicate a diagnosis of PD (low sensitivity). Hence, the AAN Practice Parameter [12] also found that there was insufficient evidence to support or refute the use of MRI in the distinguishing PD from other parkinsonian syndromes.

Single Photon Emission Computer Tomography

A well designed meta-analysis was completed on the utility of single photon emission computer tomography (SPECT) scanning in the diagnosis of PD [21]. SPECT using presynaptic tracers was able to distinguish early PD from controls (OR 60, 95% CI 13–227), PD from essential tremor (OR 210, 95% CI 79–562), and PD from vascular parkinsonism (OR 105, 95% CI 32–348), although the large confidence intervals indicate imprecision. Accuracy for both presynaptic (OR 2, 95% CI 1–4) and postsynaptic tracers (OR 19, 95% CI 9–36) was lower to distinguish PD from the other parkinsonian syndromes. SPECT is probably not useful to distinguish PD from other parkinsonian syndromes.

F-Fluorodeoxyglucose Positron Emission Tomography

In a prospective study, F-Fluorodeoxyglucose Positron emission tomography was used to differentiate MSA from PD by two blinded raters [16]. The time from symptom onset to evaluation was 2 years for the MSA group and 3.3 years for the PD group. The gold standard was clinical diagnosis by a movement disorders specialist. Patients with MSA were more likely to demonstrate glucose hypometabolism in the putamen, pons, and cerebellum compared to patients with PD. FDG-PET distinguished MSA from PD with a sensitivity of 90–95% and a specificity of 100% [12].

Meta-iodobenzylguanidine Myocardial Scintigraphy

Myocardial meta-iodobenzylguanidine (MIBG) scintigraphy assesses sympathetic nerve terminals. In a prospective study, 391 patients presenting with one or more Parkinson-like symptoms were evaluated with MIBG scintigraphy and followed longitudinally to confirm the diagnosis [22]. The eventual clinical diagnosis was 122 patients with PD, 14 patients with MSA, 7 patients with PSP, 5 patients with dementia with Lewy Bodies (DLB), 15 patients with AD, 129 patients with cerebrovascular disease, and 81 patients with other diseases (not specified). MIBG was decreased in most patients with PD (especially advanced PD), but was also decreased in a number of other disorders including AD and DLB. The sensitivity of myocardial MIBG scintigraphy to diagnose PD was 88% while the specificity was only 37%. Therefore, cardiac MIBG scintigraphy is not useful in the diagnosis of PD.

Transcranial Ultrasound

In patients with PD, transcranial ultrasound (TCS) has been reported to show increased echogenicity in the area of the substantia nigra (SN). One prospective, double-blind, cohort study of 60 undiagnosed patients with akinetic-rigid symptoms (patients with rest tremor were excluded) evaluated TCS in the diagnosis of early PD [23]. The gold standard was clinical diagnosis after 1 year. If the diagnosis was still uncertain, PET and/or SPECT were performed. Increased echogenicity of the SN on TCS differentiated PD from atypical parkinsonism with a sensitivity of 91% (95% CI 82–99) and a specificity of 82% (95% CI 64–100). The initial clinical diagnosis of patients at baseline was only 37%, which was much lower than reported in other studies. It is not clear if excluding patients with rest tremor biased the results. The AAN Practice Parameter reviewed an earlier study and concluded that there was insufficient evidence to support or refute the use of TCS for PD diagnosis [12] (Table 7.3).

Clinical Bottom Lines

In differentiating PD from other parkinsonian syndromes:

1. Use of the UK Brain Bank criteria in the clinical diagnosis of PD has a sensitivity of 90%, when compared to pathological diagnosis.
2. Early falls, poor response to levodopa, symmetrical onset, rapid progression, autonomic dysfunction, and absence of tremor are probably useful in differentiating other Parkinsonian syndromes from PD. The utility increases if several features are present.

Table 7.3 The utility of diagnostic tests to distinguish PD from other parkinsonian syndromes

Summary of diagnostic tests to distinguish PD from atypical parkinsonism

	Sensitivity (95% CI)	Specificity (95% CI)	Gold Standard	Strength of recommendation
Clinical diagnosis (MD specialist)	91% (85–97)	98% (95–100)	Pathologic diagnosis	Good
Levodopa Challenge Test	71%	81%	Clinical	Moderate – No advantage over clinical diagnosis
Olfaction testing	77% (70–85)	85% (74–85)	Clinical	Moderate – No advantage over clinical diagnosis
MRI	65–70% (for diagnosis of MSA or PSP)	77–100% (for diagnosis of MSA or PSP)	Clinical	Unknown utility for PD
SPECT	OR = 2 (1–4) – presynaptic OR = 19 (9–36) – postsynaptic		Clinical	Not useful
FDG-PET	90–95% (for MSA vs. PD)	100% (for MSA vs. PD)	Clinical	Unknown – may be useful for MSA vs. PD
MIBG	88%	37%	Clinical	Not useful
Transcranial ultrasound	91% (82–99)	82% (64–100)	Clinical + SPECT and/or PET	Unknown, insufficient evidence

3. The levodopa or apomorphine challenge is moderately sensitive and specific for confirming diagnosis of PD. There is insufficient evidence to recommend this test as more useful than clinical diagnosis.
4. Olfactory testing is moderately sensitive and specific in the diagnosis of PD. There is insufficient evidence to recommend this test as more useful than clinical diagnosis.
5. Abnormal MRI findings may be useful to diagnose PSP or MSA, but the absence of these findings does not predict a diagnosis of PD.
6. SPECT scanning is probably not useful for PD diagnosis.
7. F-FDG-PET may be useful to distinguish MSA from PD, but there is insufficient evidence to determine if F-FDG-PET is useful to distinguish PD from other parkinsonian disorders.
8. MIBG is not useful to differentiate PD from other parkinsonian syndromes.
9. There is insufficient evidence to support or refute the use of TCS in PD diagnosis.

Treatment

Clinical Questions

1. In patients with PD, are there medications that slow the progression of the disease?
2. In a patient with early onset PD, what medications are effective and well tolerated for improvement of motor symptoms?
3. In a patient with more advanced PD with motor fluctuations, what medications are effective and well tolerated for treatment of wearing off and dyskinesias?
4. In a patient with advanced PD who is developing psychosis, hallucinations, and dementia, what medications are indicated to treat these symptoms?

Treatment for Patients in the Early Stages of Parkinson's Disease

Neuroprotection

Based on one RCT, a review by the AAN found that there is good evidence that Vitamin E is not neuroprotective in Parkinson's disease [24]. Levodopa was found to be not neurotoxic based on one RCT, and possibly neuroprotective for the first 9 months. There was insufficient evidence to support the use of riluzole, coenzyme Q10, pramipexole, ropinirole, amantadine, or thalamotomy [24]. From a delayed start design RCT of rasagiline, participants treated for 12 months had less-functional decline than those treated for 6 months, although rasagiline does have symptomatic benefit. From a previous AAN guideline [25], there was good evidence to support that selegiline is not neuroprotective. The European Federation Neurological Societies (EFNS) Task Force guideline reported similar findings [26].

Symptomatic Treatment

Amantadine

The Cochrane collaboration reviewed six RCTs of amantadine as monotherapy and as adjunct treatment [27]. As the studies all contained significant methodological flaws, the authors concluded that there was insufficient evidence to support or refute the use of this medication in the symptomatic treatment of early PD. Side effects were reported as mild including dizziness, anxiety, incoordination, insomnia, nausea, headache, nightmares, confusion, constipation, and livedo reticularis, affecting approximately 5% of patients.

Anticholinergics

One Cochrane review examined the use of anticholinergics in early PD from nine double-blind, crossover studies of 5–20 weeks duration that included 221 patients [28]. Due to the heterogeneous design and incomplete data, numbers needed to treat could not be calculated. Anticholinergics were more effective than placebo in the treatment of motor symptoms, and tremor was not more responsive than other symptoms. There were significant neuropsychiatric and cognitive side effects that frequently led to withdrawal of medication.

The EFNS Task Force guideline reported similar results concluding that anticholinergics had a small effect on the motor symptoms of PD disease but no evidence to support a specific effect on tremor [26]. Frequently reported side effects included blurred vision, urinary retention, constipation, nausea, and impaired mental function.

Monoamine Oxidase B Inhibitors

A Cochrane review from 2005 included ten randomized controlled trials, of 2,422 patients, of the MAO-B inhibitors selegiline and lazabemide [29]. MAO-B inhibitors resulted in a small improvement in clinical scores on the UPDRS motor and ADL scores that were statistically but not clinically significant. There was a small treatment effect on motor fluctuations (OR 0.75; 95% CI 0.59–0.94) but not dyskinesias. There was no neuroprotective effect. Withdrawals due to side effects were greater than placebo (OR 2.36; 95% CI 1.32–4.20).

The EFNS Task Force guideline reported a small symptomatic effect of monotherapy for both selegiline and rasagiline [26]. A further five RCTs evaluating selegiline as adjunct therapy did not show beneficial effects. Selegiline was not found to prevent motor fluctuations based on one RCT and two nonrandomized studies.

Dopamine Agonists

The EFNS Task Force guideline reported that dopamine agonists (DAs) provided symptomatic improvement over placebo in four RCT studies of dihydroergocryptine, pergolide, pramipexole, and ropinirole [26]. Other DAs were reported as probably effective with lower levels of evidence. Less than 20% of participants remained on monotherapy after 5 years. DAs were found to be effective as adjunct therapy in participants already taking levodopa. There are no head to head comparisons among DA as monotherapy; in adjunct studies, it was difficult to determine differences in symptomatic effect due to methodological design.

DAs have an overall higher incidence of side effects as compared to levodopa (see below) [26]. A meta-analysis included seven cross-sectional studies of 477 patients treated with ergot dopamine agonists (pergolide or cabergoline), compared to 127 patients treated with nonergot dopamine agonists (pramipexole or ropinirole) and 364 control patients [30]. Twenty-six percent of patients on ergot dopamine agonists developed moderate to severe valvular heart disease compared to 10% in the other two groups (NNH = 6). As a result, pergolide was voluntarily withdrawn in Canada and the United States. Echocardiography screening is recommended in patients on ergot DA, but the frequency required is not known. Regression after ergot DA cessation occurs.

DAs are also associated with impulse control or reward-seeking behaviors, which include hypersexuality, compulsive spending, and pathologic gambling. Two prospective cohort studies have evaluated this adverse effect. In the first study, 297 consecutive patients with PD from a tertiary movement disorders center were screened for reward-seeking behaviors by use of a survey, and then formal psychiatric evaluation, using the DSM-IV criteria for impulse-control disorders and other standardized testing [31]. The prevalence of impulse-control behaviors was 6.1% overall in patients with PD and 13.7% among patients taking DA. A second prospective cohort study screened 272 consecutive patients from two movement disorders clinics [32]. In patients with a positive screen, the Minnesota Impulsive Disorders Interview was administered by telephone in addition to a review of the patients' clinical records. Impulse-control disorders were confirmed in 6.6%, all of whom were taking DA. From multivariate analysis the following factors were associated with impulse-control disorders: prior history of impulse-control problems, use of DA or amantadine, and higher doses of medication. Risk did not vary with the type of dopamine agonist used.

Dopamine Agonists and Levodopa

The Cochrane Collaboration reviewed the use of DA therapy in early PD [33]. From 29 studies comparing DA (as monotherapy or adjunctive therapy) to placebo or to levodopa, with 5,247 participants, DAs were more effective than placebo. Compared to levodopa, subjects on DAs were less likely to develop dyskinesias (OR 0.51, 95% CI 0.43–0.59), dystonia (OR 0.64, 95% CI 0.51–0.81), and motor fluctuations (OR 0.75, 95% CI 0.63–0.90). Symptomatic motor control was better with levodopa than DA. Those taking DAs were more likely to discontinue treatment due to adverse effects compared to participants taking levodopa (OR 2.49, 95% CI 2.08–2.98). Adverse events were more frequent in the DA groups compared to levodopa: edema (OR 3.68, 2.62–5.18), somnolence (OR 1.49, 95% 1.12–2.00), constipation (OR 1.59, 95% CI 1.11–2.28), dizziness (OR 1.45, 95% CI 1.09–1.92), hallucinations (OR 1.69,

95% CI 1.13–2.52), and nausea (OR 1.32, 95% CI 1.05–1.66). The authors concluded that motor symptoms were better controlled by levodopa, whereas motor complications were lower using DA but at the expense of increased nonmotor symptoms.

Two AAN Practice Guidelines and the EFNS Task Force Guidelines examined levodopa and DA as initial therapies and adjunctive therapies for motor fluctuations and reached similar conclusions [25, 26, 34].

Levodopa

A recent placebo-controlled RCT confirmed the symptomatic effect of levodopa in the treatment of PD symptoms and that levodopa does not result in accelerated loss of dopaminergic cells [35]. Motor fluctuations occur in approximately 40% of people after 5 years of treatment, with risk factors including younger age, longer disease duration, and levodopa dose.

In the AAN Practice Guideline from 2002, one RCT trial comparing immediate release levodopa to controlled release (CR) levodopa found no difference in effectiveness or rate of motor complications between the two groups [25]. The guideline recommended that both preparations of levodopa were equally effective in early treatment of PD.

Medication Treatment of Wearing Off in Advanced Parkinson's Disease

DAs, COMT inhibitors, and monoamine oxidase B inhibitors have all been reported to reduce wearing off in Parkinson's disease, with no benefit of one class over another [34].

Dopamine Agonists

From the AAN Practice Parameter [34] and EFNS Task Force guideline [36], based on nine placebo-controlled trials, DA consistently reduced off time in Parkinson's disease by 1.5–2 h. Levodopa doses were reduced by approximately 20% when used in conjunction with DA versus placebo. In most cases, there was an increase in dyskinesias concurrent with the improvement in off time. The authors concluded that the evidence was moderately strong for the use of DA in wearing off.

COMT Inhibitors

The AAN Practice Parameter found two well-designed RCTs of COMT inhibitors in the treatment of wearing off [34]. Although dyskinesias may be increased with COMT inhibitor administration, OFF time was reduced by approximately 1 h. Side effects included those associated with increased dopaminergic doses (nausea, somnolence, hallucinations), in addition to diarrhea. Tolcapone probably reduces off time and may be considered to reduce off time; however, tolcapone is associated with an increase in liver enzymes in 1% of the population and rare cases of fatal hepatoxicity. Tolcapone should be used with close monitoring of liver enzymes according to each country's requirements.

Both the EFNS guidelines [36] and the Cochrane Collaboration [37] had similar conclusions based on the same original articles as discussed above.

Monoamine Oxidase B Inhibitors

The AAN Practice Parameter examined monoamine oxidase B inhibitors on wearing off [34]. Based on one RCT with a weaker level of evidence, selegiline, and rasagiline reduced off time by approximately 1 h. Dyskinesias were increased with rasagiline in one study [38].

The EFNS Task Force concluded that there was no consistent evidence supporting the use of selegiline in wearing off symptoms, although there was a symptomatic benefit as monotherapy [36]. For rasagiline, the authors concluded that rasagiline was effective in reducing off time and well tolerated. In addition, based on one RCT, rasagiline was found to be equally effective to entacapone with an improvement in off time of approximately 1 h [39].

Levodopa: Various Forms of Administration

Intraduodenal levodopa reduced off time in a select group of advanced PD patients not well controlled with oral medication. Two studies of continuous intraduodenal levodopa were underpowered to conclude improvement over oral medication [36]. A randomized, crossover trial of 24 patients with motor fluctuations compared duodenal infusion therapy to oral medication [40]. Six patients dropped out of the study, five in the infusion group (unable to tolerate procedure or pump, patient pulled out tube) and one in the medical arm. Of the remaining 18 patients, there was significant improvement in motor scores and quality of life in the duodenal infusion arm compared to conventional oral therapy.

Medication Treatment of Dyskinesias in Advanced Parkinson's Disease

Amantadine

When reviewed by the AAN Practice Parameter, amantadine was reported to be possibly effective in the reduction of dyskinesia with a moderate level of evidence based on one RCT of short duration treatment (3 weeks) [34]. No adverse effects were reported from this study. The EFNS Task Force guideline concluded that amantadine reduces dyskinesias but the benefit may last only 3–8 months [36]. A Cochrane review evaluated three RCTs of amantadine in the treatment of dyskinesia [41]. Due to methodological flaws in these studies (short duration of treatment, no washout between crossover arm in two studies, combining data from both arms, no quality of life or patient satisfaction scores, outcomes assessments not well described or validated), the authors concluded that there was insufficient evidence to support or refute the use of amantadine in the treatment of dyskinesias.

Clozapine

The AAN Practice Parameter reported that there was insufficient evident to support or refute the use of clozapine for treatment of dyskinesias [34]. By contrast, the EFNS Task Force guideline, since their methodology incorporated expert consensus, concluded that the level of evidence was sufficient to conclude that clozapine probably reduces dyskinesias [36]. Both practice guidelines cautioned about the potential for toxicity due to agranulocytosis and the need for careful monitoring of blood cell counts.

Surgical Treatment of Motor Fluctuations and Dyskinesias

Surgical studies for the treatment of PD are challenging to interpret as assessment must be blinded to provide the highest class of evidence. Hence, despite anecdotal evidence of striking benefits, the strength of evidence results in weak conclusions such as possibly or probably effective in relieving the motor symptoms of PD. Based on four large prospective cohort studies, the AAN Practice Parameter concluded that deep brain stimulation of the subthalamic nucleus (DBS-STN) is possibly effective in improving motor function as well as in reducing off time, dyskinesias, and daily levodopa dose [34]. Adverse effects were examined separately, based on data from 360 patients in a large number of studies. Adverse effects included surgically related effects, hardware-related effects, and stimulation-related effects. There was a 2.8% risk of permanent disability secondary to infection, hemorrhage, cerebrospinal leak, and death in 0.6% due to pulmonary embolism and aspiration pneumonia. Stimulation-related effects that typically resolve with programming changes, include paresthesia, dysarthria, eyelid-opening apraxia, hemiballismus, dizziness, dyskinesia, and facial contractions.

There was only one large prospective study of globus pallidus stimulation. The authors concluded that there was insufficient evidence to recommend or refute the use of globus pallidus stimulation for motor fluctuations in PD because of the degree of risk–benefit ratio [34].

The EFNS Task Force guideline, based on a meta-analysis of 20 studies of DBS-STN surgery, concluded that the average improvement in motor scores was 53% at

1 year, with some deterioration by 5 years [36]. From large prospective studies, reductions in levodopa dosage of 50–60%, improvement in off time of 60%, and decreased dyskinesias of 60–75% were reported. Psychiatric side effects occurred in 10% following surgery, although it is not clear if these were related to the surgery or the underlying disease process. In older patients and those with preexisting cognitive impairments, there was an increased risk of further cognitive deterioration following surgery.

Since these guidelines were published, two large and one small RCT were published. One large multicentered unblinded RCT with 156 participants compared DBS-STN versus best medical treatment in advanced PD [42]. Data were analyzed in a pair-wise comparison, so it is not possible to report risk reductions or numbers needed to treat. The primary outcomes were quality of life and improvement in motor scores. Significantly more pairs had improvements in favor of surgery for both outcomes. Serious adverse events occurred in 13% in the surgery group versus 4% in the medication group. There were three fatalities in the surgical group from intraoperative intracerebral hemorrhage, suicide at 5 months after surgery, and pneumonia 6 weeks after surgery. In the medical group, one person died while driving during a psychotic episode. Assessment of cognition and behavior found no difference in cognition between groups; however, the surgical group had significantly lower scores on verbal fluency and reading time than the medical group. Additionally, 13% of the surgery group developed severe psychiatric adverse events including suicide, depression, psychosis, and apathy. In the medical group, 10% developed severe psychiatric adverse events including death (secondary to a motor vehicle collision during a psychotic episode) and psychosis.

In patients with advanced PD with motor fluctuations, a RCT using blinded assessment evaluated the best medical management ($n=134$) versus DBS-STN ($n=60$) and DBS-globus pallidus (GP) ($n=60$) [43]. Patients were followed for 6 months. Meaningful motor improvement occurred in 71% in the surgery group versus 32% in the medical group. Results were similar when stratified by age. Quality of life measures improved in the surgical group. Neuropsychological testing demonstrated a significant decline from baseline in the surgery group for working memory, processing speed, phonemic fluency, and delayed recall. Adverse events occurred more frequently in the surgery group, with a significant increase in falls, gait disturbance, depression, and dystonia compared to the medical group. Surgical site infections and pain occurred in 9% of patients in the surgical group. One patient in the surgical group died secondary to an intracerebral hemorrhage. Serious adverse events occurred in 40% of the surgical group versus 11% of the medical group (RR 3.8, 95% CI 2.3–6.3). The majority of adverse events had reversed by 6 months.

A nonblinded, randomized, RCT evaluated the use of DBS-STN versus best medical care in 20 young patients (less than 55 years) with early Parkinson's disease of 5–10 years duration [44]. Motor scores and activity of daily living scores OFF medication improved, but the best ON state did not improve. Dyskinesias and levodopa dose significantly reduced while quality of life scores improved at 18 months in the surgical group. Nine patients (90%) in the surgery group and three (30%) in the medication group had transient psychiatric symptoms that resolved by

18 months. One patient in the surgical group (10%) developed a somatoform disorder that had not resolved by 18 months. There was no change in cognitive functioning between groups.

Clinical Bottom Lines

In the treatment of early PD

1. There is insufficient evidence to support any pharmacological agents as being neuroprotective.
2. There is insufficient evidence to support or refute amantadine as monotherapy for early symptomatic treatment.
3. Anticholinergics have a small symptomatic effect in the treatment of Parkinson's disease, but adverse effects are common and may limit use. There was no evidence to support the use of anticholinergics specifically for the treatment of tremor.
4. Monoamine oxidase B inhibitors had a small effect on the motor symptoms and wearing off symptoms of PD.
5. Dopamine agonists and levodopa are both effective in the treatment of motor symptoms in PD. Levodopa provides superior motor benefit to dopamine agonists. From comparative studies, dopamine agonists were less likely to cause motor fluctuations, but more likely to cause nonmotor side effects, as compared to levodopa.
6. There is an increased risk of valvular heart disease with ergot dopamine agonists (cabergoline and pergolide), compared to nonergot dopamine agonists (pramipexole and ropinirole), NNH=6. Bromocriptine, also an ergot dopamine agonist, likely has the same risk, although no studies have specifically looked at bromocriptine.
7. Use of dopamine agonist and history of previous impulse-control behaviors are associated with an increase lifetime risk of development of impulse-control disorders.
8. There was no difference in effectiveness or side effect profile between immediate release levodopa and CR levodopa.

In the treatment of more advanced PD with motor fluctuations and dyskinesias:

9. Dopamine agonists, entacapone, and rasagiline are effective in reducing off time, but may worsen dyskinesias, when used with levodopa. There is no evidence to support the use of one medication over the other. Tolcapone is also effective in reducing off time, but the potential for hepatotoxicity requires close monitoring and this medication should be used with caution.
10. Amantadine is possibly effective in the reducing dyskinesias, but the effect may only persist for a few months.
11. DBS-STN is effective in improving motor fluctuations, reducing dyskinesias, and decreasing daily medication dosages in advanced PD. This procedure is appropriate for a carefully selected group of individuals. Adverse effects include surgical, device, and stimulation-related events. Psychiatric events may occur more frequently following surgery.

Summary

The incidence and prevalence of PD is well established based on a number of well-designed epidemiology studies. Etiologies of PD are less well established although there are links to genetic and environmental factors. Diagnosis of PD rest on clinical diagnosis; there is no evidence to support laboratory or radiological investigations as being more useful than clinical diagnosis. Therapy options have been well studied for early treatment of PD. More research is needed for the treatment of advanced PD, particularly the nonmotor manifestations.

Essential Tremor

Introduction

Essential tremor (ET) is the most common movement disorder being 20 times more common than Parkinson's disease [45]. The diagnosis of ET is based on clinical criteria including postural and kinetic tremor, which can be present in the arms, head, and/or voice [46]. Secondary causes of tremor such as medications and neurodegenerative disorders must be excluded. From a diagnostic standpoint, difficulties in determining incidence and prevalence rates exist due to the lack of a definitive diagnostic test, and presence of tremor associated with other disorders.

Clinical Scenario

A 70-year-old man presents with a 5-year history of bilateral action arm tremor. Apart from the tremor, the neurological examination is normal and he meets the diagnosis of ET. The patient inquires about the underlying etiologies and treatment options for this disorder.

Epidemiology

Clinical Questions

1. What is the incidence and prevalence of ET?
2. Are there risk factors for the development of ET?

Incidence and Prevalence of ET

The reported prevalence of ET varies widely due to diagnostic challenges listed above, differences in study designs (community based or service based, diagnosis confirmed or self-report), and differences in study populations (gender, age, ethnicity, population size) [47]. One meta-analysis, which included five studies with well-defined diagnostic criteria for ET, the presence of kinetic tremor, and community-based samples, was reviewed [45]. The prevalence of ET for all age groups was found to range from 4.1 to 39.2/1,000. For persons over 60 years, the prevalence ranged from 13 to 50.5/1,000.

More recent well-designed prospective community studies confirmed that prevalence varies by country and age. From Singapore [48], the prevalence was found to be 2.37/1,000 in adults over 50. The prevalence was three times greater for men, increased with age, and differed among various ethnic groups. In Spain, a similar study design found a prevalence of ET of 40/1,000 in adults over 65 years [49]. An American study found the prevalence rate for individuals over 65 years of age to be 48/1,000 (95% CI 42–54) [50]. When stratified by age, the rates varied from 37/1,000 at 65–69 years up to 73/1,000 over 85 years. When stratified by gender, the rates were 46/1,000 in men and 50/1,000 in women. Tremor location was: 84.8% limb; 8.2% head and limb; 4.3% limb and voice; 1.2% head, limb and voice; and 1.6% isolated head tremor. At least one other family member had tremor in 34% of cases [50].

Two studies of ET incidence were retrieved. A clinic-based, retrospective study of medical records over a 45-year period found an incidence of 23.7/100,000 person years [51]. Due to referral bias to a specialized neurology clinic, this figure likely underestimates the true incidence in the general population. A recent community-based study from Spain reported an incidence to be 616/100,000 person years for individuals over 65 years. Incidence increased with increasing age in both studies [52].

Risk Factors for the Development of ET: Genetics and Environment

Both genetic and environment factors appear to have a role in the development of ET. The evidence for genetics is somewhat conflicting. A review of 13 studies of family aggregations of tremor found great variability among reported rates of family history of tremor, ranging from 17 to 100% [53]. In a large twin study, 2,448 twin pairs over 70 years were screened for ET by an interview and Archimedes spiral test [54]. All 109 twin pairs with a positive screening test were evaluated by a movement disorders specialist blinded to the diagnosis of the other twin. Established clinical criteria were used for diagnosing definite, probable, and possible ET. Using the definite and probable ET group, concordance rates were 0.93 for monozygotic twins and 0.29 for dizygotic twins. The estimate of heritability was

99% (95% CI 90–100). A smaller study including only 16 twin pairs also found an increased concordance with monozygotic twins, but the findings were not statistically significant, possibly due to the small sample size [55]. The twin studies suggest a significant genetic link, although since concordance was not 100%, environmental factors may play a role. Alternatively, there may be decreased penetrance. One study examined genetic factors relating to age of onset of ET in 193 cases [56]. Age of onset was lower in patients with a family history of ET (40.9 ± 22 years) compared to patients with no family history of ET (57.3 ± 18.4 years).

Studies of linkage analysis in familial cases have identified four genetic loci, on chromosomes 2, 3, 5, and 6 [57–60]. Other families have not been linked to these loci suggesting genetic heterogeneity [61].

There are few controlled studies evaluating environmental exposures in the development of ET. One case-control study of 100 patients with ET and 143 age-matched controls evaluated serum lead levels and lead exposure finding a significant increase in serum lead levels in patients with ET compared to controls (OR = 1.19, 95% CI 1.03–1.37) [62]. There was no difference in lead exposure between groups. Another case-control study of 150 patients with ET and 150 matched controls evaluated serum harmane levels, a beta-alkaloid carboline that occurs naturally in meat (especially when cooked at high temperature for long periods of time) [63]. Elevation in serum harmane may be due to increased meat consumption or an inherent lack of ability to metabolize it. Mean log serum harmane level was 50% higher in cases than controls. Interestingly, the serum harmane levels were highest in cases of familial ET.

Clinical Bottom Lines

1. From community-based studies, the prevalence of essential tremor ranges from 3 to 48/1,000 in adults over 50 years of age.
2. From one community-based study, the incidence of essential tremor is 616/100,000 person years in adults over 65 years of age.
3. Both incidence and prevalence increase with age. Men and women are probably equally affected.
4. Given the high concordance of ET with monozygotic twins, genetics likely plays a significant role. Genetic heterogeneity exists.
5. Unknown environmental factors may play a role in the development of ET.

Diagnosis

Clinical Questions

1. What clinical features are useful in the diagnosis of Essential Tremor (ET)?
2. What, in any, investigational tests are sensitive and specificity to confirm the diagnosis of ET?

Table 7.4 Consensus Statement of the Movement Disorders Society on Tremor [46]

Inclusion criteria	Exclusion criteria
1. Bilateral postural tremor with or without kinetic tremor	1. Other abnormal neurological signs
2. Tremor involves hand and forearms, and must be visible and persistent	2. Presence of known causes of increased physiological tremor
3. Duration greater than 5 years	3. Concurrent or recent exposure to tremorogenic drugs or presence of a drug withdrawal state
	4. Trauma to the nervous system within 3 months before onset of tremor
	5. Historical or clinical evidence of psychogenic origins
	6. Evidence of sudden onset or stepwise deterioration

Diagnosis of Essential Tremor

There are multiple criteria for diagnosis of ET [47]. The Consensus Statement of Movement Disorders Society on Tremor criteria [46] for definite ET are most commonly used (Table 7.4).

As ET lacks a neuropathological diagnosis, and biochemical and genetic markers are not available, it is difficult to assess diagnostic tests in ET and not surprisingly, the literature on this topic is sparse.

Electrophysiological evaluations including quantitative computerized tremor analysis with accelerometry and electromyography are used in research studies. One double-blind, prospective study of 54 patients with undifferentiated tremor underwent diagnosis by clinical and electrophysiological criteria. Results demonstrated a high concordance rate of 94% between diagnostic methods [64]. A second double-blind, prospective study of 300 patients with postural tremor found electrophysiological criteria had a 98% sensitivity and 82% specificity compared with clinical criteria [65]. The results of these two studies are difficult to interpret in the absence of a gold standard diagnostic test.

The main differential diagnoses in ET are Parkinson's disease, dystonic tremor, and enhanced physiological tremor. SPECT scanning (see PD "Diagnosis" section) has been studied to differentiate ET and PD, but shown to be not helpful given very wide confidence intervals [21].

Clinical Bottom Lines

In the clinical diagnosis of ET

1. Diagnosis of ET is based on clinical criteria. There is no pathological or laboratory-based diagnosis. The lack of a gold standard makes assessment of any diagnostic tools problematic.

2. Electrophysiological tests (accelerometry and EMG) demonstrate good agreement with clinical criteria. The additional benefit of electrophysiology is questionable and not typically used in a clinical setting for diagnosis.
3. Neuroimaging techniques are probably not useful in the diagnosis of ET.

Treatment

Clinical Questions

1. In patients with ET, what medications are effective and well tolerated to improve the tremor?
2. In patients with ET, what is the efficacy and safety of thalamic stimulation and thalamotomy to improve tremor?

Medical Treatment of Essential Tremor

Beta Blockers

The AAN Practice Parameter reviewed twelve well-designed RCTs and all demonstrated benefit of propranolol (mean dose 180 mg/day, range 60–320) in the treatment of limb tremor [66]. The studies reported a 50% improvement on both clinical rating scales and accelerometry. Side effects included fatigue, lightheadedness, impotence, and bradycardia in 12–66% of patients. There was good evidence that propranolol long acting (LA) was equivalent to the regular formulation. There was less evidence to support the efficacy of propranolol in the treatment of head tremor; however, propranolol should still be considered given the lack of specific therapies for head tremor. In terms of long-term efficacy, two open label studies of propranolol reported sustained treatment effects in 40–60% of patients for up to 1 year, although dose escalations were frequently required.

Based on lower levels of evidence, three other beta blockers were reported to be probably effect in the treatment of limb tremor: sotalol, atenolol, and nadolol. Pindolol did not reduce limb tremor based on one well-designed RCT [66].

Antiepileptics

The AAN Practice Parameter found there was good evidence to support the use of primidone (mean dose 480 mg/day, range 50–1,000 mg) in the treatment of limb tremor [66]. Four well-designed RCTs as well as eight studies with lower levels of evidence reported a 50% tremor improvement based on clinical rating scales and accelerometry. Acute adverse effects, including sedation, drowsiness, fatigue, nausea, vomiting, ataxia, confusion, and dizziness occurred with a moderate to high frequency. Based on two open-label and one double-blind study, primidone had a sustained effect in tremor reduction in 50% of patients for at least 1 year. Based on three comparative trials, primidone and propranolol resulted in similar improvement in limb tremor. The only double-blind comparative trial reported greater initial side effects with primidone. In addition, based on two studies of moderate level of evidence, the combination of primidone and propranolol resulted in a small additional improvement over monotherapy.

One placebo-controlled trial using a clinical rating scale showed gabapentin-reduced limb tremor by 30% with a 77% improvement in accelerometry [66]. However, it was not effective as adjunct treatment.

Pregabalin, an isomer of gabapentin, was studied in a placebo-controlled, double-blind RCT in 22 patients with ET [67]. Using the Clinical Global Impression score, 67% of patients on pregabalin reported improvement compared with 20% on placebo. The pregabalin group had improved on accelerometry; however, the total clinical rating scales scores for tremor were not different between groups. Withdrawals for side effects were higher in the treatment group compared to the placebo group, although this was not statistically significant, 27% versus 9%. (NNH = 6, 95% CI −2 to 8, NS). Given the mixed results and high number of withdrawals, there is insufficient evidence to support or refute the use of pregabalin based on this study.

The AAN Practice Parameter recommended that topiramate should be considered for treatment of ET [66]. In one double-blind, placebo-controlled trial, patients on topiramate reported an improvement in the clinical rating scale; however, 40% of patients in the treatment group withdrew due to side effects. These included appetite suppression, weight loss, paresthesia, and impaired concentration. Since that practice parameter was published, a multicenter, placebo-controlled, double blinded RCT was conducted in 208 patients with moderate to severe ET [68]. Patients in the topiramate group had greater improvement in the clinical rating scale compared to placebo. In addition, 69% of patients on topiramate reported a "good to very good" outcome compared to 15% in the placebo group (NNT = 2, 95% CI 1–2). Withdrawal due to side effects was significantly higher in the treatment group than placebo group, 31.9% versus 9.5% (NNH = 5, 95% CI 3–8).

Levetiracetam and zonisamide are probably not effective in reducing tremor based on two small randomized placebo-controlled, double blind studies and two open-label studies (levetiracetam) and one randomized double-blind, placebo-controlled (zonisamide) [69, 70].

Benzodiazepines

The AAN Practice Parameter reviewed two randomized placebo-controlled studies of alprazolam in the treatment of ET [66]. Both studies reported a 30% improvement on a clinical rating scale. Side effects included mild sedation and fatigue. The authors reported that alprazolam was probably effective in the treatment of ET, but cautioned that benzodiazepine risk of dependency required careful use. The short half-life and short dose response curve predispose to rebound effects.

In two double-blind studies of clonazepam, tremor improved significantly in one study and minimally in the second study [66]. Drowsiness was reported in 40% of patients in the second study.

Neuroleptics

Clozapine reduced tremor on clinical rating scales and accelerometry by about 50% in two double-blind studies [66]. Caution should be used with administration due to the potential side effect of agranulocytosis. Sedation was also reported as a significant side effect.

A recent randomized, double-blind, crossover trial of 38 patients comparing propranolol to olanzapine for ET found them to be equally efficacious on the clinical rating scale [71]. Improvement on a global impression scale was reported in 87% of patients on olanzapine and 63% of patients on propranolol. Olanzapine side effects included sedation, fatigue, dizziness, and nausea. The risk of parkinsonism and tardive dyskinesia, particularly in the older population, needs to be considered with olanzapine.

Botulinum Toxin Chemodenervation

The best evidence for botulinum toxin A in ET comes from two placebo-controlled studies of 25 and 133 patients with moderate to severe hand tremor [72]. The smaller study found a 50% absolute risk reduction in patient self-reported tremor severity in the botulinum toxin group compared to placebo, although there was no significant difference in the clinical rating scale scores between groups. All patients treated with botulinum toxin reported some degree of finger weakness. The larger study found improvement in postural tremor and minimal improvement in kinetic tremor in the botulinum toxin group. The AAN Practice Parameter concluded that botulinum toxin was modestly effective in reducing hand tremor, but the side effects of hand weakness may outweigh the benefits.

The AAN Practice Parameter concluded that there was insufficient evidence to support or refute the use of botulinum toxin in the treatment of head or vocal tremor [72] (Table 7.5).

Surgical Treatment of Essential Tremor

The AAN Practice Parameter completed an extensive review of thalamotomy and thalamic deep brain stimulation (DBS) surgery for treatment of ET [66]. These procedures are recommended for severe, medication refractory essential tremor. Both procedures target the ventral intermediate (VIM) nucleus of the thalamus.

Table 7.5 Pharmacological treatment of essential tremor

	Useful for tremor treatment	Strength of evidence	Side effects reported
Beta-blockers			
Propranolol	YES	Strong	Chronic – fatigue, impotence, lightheadedness, bradycardia
Sotalol	Probably	Moderate	
Atenolol	Probably	Moderate	
Nadolol	Possibly	Weak	
Pindolol	NO	Moderate	
Antiepileptics			
Primidone	YES	Strong	Acute – sedation, nausea, vomiting, ataxia, confusion, dizziness, acute toxic reaction
Topiramate	YES	Strong	Appetite suppression, weight loss, paraesthesias, impaired concentration
Gabapentin	Probably	Moderate	Sedation
Pregabalin	Unknown		
Levetiracetam	NO	Strong	
Zonisamide	NO	Moderate	
Benzodiazepines			
Alprazolam	Probably	Moderate	Dependency, Sedation
Clonazepam	Possibly	Weak	
Neuroleptics			
Clozapine	Probably	Moderate	Agranulocytosis, sedation
Olanzapine	Probably	Moderate	Sedation, fatigue, dizziness, nausea
Botulinum toxin			
Hand Tremor	Possibly	Moderate	Hand weakness, bruising
Head tremor	Unknown		
Vocal tremor	Unknown		

Older literature documents a high frequency of side effects with bilateral thalamotomy (severe dysarthria, dysphonia, and confusion), and therefore unilateral thalamotomy is recommended. Using DBS, bilateral thalamic stimulation, however is safe. Both unilateral thalamotomy and thalamic stimulation were equal in efficacy, but the perioperative side effect profile was higher in unilateral thalamotomy. Tremor improvement following either procedure was 60–90%. All thalamotomy studies were open label. By contrast, DBS can be assessed by blinded assessments since the stimulator can be turned on or off.

Adverse effects of unilateral thalamotomy occur in 14–47% of patients. Two studies reported a 16% occurrence of permanent neurological effects of hemiparesis and speech difficulty. Other transient sequelae include speech dysarthria, motor weakness, cognitive deficit, confusion, somnolence, and facial paresis. Adverse effects of thalamic DBS occurred at a lower rate (18%). In addition, equipment-related and stimulation-related effects can occur. The adverse effects are described in more detail in the PD section.

Clinical Bottom Lines

In the treatment of ET

1. There is good evidence to support the use of propranolol in the management of limb tremor. Propranolol may be useful in the treatment of head tremor. Long acting propranolol is as effective as convention propranolol.
2. There is good evidence to support the use of primidone in the management of limb tremor. Acute side effects may limit use.
3. Primidone and propranolol are equally effective in the treatment of limb tremor. Combination therapy may provide a small added benefit.
4. Based on lower levels of evidence, sotalol, atenolol, and nadolol are probably effective in reducing limb tremor; however, pindolol is probably not effective.
5. Based on good evidence, topiramate is effective in managing moderate to severe limb tremor. Side effects may limit use.
6. Gabapentin is probably effective in treating limb tremor based on moderate evidence.
7. There is insufficient evidence to support or refute the use of pregabalin.
8. Levetiracetam and zonisamide are probably not effective in the treatment of tremor.
9. Based on moderate evidence, alprazolam and clonazepam are probably effective in treating limb tremor. The evidence is weaker for clonazepam and side effects of sedation were common. Due to the risk of dependency and tolerance, benzo-diazepines should be used with caution.
10. Clozapine and olanzapine are probably effective in reducing tremor. Adverse effects, particularly agranulocytosis for clozapine and extrapyramidal side effects for olanzapine may restrict use.
11. Botulinum toxin may be modestly effective in the treatment of limb tremor, although resulting hand weakness may limit use.
12. There is insufficient evidence to support or refute the use of botulinum toxin in head or voice tremor.
13. Unilateral thalamotomy and thalamic stimulation surgery (unilateral or bilateral) are both effective in the treatment of severe, medication refractory limb tremor. Permanent neurological sequelae are higher with unilateral thalamotomy. Surgery is indicated for a highly selected group of patients. Surgery and stimu-lator-related side effects must be considered in the risk–benefit decision.

Summary

ET is a common movement disorder that increases with increasing age. Genetics play a significant role in etiology, while less is known about environmental factors. ET is a clinical diagnosis and more research is needed in this area. There are a num-ber of medications used to treat ET, although the degree of clinical improvement and side effect profile often limit their effectiveness.

Primary Dystonia

Introduction

Dystonia is defined as a syndrome of sustained muscle contractions causing repetitive twisting or abnormal postures [73]. Dystonia may be primary or secondary (to a variety of toxic, metabolic, traumatic, and infectious processes affecting basal ganglia function). By definition, primary dystonia is not associated with other neurological abnormalities, and the diagnosis is clinical. There are no associated pathological or serological abnormalities.

Clinical Scenario

A 40-year old woman presents with signs and symptoms of cervical dystonia. Her neurological examination is otherwise normal. She inquires about diagnostic tests and treatment options for this disorder.

Epidemiology

Clinical Questions

1. What is the incidence and prevalence of primary dystonia?
2. Are there risk factors for the development of primary dystonia?

Incidence and Prevalence of Primary Dystonia

As primary dystonia is a clinical diagnosis, studies of incidence and prevalence are challenging.

One well-designed community-based study examined the incidence of primary dystonia [74] using chart review from Rochester, Minnesota over a 32-year period. From this study, the incidence of early-onset, generalized dystonia was 2 million person years and the incidence of late-onset, focal dystonia was 24 million person years.

One well-designed systematic review of epidemiology studies in dystonia examined potential biases to determine a more accurate report of prevalence of primary dystonia [75]. All studies were reviewed and validity evaluated based on the following criteria: diagnosis established by neurological and nonneurological services, specific diagnostic criteria used, dystonia severity graded, all ages included, affected relatives included, and all types of dystonia included. Three studies of early-onset dystonia and five studies of late-onset dystonia were included. From these combined studies, the prevalence of primary early-onset primary dystonia was 24 million in Northern England and 44 and 50 million in the Ashkenazi Jewish population in Israel and New York, respectively. The prevalence of late-onset primary dystonia was 101, 133, 136, 254, and 430 million from studies in Japan, Italy, Serbia, Norway, and Northern England, respectively. Cervical dystonia was the most common form of late-onset focal dystonia in all countries except Japan and Italy, where blepharospasm was more common. Cervical dystonia may be more common in women.

A meta-analysis of 83 case series published over the last 25 years of 5,057 cases of primary dystonia found that dystonia presents in a caudal–rostral pattern related to age of onset [76]. DYT1 dystonia presented at a mean of 11 years (95% CI 10–12) and most frequently involved the foot, writer's cramp presented at a mean of 38.4 years (95% CI 37–40), cervical dystonia at a mean of 40.8 years (95% CI 40–41), spasmodic dysphonia at a mean age of 43 years (9% CI 42–44), and blepharospasm at a mean age of 55.7 years (95% CI 55–56).

Etiological Factors: Genetics and Environment

The etiology in most cases of primary dystonia is not known. In early-onset primary dystonia, the DYT1 gene mutation (a deletion in the Torsin A gene located on chromosome 9q34) is associated with an autosomal dominant inheritance pattern with incomplete penetrance and variable phenotype [77, 78]. This gene mutation occurs more commonly in the Ashkenazi Jewish population likely due to a founder effect [79].

One study screened 256 consecutive patients with both early and late-onset primary dystonia for the DYT1 gene mutation. Six patients carried the gene mutation. Two presented with generalized dystonia, while four presented with cranial–cervical dystonia or writer's cramp [78]. The mean age of onset of dystonia in the DYT1 positive patients was 15 years (range 7–41). Presentation within a single family can vary widely.

In a literature review of 13 families with late-onset primary dystonia, eight of the families had phenotypic variability in type of dystonia while five presented with consistent phenotype in affected members [80]. Genetic tests were performed in ten of the families and of these, three families were found to carry gene mutations linked to dystonia (DYT1, chromosome 9q34 and DYT7, chromosome 18p). Based on this review, in the majority of cases of late-onset dystonia, the pattern of inheritance is not clear and different gene mutations likely are causative.

Case-control studies indicate there may be both environmental and hereditary risk factors related to the development of primary dystonia. One multicentered case-control trial of 202 patients with primary dystonia and 202 controls evaluated risk factors including lifestyle factors, education, concurrent disease states, toxic exposures, trauma, and family history of dystonia or other movement disorders [81]. From multivariate analysis, eye diseases (blepharitis and keratoconjunctivitis) (OR 3.11, 95% CI 1.38–7.02), head trauma with loss of consciousness (OR 3.2, 95% CI 1.04–10.1), neck or trunk trauma (OR 7.84, 95% CI 1.35–45.7), family history of dystonia (OR 10.9, 95% CI 1.39–84.7), and family history of tremor (OR 5.66, 95% CI 1.81–17.7) were independent risk factors for the development of primary dystonia. Current smoking (OR 0.51, 95% CI 0.29–0.89) and hypertension (OR 0.36, 95% CI 0.16–0.65) were protective factors for the development of dystonia. Among cases, history of eye diseases was significantly higher among patients with blepharospasm compared to other types of dystonia (25.4% versus 10%). Neck or trunk trauma over the preceding 7 years was significantly higher among patients with cervical dystonia than other types (12% versus 3.5%). The authors concluded that injury to the affected body part may be linked to later development of dystonia. Given that the data were collected by retrospective patient reports, the wide confidence intervals, and the protracted time from injury to development of dystonia, the causation is unclear and the authors' conclusions are not substantiated by the evidence presented.

A second case-control study examined the risk of developing cervical dystonia for those with a previous diagnosis of scoliosis in 72 cases of cervical dystonia and 144 neurologic controls [82]. The authors found a history of scoliosis in puberty increased the risk of development of cervical dystonia on multivariate analysis (OR 6.8, 95% CI 1.5–29.7) and that a family history of dystonia was an independent risk factor for development of cervical dystonia (OR 11.7, 95% CI 1.3–103). Confidence intervals were wide, decreasing the certainty of the findings.

A third multicentered case-control study of 165 cases and 180 matched controls examined the risk of eye disease for the development of blepharospasm [83]. Logistic regression analysis found a significant independent association of reported ocular symptoms (conjunctivitis and dry eye syndrome) occurring at the time of onset of blepharospasm symptoms (OR 3.3, 95% CI 1.95–5.56).

Clinical Bottom Lines

1. Based on moderate evidence, the prevalence of early-onset primary dystonia (less than 20 years) ranges from 24 to 50 million and the prevalence of late-onset primary dystonia (greater than 20 years) ranges from 101 to 430 million. Cervical dystonia may occur more frequently, but this was not found in all studies.
2. Based on good evidence, the presenting phenotype of primary dystonia is related to age of onset.

3. The DYT1 gene mutation is an established cause of primary dystonia in a small number of cases. The population frequency depends on ethnic origin. The mode of inheritance is autosomal dominant with reduced penetrance (30–40%) and variable phenotype.
4. In late-onset primary dystonia, genetics may have a small role in the development of dystonia, based on weak evidence.
5. Environmental triggers of previous injury may be risk factors for the development of cervical dystonia and blepharospasm. The evidence is stronger for blepharospasm.

Diagnosis

Clinical Questions

1. What clinical guidelines are useful to recommend genetic testing for the DYT1 mutation?
2. What, in any, investigational tests are sensitive and specificity to confirm the diagnosis of Primary Dystonia?

Diagnosis of Primary Dystonia

The EFNS Task Force Guideline reviewed the evidence for diagnosis of primary dystonia [84]. As there are no well-controlled studies evaluating clinical criteria, the diagnosis relies on criteria based on descriptive case series and expert opinion.

The most common genetic cause of primary generalized dystonia is the DYT-1 mutation on Chromosome 9q34. Several studies attempted to identify clinical features that may predict the presence of the DYT-1 mutation and, therefore, guide genetic testing. Using a select population of 267 individuals with primary generalized dystonia (170 younger clinic patients and 87 affected carriers of patients with the DYT-1 mutation), a cut-off of age of onset under 26 years had a sensitivity of 100% and a specificity of 43% in the non-Ashkenazi Jewish population and a specificity of 63% in the Ashkenazi Jewish population to predict the presence of the DYT1 mutation [85]. The authors concluded that all individuals with primary dystonia under 26 years should undergo genetic testing.

Although a number of other genes have been determined to cause and or be associated with primary dystonia, genetic testing is not clinically available, and only performed in research settings [86, 87].

Based on the EFNS Task Force guidelines [84] and a thorough review of the literature, there are no electrophysiological or neuroimaging tests that have been assessed in controlled studies to accurately diagnose dystonia.

Clinical Bottom Lines

In the diagnosis of Primary Dystonia

1. The diagnosis is based on clinical criteria. There is no pathological or laboratory-based gold standard for diagnosis. The lack of a gold standard makes assessment of any diagnostic tools problematic.
2. Genetic testing for the DYT1 mutation may be recommended in individuals presenting with dystonia under the age of 26 years.
3. Neuroimaging techniques and electrophysiological studies are not useful in the diagnosis of primary dystonia.

Treatment

Clinical Questions

1. In patients with primary dystonia, what pharmacological therapies are effective and well tolerated to improve symptoms?
2. What is the efficacy and safety of neurosurgery – pallidal stimulation and pallidotomy – in the treatment of primary dystonia?

Medical Treatment for Patients with Primary Focal Dystonia

Medical treatment for patients with adult onset primary focal dystonia (cervical dystonia, blepharospasm, writer's cramp) includes oral medication and intramuscular botulinum toxin injections.

Intramuscular Injections of Botulinum Toxin: Cervical Dystonia

A Cochrane systematic review examined the use of botulinum toxin A in cervical dystonia [88]. Thirteen well-designed, double-blind, placebo-controlled, randomized trials included 680 patients. Clinical rating scale scores improved with botulinum toxin compared to placebo with a number needed to treat (NNT) of 3 (95% CI 3–4). Adverse events were transient and mild to moderate including dysphagia [number needed to harm (NNH) of 10, 95% CI 8–14], neck weakness (NNH 8, 95% CI 7–10), and dry or sore throat (NNH 10, 95% CI 7–21). A second Cochrane paper reviewed botulinum toxin B in the treatment of cervical dystonia [89]. Three well-designed double-blind, placebo-controlled trials randomized a total of 308 patients. Botulinum toxin B was found to result in improvement in cervical dystonia over placebo in clinical rating scales with a NNT of 3 (95% CI 2–6). Adverse events were transient and included dysphagia (NNH 8, 95% CI 7–11) and dry mouth (NNH 6, 95% CI 6–8).

Similarly, the AAN Practice Parameter [72] and a meta-analysis [90] concluded that botulinum toxin was effective and well tolerated in the treatment of cervical dystonia based on strong evidence and recommend that botulinum toxin should be used for the treatment of cervical dystonia.

Two double-blind, RCTs have compared botulinum toxin A to toxin B in the treatment of cervical dystonia. In the first study of 139 subjects, both serotypes demonstrated improvement in clinical rating scales at 4 weeks with no significant difference between groups for treatment effect or duration of effect [91]. Toxin B group had a higher rate of dysphagia (48% versus 19%) and dry mouth (80% versus 41%) compared to toxin A. In the second similar design RCT of 111 subjects, no difference was found in treatment effect, duration of effect, or number of adverse events [92]. Mild dry mouth occurred more frequently in the botulinum toxin B group at 32% versus 6% in the toxin A group.

Based on open label studies, botulinum toxin has sustained efficacy for cervical dystonia in up to 67% of patients for up to 10 years [90, 93, 94].

Intramuscular Injections of Botulinum Toxin: Blepharospasm

From a meta-analysis of three double-blind and one single-blind RCT of 73 patients, botulinum toxin A was reported to be probably effective in the treatment of blepharospasm [90]. The AAN Practice Parameter authors also concluded that botulinum toxin was probably effective in the treatment of blepharospasm and that adverse effects were generally mild and transient including blurred vision, tearing, ptosis, and bruising [72]. While the Cochrane review reported the evidence was weak due to small sample sizes and methodological problems (variable and poorly defined outcomes, different types of dystonia included, combination of open and blind evaluations), the authors concluded that botulinum toxin was probably effective and safe in the treatment of blepharospasm [95]. The authors also concluded that due to the high rate of efficacy (90%), it is unlikely that further placebo-controlled studies would be done due to ethical concerns.

Intramuscular Injections of Botulinum Toxin: Writer's Cramp (Focal Task-Specific Writing Dystonia)

A meta-analysis of two small placebo-controlled trials demonstrated improvement in hand dystonia with intramuscular botulinum toxin injection [90]. A larger double-blind, RCT of 40 patients with writer's cramp evaluating botulinum toxin was completed [96]. Outcome measures included patient satisfaction (desire to continue treatment) at 3 months and a clinical rating scale evaluated at 2 and 3 months. Subject retention was 100%. Seventy percent of patients in the treatment group versus 32% in the placebo group reported satisfaction with treatment and wished to continue [NNT 3 (95% CI 3–11)]. There was improvement of clinical rating scales in the treatment group. Hand weakness was transient but occurred in 90% of the botulinum toxin group versus 10% of the placebo group [NNH 1.3 (95% CI 1–2)].

An AAN Practice Parameter [72] concluded that botulinum toxin was probably effective for this indication based on the trial described above as well as three smaller placebo-controlled trials of moderate levels of evidence.

Trihexyphenidyl

A review of oral medications for treatment of primary dystonia in adults found a paucity of controlled trails. One double-blind, randomized, placebo-controlled trial evaluated trihexyphenidyl in children and young people with generalized dystonia (see below), but little evidence exists for the use in focal dystonia in the adult population. One double-blind crossover trial in adults with cranial dystonia found no treatment benefit for trihexyphenidyl over placebo [90].

A meta-analysis [90], AAN Practice Parameter [72], and Cochrane collaboration [97] reviewed the evidence comparing botulinum toxin to trihexyphenidyl in adults with cervical dystonia. From one double-blind, RCT botulinum toxin was more efficacious and better tolerated than trihexyphenidyl, with 72% meaningful improvement in the botulinum group on the clinical rating scale versus 38% improvement in the trihexyphenidyl group (NNT 3). Adverse events occurred more frequently in the trihexyphenidyl group including dry mouth (78%, NNH 2), forgetfulness (48%, NNH 4), and fatigue (22%, NNH 5) [98].

Other Oral Medications

No RCT studies were found evaluating other treatments such as tetrabenazine and neuroleptics.

Medication Treatment for Primary Generalized Dystonia

The use of oral medication and intrathecal baclofen were reviewed in primary generalized dystonia presenting in childhood or early adulthood.

Trihexyphenidyl

From a meta-analysis review, one double-blind, RCT evaluated younger patients [mean age 18.9 years (range 9–32)] with segmental and generalized dystonia treated with trihexyphenidyl [90]. The treatment group demonstrated improvement over placebo. Trihexyphenidyl was better tolerated and more effective in children than adults.

Other Oral Medications

There are no controlled trials supporting the use of levodopa for treatment of generalized primary dystonia [90].

The dopamine agonist, lisuride, was studied in two placebo-controlled randomized trials and found to be probably ineffective in the treatment of either generalized or focal dystonia [99, 100].

There is insufficient evidence to support or refute the use of any other oral medications in the treatment of generalized or focal dystonia [90].

Intrathecal Baclofen

Based on a meta-analysis [90] and review of the literature, only cases series have been published on the use of intrathecal baclofen in generalized dystonia. In a retrospective study of 14 subjects using intrathecal baclofen pumps, a blinded rater found that only 36% of patients demonstrated improvement in dystonia on objective criteria.

Surgical Treatment of Primary Dystonia: Pallidal Stimulation

Pallidal stimulation surgery is indicated for a select group of medication refractory patients with moderate to severe dystonia. Perioperative and hardware-related adverse effects must be considered in the risk–benefit ratio.

One randomized, double-blind, sham-stimulation controlled study assessed pallidal stimulation in the treatment of primary dystonia [101]. Forty patients with primary dystonia [16 patient with segmental dystonia (49 ± 13.5 years) and 24 patients with generalized dystonia (34 ± 10 years)], underwent surgical placement of the pallidal neurostimulator. Following surgery, patients were randomized to stimulation or no stimulation groups. Blinded outcome assessments occurred at 3 months and included clinical rating scales of dystonia, disability scales, and quality of life measurements. There was a significant improvement on all assessment scales in the stimulation group at 3 months. A positive response to treatment, defined as a greater than 25% reduction in motor scores, occurred in 75% of the stimulation group versus 15% of the sham stimulation group (NNT 2, 95% CI 1–3). Adverse events in the first 3 months were transient and occurred in 25% of the stimulation group and 15% of the sham group. There were an equal number of severe adverse events (infection and lead displacement) between groups.

Two single-blind trials assessed pallidal stimulation treatment of primary dystonia. The first study evaluated 22 patients (30 years, range 14–54) with primary generalized dystonia in a prospective trial of pallidal stimulation [102]. Videotapes of all patients were evaluated by a blinded rater using a clinical rating scale at baseline, 3 months, and 12 months. Cognition, mood, and quality of life assessments were completed at baseline and 12 months. Dystonia as measured by videotaped rating of a clinical rating scale (Burke–Fahn–Marsden Dystonia rating scale) improved at 3 months compared to baseline and remained stable to 12 months. Quality of life measures improved at 12 months while mood and cognition were unchanged. There were five adverse events, all of which resolved by 12 months. A similar study design was used for assessment of pallidal stimulation in ten patients with medically refractory cervical dystonia [103]. Outcomes were assessed by the clinical rating scale of dystonia (Toronto Western Spasmodic Torticollis Rating Scale), neuropsychological testing, and quality of life scale (Short Form-36). Two independent blinded raters evaluated dystonia from videotapes of the clinical rating scale done at baseline and 12 months. Patients showed improvement in dystonia scores, quality of life scales, and depression scores from baseline. Transient adverse events occurred in four patients. Two patients demonstrated minor changes in verbal memory and fluency on neuropsychological testing that had not resolved at 12 month follow-up.

Longer term efficacy was assessed in one study of 22 patients with primary generalized dystonia at 1 year and 3 years after pallidal stimulation using blinded rating of the videotaped clinical rating scale (Burke–Fahn–Marsden dystonia scale) [104]. Motor benefit was sustained at 1 and 3 year assessments. A second study of ten patients treated with pallidal stimulation for cervical dystonia were followed and assessed at 32 ± 20 months [105]. Follow up assessment was unblinded. Motor improvements in dystonia seen at 6 months postoperatively were sustained to the last follow up visit.

Clinical Bottom Lines

In the Treatment of Primary Dystonia

1. There is good evidence to support the use of botulinum toxin types A and B for the treatment of cervical dystonia. Adverse effects, including dysphagia and dry mouth, are transient and mild to moderate in nature. Treatment benefit with regular treatments (typically every 3–4 months) may be sustained in the majority of patients at least to 5 years.
2. Based on one comparative trial, botulinum toxin A is probably more effective and better tolerated than trihexyphenidyl for the treatment of cervical dystonia.
3. Based on small studies with lower levels of evidence, botulinum toxin A is probably effective in the treatment of blepharospasm.
4. Botulinum toxin A is probably effective in the treatment of writer's cramp. Hand weakness is a common but transient side effect.
5. Trihexyphenidyl is probably effective in the treatment of childhood onset generalized dystonia.
6. There is insufficient evidence to support or refute the use of any other oral medications in the treatment of generalized or focal dystonia.
7. There is insufficient evidence to support the use of intrathecal baclofen in the treatment of primary dystonia.
8. In patients with medically refractory generalized and cervical dystonia, pallidal stimulation surgery is effective in reducing dystonia. This effect may be sustained for up to 3 years or longer. Adverse effects were both surgical and stimulation related. This procedure is indicated for a highly select group of patients in experienced centers with appropriate preoperative and postoperative assessments.

Summary

Primary dystonia is a heterogeneous disorder affecting all age groups. There is good evidence to support that body distribution is linked to age of onset. Diagnosis rests in clinical evaluation. Genetics play a small role in etiology and genetic screening is for recommended for younger onset cases. Botulinum toxin is well established as an effective and well-tolerated treatment for focal dystonia. There is less evidence for the use of trihexyphenidyl in the treatment of childhood onset generalized dystonia. No other medication treatments are established.

Search Strategies

Parkinson's Disease

Epidemiology

MEDLINE database was searched since its inception to January of 2009. Medical Subject Heading (MeSH) terms and text words *Parkinson's disease, epidemiology,* and (*etiology OR risk factors OR prevalence OR incidence*) were combined with the Boolean "AND". Limits of "human," "English," "meta-analysis," and "practice guidelines" were applied. This resulted in 85 citations. The citations and abstracts of these were reviewed for relevance and 14 articles were chosen for review. Reference lists of review articles were also screened for any relevant articles.

Six meta-analyses and one case-control study dealing with incidence, prevalence, and risk factors were included as they represented the highest level of evidence.

Diagnosis

MEDLINE database was searched since its inception to January of 2009. MeSH terms and text words *Parkinson's disease* and *diagnosis* were searched and combined using the Boolean "AND." After limiting the retrieval to "English," "human," and "practice guidelines" a final set of 16 citations were obtained. From this search, all citations and abstracts were searched for relevance to the clinical question revealing four articles. All four articles were reviewed and included if they met the following criteria: address a focused clinical question, contain a thorough search of the litera-ture, and assess the validity of the studies.

A second search was conducted using the MeSH terms and text words *Parkinson's disease* and *diagnosis* and (*sensitivity OR specificity*) and (*physical examination OR magnetic resonance imaging OR positron-emission tomography OR ultrasonography OR olfactory OR SPECT OR growth hormone OR cardiac MIBG OR physical examination OR diagnostic tests*) and combined using the Boolean "AND." After limiting the retrieval to "English" and "human" a final set of 470 citations were obtained, of which 63 articles were selected and reviewed; they were included if they contributed new information not reported in the meta-analysis or systematic practice guidelines, and if they met the following criteria: appropriate spectrum of patients included, presence of a defined gold standard (autopsy or the surrogate marker of clinical diagnosis), diagnostic test was compared to the gold standard in a blinded fashion, and greater than ten participants in the each cohort.

Cochrane Database was searched from inception to January 2009 for the term *Parkinson's disease* and *diagnosis* revealing no additional reviews.

One practice parameter, two systematic reviews, one critically appraised topic, and eleven additional cohort or case-control studies fulfilled criteria.

Treatment

MEDLINE database was searched since its inception to January of 2009. MeSH terms and text words *Parkinson's disease* and (*therapy OR therapeutics*) were searched and combined using the Boolean "AND." After limiting the retrieval to "English," "human," and ("meta-analysis" OR "practice guidelines") a final set of 77 citations were obtained. From this search, all citations and abstracts were searched for relevance to the clinical question revealing 35 articles. All 35 articles were reviewed and included if they met the following criteria: addressed a focused clinical question, contained a thorough search of the literature, and assessed the validity of the studies.

The same search using the limit "randomized controlled trial" and "the last 5 years" was searched to reveal any new therapy studies that may have been published since the most recent meta-analysis and practice guidelines. This search revealing 285 citations that were reviewed and 70 citations were chosen from this group. The abstracts of these articles were reviewed for relevance. Thirty five articles were chosen for formal review and included if they contributed new information not reported in the meta-analysis or systematic practice guidelines, and if they met the following criteria: concealed randomization, blinding of outcomes, patient losses less than 20%, and at least 20 participants.

Cochrane Database was searched from inception to January 2009 for the term *Parkinson's disease* revealing an additional four reviews.

For medication treatment in the early stages of PD, three Cochrane systematic reviews, one meta-analysis, and three well-designed practice parameters fulfilled criteria for inclusion. For medication treatment of the motor fluctuations and dyskinesias in PD, two Cochrane systematic reviews and two practice parameters fulfilled criteria. For surgical treatment of motor fluctuations and dyskinesias, two practice parameters, one meta-analysis, and three recent RCT fulfilled criteria. For treatment of depression, psychosis, and dementia in PD, one practice parameter, three meta-analyses, and one recent RCT met criteria.

Essential Tremor

Epidemiology

MEDLINE database was searched since its inception to January of 2009. MeSH and text words *essential tremor, epidemiology*, and (*etiology OR risk factors OR prevalence OR incidence*) was combined with the Boolean "AND." Limits of "human" and "English" were applied. This resulted in 180 citations. The citations and abstracts of these were reviewed for relevance and 73 articles were chosen for review. Reference lists of review articles were also screened for any relevant articles.

One meta-analysis and 13 case-control or cohort studies were included as they represented the highest level of evidence.

Diagnosis

MEDLINE database was searched since its inception to January of 2009. MeSH terms and text words *essential tremor* and *diagnosis* were searched and combined using the Boolean "AND." The search limits "English," "human," and "practice guidelines" were included. No citations were found.

A second search was conducted using the MeSH terms and text words *essential tremor, diagnosis, diagnostic tests*, and (*sensitivity OR specificity*) and combined using the Boolean "AND." After limiting the retrieval to "English" and "human," a final set of 57 citations were obtained. From this search, all citations and abstracts were searched for relevance to the clinical question revealing 13 articles. All 13 articles were reviewed and included if they met the following criteria: appropriate spectrum of patients included, presence of a defined gold standard (autopsy or the surrogate marker of clinical diagnosis), diagnostic test was compared to the gold standard in a blinded fashion, and greater than ten participants in each cohort.

A third search using the term *accuracy* in place of *diagnostic tests, sensitivity*, and *specificity* was conducted. Two additional articles were found and reviewed.

Cochrane Database was searched from inception to January 2009 for the term *tremor* and *diagnosis* revealing no additional reviews.

One retrospective study and two double-blind, prospective trials fulfilled criteria for inclusion.

Treatment

MEDLINE database was searched since its inception to January of 2009. MeSH terms and text words (*tremor OR essential tremor*) and (*therapy OR therapeutics*) were searched and combined using the Boolean "AND." After limiting the retrieval to "English," "human," and ("meta-analysis" OR "practice guidelines") a final set of three citations were obtained. From this search, all citations and abstracts were searched for relevance to the clinical question revealing two practice parameters. These two systematic reviews were included as they met the following criteria: address a focused clinical question, contain a thorough search of the literature, and assess the validity of the studies.

The same search using the limits "randomized controlled trial" and "the last 10 years" was searched to reveal any new therapy studies that may have been published since the most recent practice guidelines. This search revealing 167 citations that were reviewed for relevance to the clinical question; 30 citations were chosen from this group. The abstracts of these articles were reviewed for relevance. Twenty one articles were chosen for formal review and included if they contributed new information not reported in the systematic practice guidelines, and if they met the following criteria: concealed randomization, blinding of outcomes, patient lost to follow-up less than 20%, and at least 20 participants.

Cochrane Database was searched from inception to January 2009 for the term *tremor* revealing no additional reviews.

Two well-designed practice parameters and eight randomized controlled trials fulfilled criteria for inclusion.

Dystonia

Epidemiology

MEDLINE database was searched since its inception to January of 2009. MeSH and text words (*primary dystonia OR dystonic disorders*), *epidemiology*, (*etiology OR risk factors OR prevalence OR incidence*) was combined with the Boolean "AND." Limits of "human" and "English" were applied. This resulted in 217 citations. The citations and abstracts were reviewed for relevance and 44 articles chosen for review. Reference lists of review articles were also screened for relevant articles.

One meta-analysis plus eight case-control and cohort studies were included as they represented the highest level of evidence.

Diagnosis

MEDLINE database was searched since its inception to January of 2009. MeSH terms and text words (*primary dystonia OR dystonic disorders*) and *diagnosis* were searched and combined using the Boolean "AND." The search limits "English" and "human" and "practice guidelines" were included. One citation was found.

A second search was conducted using the MeSH terms and text words (*primary dystonia OR dystonic disorders*), *diagnosis*, and (*diagnostic tests OR sensitivity OR specificity*) combined using the Boolean "AND." After limiting the retrieval to "English" and "human" a final set of 71 citations were obtained. All citations and abstracts were searched for relevance to the clinical question revealing five articles. All five articles were reviewed and included if they met the following criteria:

appropriate spectrum of patients included, presence of a defined gold standard (autopsy or the surrogate marker of clinical diagnosis), diagnostic test was compared to the gold standard in a blinded fashion, and greater than ten participants in the each cohort.

A third search using the term *accuracy* in place of (*diagnostic tests OR sensitivity OR specificity*) was conducted. No additional articles were found.

Cochrane Database was searched from inception to January 2009 for the term *primary dystonia* and *diagnosis* revealing no additional reviews.

One practice guideline and two case-control studies fulfilled criteria for inclusion.

Treatment

MEDLINE database was searched since its inception to January of 2009. MeSH terms and text words (*dystonic disorders OR primary dystonia*) and (*therapy OR therapeutics*) were searched and combined using the Boolean "AND." After limiting the retrieval to "English," "human," and (meta-analysis OR practice guidelines), a final set of 13 citations were obtained. From this search, all citations and abstracts were searched for relevance to the clinical question revealing one practice parameter and three meta-analyses. These four systematic reviews were included as they met the following criteria: address a focused clinical question, contain a thorough search of the literature, and assess the validity of the studies.

The same search using the limits (randomized controlled trial OR clinical trial) instead of (meta-analysis OR practice guidelines) was conducted to reveal any new therapeutic studies that may have been published since the most recent practice guidelines and meta-analysis. This search revealed 208 citations, which were reviewed for relevance to the clinical question; 53 citations were chosen from this group. The abstracts of these articles were reviewed for relevance. Nineteen articles were chosen for formal review and included if they contributed new information not reported in the systematic reviews and if they met the following criteria: concealed randomization, blinding of outcomes, patient lost to follow-up less than 20%, and at least 20 participants.

Cochrane Database was searched from inception to January 2009 for the term *primary dystonia* revealing three additional reviews.

One well-designed practice parameter, six meta-analyses and ten controlled trials fulfilled criteria for inclusion.

References

1. Forno LS. Neuropathology of Parkinson's disease. J Neuropathol Exp Neurol. 1996;55(3):259–72.
2. Hughes AJ, Daniel SE, Kilford L, Lees AJ. Accuracy of clinical diagnosis of idiopathic Parkinson's disease: a clinico-pathological study of 100 cases. J Neurol Neurosurg Psychiatry. 1992;55(3):181–4.

3. Hirtz D, Thurman DJ, Gwinn-Hardy K, Mohamed M, Chaudhuri AR, Zalutsky R. How common are the "common" neurologic disorders? Neurology. 2007;68(5):326–37.
4. Thacker EL, Ascherio A. Familial aggregation of Parkinson's disease: a meta-analysis. Mov Disord. 2008;23(8):1174–83.
5. Priyadarshi A, Khuder SA, Schaub EA, Shrivastava S. A meta-analysis of Parkinson's disease and exposure to pesticides. Neurotoxicology. 2000;21(4):435–40.
6. Firestone JA, Smith-Weller T, Franklin G, Swanson P, Longstreth Jr WT, Checkoway H. Pesticides and risk of Parkinson disease: a population-based case-control study. Arch Neurol. 2005;62(1):91–5.
7. Lai BC, Marion SA, Teschke K, Tsui JK. Occupational and environmental risk factors for Parkinson's disease. Parkinson Relat Disord. 2002;8(5):297–309.
8. Hernan MA, Takkouche B, Caamano-Isorna F, Gestal-Otero JJ. A meta-analysis of coffee drinking, cigarette smoking, and the risk of Parkinson's disease. Ann Neurol. 2002;52(3):276–84.
9. de Lau LM, Breteler MM. Epidemiology of Parkinson's disease. Lancet Neurol. 2006;5(6):525–35.
10. Allam MF, Campbell MJ, Hofman A, Del Castillo AS, Fernandez-Crehuet Navajas R. Smoking and Parkinson's disease: systematic review of prospective studies. Mov Disord. 2004;19(6):614–21.
11. Hughes AJ, Daniel SE, Ben-Shlomo Y, Lees AJ. The accuracy of diagnosis of parkinsonian syndromes in a specialist movement disorder service. Brain. 2002;125(Pt 4):861–70.
12. Suchowersky O, Reich S, Perlmutter J, Zesiewicz T, Gronseth G, Weiner WJ. Practice Parameter: Diagnosis and prognosis of new onset Parkinson disease (an evidence-based review). Report of the Quality Standards Subcommittee of the American Academy of Neurology. Neurology. 2006;66:968–75.
13. Hughes AJ, Daniel SE, Lees AJ. Improved accuracy of clinical diagnosis of Lewy body Parkinson's disease. Neurology. 2001;57(8):1497–9.
14. Clarke CE, Davies P. Systematic review of acute levodopa and apomorphine challenge tests in the diagnosis of idiopathic Parkinson's disease. J Neurol Neurosurg Psychiatry. 2000;69(5):590–4.
15. McKinnon JH, Demaerschalk BM, Caviness JN, Wellik KE, Adler CH, Wingerchuk DM. Sniffing out Parkinson disease: can olfactory testing differentiate parkinsonian disorders? Neurologist. 2007;13(6):382–5.
16. Kwon KY, Choi CG, Kim JS, Lee MC, Chung SJ. Comparison of brain MRI and 18 F-FDG PET in the differential diagnosis of multiple system atrophy from Parkinson's disease. Mov Disord. 2007;22(16):2352–8.
17. von Lewinski F, Werner C, Jorn T, Mohr A, Sixel-Doring F, Trenkwalder C. T2*-weighted MRI in diagnosis of multiple system atrophy. A practical approach for clinicians. J Neurol. 2007;254(9):1184–8.
18. Nicoletti G, Lodi R, Condino F, et al. Apparent diffusion coefficient measurements of the middle cerebellar peduncle differentiate the Parkinson variant of MSA from Parkinson's disease and progressive supranuclear palsy. Brain. 2006;129(Pt 10):2679–87.
19. Righini A, Antonini A, De Notaris R, et al. MR imaging of the superior profile of the midbrain: differential diagnosis between progressive supranuclear palsy and Parkinson disease. Am J Neuroradiol. 2004;25(6):927–32.
20. Quattrone A, Nicoletti G, Messina D, et al. MR imaging index for differentiation of progressive supranuclear palsy from Parkinson disease and the Parkinson variant of multiple system atrophy. Radiology. 2008;246(1):214–21.
21. Vlaar AM, van Kroonenburgh MJ, Kessels AG, Weber WE. Meta-analysis of the literature on diagnostic accuracy of SPECT in parkinsonian syndromes. BMC Neurol. 2007;7:27.
22. Nagayama H, Hamamoto M, Ueda M, Nagashima J, Katayama Y. Reliability of MIBG myocardial scintigraphy in the diagnosis of Parkinson's disease. J Neurol Neurosurg Psychiatry. 2005;76(2):249–51.
23. Gaenslen A, Unmuth B, Godau J, et al. The specificity and sensitivity of transcranial ultrasound in the differential diagnosis of Parkinson's disease: a prospective blinded study. Lancet Neurol. 2008;7(5):417–24.

24. Suchowersky O, Gronseth G, Perlmutter J, Reich S, Zesiewicz T, Weiner WJ. Practice Parameter: Neuroprotective strategies and alternative therapies for Parkinson disease (an evidence-based review). Report of the Quality Standards Subcommittee of the American Academy of Neurology. Neurology. 2006;66:976–82.

25. Miyasaki JM, Martin W, Suchowersky O, Weiner WJ, Lang AE. Practice parameter: initiation of treatment for Parkinson's disease: an evidence-based review: report of the Quality Standards Subcommittee of the American Academy of Neurology. Neurology. 2002;58(1):11–7.

26. Horstink M, Tolosa E, Bonuccelli U, et al. Review of the therapeutic management of Parkinson's disease. Report of a joint task force of the European Federation of Neurological Societies and the Movement Disorder Society-European Section. Part I: early (uncomplicated) Parkinson's disease. Eur J Neurol. 2006;13(11):1170–85.

27. Crosby N, Deane KH, Clarke CE. Amantadine in Parkinson's disease. Cochrane Database Syst Rev. 2003(1):CD003468.

28. Katzenschlager R, Sampaio C, Costa J, Lees A. Anticholinergics for symptomatic management of Parkinson's disease. Cochrane Database Syst Rev. 2002(3):CD003735.

29. Macleod AD, Counsell CE, Ives N, Stowe R. Monoamine oxidase B inhibitors for early Parkinson's disease. Cochrane Database Syst Rev. 2005(3):CD004898.

30. Simonis G, Fuhrmann JT, Strasser RH. Meta-analysis of heart valve abnormalities in Parkinson's disease patients treated with dopamine agonists. Mov Disord. 2007;22(13):1936–42.

31. Voon V, Hassan K, Zurowski M, et al. Prevalence of repetitive and reward-seeking behaviors in Parkinson disease. Neurology. 2006;67(7):1254–7.

32. Weintraub D, Siderowf AD, Potenza MN, et al. Association of dopamine agonist use with impulse control disorders in Parkinson disease. Arch Neurol. 2006;63(7):969–73.

33. Stowe RL, Ives NJ, Clarke C, et al. Dopamine agonist therapy in early Parkinson's disease. Cochrane Database Syst Rev. 2008(2):CD006564.

34. Pahwa R, Factor SA, Lyons KE, et al. Practice Parameter: treatment of Parkinson disease with motor fluctuations and dyskinesia (an evidence-based review): report of the Quality Standards Subcommittee of the American Academy of Neurology. Neurology. 2006;66(7):983–95.

35. Fahn S, Oakes D, Shoulson I, et al. Levodopa and the progression of Parkinson's disease. N Engl J Med. 2004;351(24):2498–508.

36. Horstink M, Tolosa E, Bonuccelli U, et al. Review of the therapeutic management of Parkinson's disease. Report of a joint task force of the European Federation of Neurological Societies (EFNS) and the Movement Disorder Society-European Section (MDS-ES). Part II: late (complicated) Parkinson's disease. Eur J Neurol. 2006;13(11):1186–202.

37. Deane KH, Spieker S, Clarke CE. Catechol-O-methyltransferase inhibitors for levodopa-induced complications in Parkinson's disease. Cochrane Database Syst Rev. 2004(4):CD004554.

38. Rascol O. Rasagiline in the pharmacotherapy of Parkinson's disease–a review. Expert Opin Pharmacother. 2005;6(12):2061–75.

39. Rascol O, Brooks DJ, Melamed E, et al. Rasagiline as an adjunct to levodopa in patients with Parkinson's disease and motor fluctuations (LARGO, Lasting effect in Adjunct therapy with Rasagiline Given Once daily, study): a randomised, double-blind, parallel-group trial. Lancet. 2005;365(9463):947–54.

40. Nyholm D, Nilsson Remahl AI, Dizdar N, et al. Duodenal levodopa infusion monotherapy vs oral polypharmacy in advanced Parkinson disease. Neurology. 2005;64(2):216–23.

41. Crosby NJ, Deane KH, Clarke CE. Amantadine for dyskinesia in Parkinson's disease. Cochrane Database Syst Rev. 2003(2):CD003467.

42. Deuschl G, Schade-Brittinger C, Krack P, et al. A randomized trial of deep-brain stimulation for Parkinson's disease. N Engl J Med. 2006;355(9):896–908.

43. Weaver FM, Follett K, Stern M, et al. Bilateral deep brain stimulation vs best medical therapy for patients with advanced Parkinson disease: a randomized controlled trial. JAMA. 2009; 301(1):63–73.

44. Schupbach WM, Maltete D, Houeto JL, et al. Neurosurgery at an earlier stage of Parkinson disease: a randomized, controlled trial. Neurology. 2007;68(4):267–71.

45. Louis ED, Ottman R, Hauser WA. How common is the most common adult movement disorder? estimates of the prevalence of essential tremor throughout the world. Mov Disord. 1998; 13(1):5–10.
46. Deuschl G, Bain P, Brin M. Consensus statement of the Movement Disorder Society on Tremor. Ad Hoc Scientific Committee. Mov Disord. 1998;13(Suppl 3):2–23.
47. Louis ED. Essential tremor. Lancet Neurol. 2005;4(2):100–10.
48. Tan LC, Venketasubramanian N, Ramasamy V, Gao W, Saw SM. Prevalence of essential tremor in Singapore: a study on three races in an Asian country. Parkinsonism Relat Disord. 2005;11(4):233–9.
49. Bergareche A, De La Puente E, Lopez De Munain A, et al. Prevalence of essential tremor: a door-to-door survey in bidasoa, spain. Neuroepidemiology. 2001;20(2):125–8.
50. Louis ED, Ottman R, Ford B, et al. The Washington Heights-Inwood Genetic Study of Essential Tremor: methodologic issues in essential-tremor research. Neuroepidemiology. 1997;16(3):124–33.
51. Rajput AH, Offord KP, Beard CM, Kurland LT. Essential tremor in Rochester, Minnesota: a 45-year study. J Neurol Neurosurg Psychiatry. 1984;47(5):466–70.
52. Benito-Leon J, Bermejo-Pareja F, Louis ED. Incidence of essential tremor in three elderly populations of central Spain. Neurology. 2005;64(10):1721–5.
53. Louis ED, Ottman R. How familial is familial tremor? The genetic epidemiology of essential tremor. Neurology. 1996;46(5):1200–5.
54. Lorenz D, Frederiksen H, Moises H, Kopper F, Deuschl G, Christensen K. High concordance for essential tremor in monozygotic twins of old age. Neurology. 2004;62(2):208–11.
55. Tanner CM, Goldman SM, Lyons KE, et al. Essential tremor in twins: an assessment of genetic vs environmental determinants of etiology. Neurology. 2001;57(8):1389–91.
56. Louis ED, Ottman R. Study of possible factors associated with age of onset in essential tremor. Mov Disord. 2006;21(11):1980–6.
57. Higgins JJ, Pho LT, Nee LE. A gene (ETM) for essential tremor maps to chromosome 2p22-p25. Mov Disord. 1997;12(6):859–64.
58. Gulcher JR, Jonsson P, Kong A, et al. Mapping of a familial essential tremor gene, FET1, to chromosome 3q13. Nat Genet. 1997;17(1):84–7.
59. Shatunov A, Sambuughin N, Jankovic J, et al. Genomewide scans in North American families reveal genetic linkage of essential tremor to a region on chromosome 6p23. Brain. 2006;129(Pt 9): 2318–31.
60. Blair MA, Ma S, Phibbs F, et al. Reappraisal of the role of the DRD3 gene in essential tremor. Parkinsonism Relat Disord. 2008;14(6):471–5.
61. Tan EK, Prakash KM, Fook-Chong S, et al. DRD3 variant and risk of essential tremor. Neurology. 2007;68(10):790–1.
62. Louis ED, Jurewicz EC, Applegate L, et al. Association between essential tremor and blood lead concentration. Environ Health Perspect. 2003;111(14):1707–11.
63. Louis ED, Jiang W, Pellegrino KM, et al. Elevated blood harmane (1-methyl-9 H-pyrido[3,4-b] indole) concentrations in essential tremor. Neurotoxicology. 2008;29(2):294–300.
64. Louis ED, Pullman SL. Comparison of clinical vs. electrophysiological methods of diagnosing of essential tremor. Mov Disord. 2001;16(4):668–73.
65. Gironell A, Kulisevsky J, Pascual-Sedano B, Barbanoj M. Routine neurophysiologic tremor analysis as a diagnostic tool for essential tremor: a prospective study. J Clin Neurophysiol. 2004;21(6):446–50.
66. Zesiewicz TA, Elble R, Louis ED, et al. Practice parameter: therapies for essential tremor: report of the Quality Standards Subcommittee of the American Academy of Neurology. Neurology. 2005;64(12):2008–20.
67. Zesiewicz TA, Ward CL, Hauser RA, et al. A pilot, double-blind, placebo-controlled trial of pregabalin (Lyrica) in the treatment of essential tremor. Mov Disord. 2007;22(11):1660–3.
68. Ondo WG, Jankovic J, Connor GS, et al. Topiramate in essential tremor: a double-blind, placebo-controlled trial. Neurology. 2006;66(5):672–7.

69. Elble RJ, Lyons KE, Pahwa R. Levetiracetam is not effective for essential tremor. Clin Neuropharmacol. 2007;30(6):350–6.
70. Handforth A, Martin FC. Pilot efficacy and tolerability: a randomized, placebo-controlled trial of levetiracetam for essential tremor. Mov Disord. 2004;19(10):1215–21.
71. Yetimalar Y, Irtman G, Kurt T, Basoglu M. Olanzapine versus propranolol in essential tremor. Clin Neurol Neurosurg. 2005;108(1):32–5.
72. Simpson DM, Blitzer A, Brashear A, et al. Assessment: Botulinum neurotoxin for the treatment of movement disorders (an evidence-based review): report of the Therapeutics and Technology Assessment Subcommittee of the American Academy of Neurology. Neurology. 2008;70(19):1699–706.
73. Fahn S. Concept and classification of dystonia. Adv Neurol. 1988;50:1–8.
74. Nutt JG, Muenter MD, Aronson A, Kurland LT, Melton 3rd LJ. Epidemiology of focal and generalized dystonia in Rochester, Minnesota. Mov Disord. 1988;3(3):188–94.
75. Defazio G, Abbruzzese G, Livrea P, Berardelli A. Epidemiology of primary dystonia. Lancet Neurol. 2004;3(11):673–8.
76. O'Riordan S, Raymond D, Lynch T, et al. Age at onset as a factor in determining the phenotype of primary torsion dystonia. Neurology. 2004;63(8):1423–6.
77. Bressman S. Genetics of dystonia. J Neural Transm Suppl. 2006;70:489–95.
78. Grundmann K, Laubis-Herrmann U, Bauer I, et al. Frequency and phenotypic variability of the GAG deletion of the DYT1 gene in an unselected group of patients with dystonia. Arch Neurol. 2003;60(9):1266–70.
79. Bressman SB, de Leon D, Kramer PL, et al. Dystonia in Ashkenazi Jews: clinical characterization of a founder mutation. Ann Neurol. 1994;36(5):771–7.
80. Defazio G, Berardelli A, Hallett M. Do primary adult-onset focal dystonias share aetiological factors? Brain. 2007;130(Pt 5):1183–93.
81. Defazio G, Berardelli A, Abbruzzese G, et al. Possible risk factors for primary adult onset dystonia: a case-control investigation by the Italian Movement Disorders Study Group. J Neurol Neurosurg Psychiatry. 1998;64(1):25–32.
82. Defazio G, Abbruzzese G, Girlanda P, et al. Primary cervical dystonia and scoliosis: a multicenter case-control study. Neurology. 2003;60(6):1012–5.
83. Martino D, Defazio G, Alessio G, et al. Relationship between eye symptoms and blepharospasm: a multicenter case-control study. Mov Disord. 2005;20(12):1564–70.
84. Albanese A, Barnes MP, Bhatia KP, et al. A systematic review on the diagnosis and treatment of primary (idiopathic) dystonia and dystonia plus syndromes: report of an EFNS/MDS-ES Task Force. Eur J Neurol. 2006;13(5):433–44.
85. Bressman SB, Sabatti C, Raymond D, et al. The DYT1 phenotype and guidelines for diagnostic testing. Neurology. 2000;54(9):1746–52.
86. Bressman SB. Genetics of dystonia: an overview. Parkinson Relat Disord. 2007;13 Suppl 3:S347–55.
87. de Carvalho Aguiar PM, Ozelius LJ. Classification and genetics of dystonia. Lancet Neurol. 2002;1(5):316–25.
88. Costa J, Espirito-Santo C, Borges A, et al. Botulinum toxin type A therapy for cervical dystonia. Cochrane Database Syst Rev. 2005(1):CD003633.
89. Costa J, Espirito-Santo C, Borges A, et al. Botulinum toxin type B for cervical dystonia. Cochrane Database Syst Rev. 2005(1):CD004315.
90. Balash Y, Giladi N. Efficacy of pharmacological treatment of dystonia: evidence-based review including meta-analysis of the effect of botulinum toxin and other cure options. Eur J Neurol. 2004;11(6):361–70.
91. Comella CL, Jankovic J, Shannon KM, et al. Comparison of botulinum toxin serotypes A and B for the treatment of cervical dystonia. Neurology. 2005;65(9):1423–9.
92. Pappert EJ, Germanson T. Botulinum toxin type B vs. type A in toxin-naive patients with cervical dystonia: randomized, double-blind, noninferiority trial. Mov Disord. 2008;23(4):510–7.

93. Skogseid IM, Kerty E. The course of cervical dystonia and patient satisfaction with long-term botulinum toxin A treatment. Eur J Neurol. 2005;12(3):163–70.
94. Berman B, Seeberger L, Kumar R. Long-term safety, efficacy, dosing, and development of resistance with botulinum toxin type B in cervical dystonia. Mov Disord. 2005;20(2):233–7.
95. Costa J, Espirito-Santo C, Borges A, et al. Botulinum toxin type A therapy for blepharospasm. Cochrane Database Syst Rev. 2005(1):CD004900.
96. Kruisdijk JJ, Koelman JH, Ongerboer de Visser BW, De Haan RJ, Speelman JD. Botulinum toxin for writer's cramp: a randomised, placebo-controlled trial and 1-year follow-up. J Neurol Neurosurg Psychiatry. 2007;78(3):264–70.
97. Costa J, Espirito-Santo C, Borges A, Ferreira JJ, Coelho M, Sampaio C. Botulinum toxin type A versus anticholinergics for cervical dystonia. Cochrane Database Syst Rev. 2005(1): CD004312.
98. Brans JW, Lindeboom R, Snoek JW, et al. Botulinum toxin versus trihexyphenidyl in cervical dystonia: a prospective, randomized, double-blind controlled trial. Neurology. 1996;46(4): 1066–72.
99. Nutt JG, Hammerstad JP, Carter JH, de Garmo PL. Lisuride treatment of focal dystonias. Neurology. 1985;35(8):1242–3.
100. Quinn NP, Lang AE, Sheehy MP, Marsden CD. Lisuride in dystonia. Neurology. 1985; 35(5):766–9.
101. Kupsch A, Benecke R, Muller J, et al. Pallidal deep-brain stimulation in primary generalized or segmental dystonia. N Engl J Med. 2006;355(19):1978–90.
102. Vidailhet M, Vercueil L, Houeto JL, et al. Bilateral deep-brain stimulation of the globus pallidus in primary generalized dystonia. N Engl J Med. 2005;352(5):459–67.
103. Kiss ZH, Doig-Beyaert K, Eliasziw M, Tsui J, Haffenden A, Suchowersky O. The Canadian multicentre study of deep brain stimulation for cervical dystonia. Brain. 2007;130(Pt 11): 2879–86.
104. Vidailhet M, Vercueil L, Houeto JL, et al. Bilateral, pallidal, deep-brain stimulation in primary generalised dystonia: a prospective 3 year follow-up study. Lancet Neurol. 2007;6(3): 223–9.
105. Hung SW, Hamani C, Lozano AM, et al. Long-term outcome of bilateral pallidal deep brain stimulation for primary cervical dystonia. Neurology. 2007;68(6):457–9.

Chapter 8
Cognitive and Behavioral Neurology

Elizabeth Finger and Kirk R. Daffner

Keywords Neurodegeneration • Neurodegenerative disease • Dementia • Alzheimer's disease • Dementia with Lewy bodies • Frontotemporal dementia • Pick's disease • Vascular dementia • Cognitive neurology • Behavioral neurology

Alzheimer's Disease

Alzheimer's disease (AD) is a progressive neurodegenerative disorder known to be the most common cause of dementia. It features insidious onset and gradual progression of deficits in short-term memory, and commonly includes deficits in executive functioning, apraxia or aphasia.

Epidemiology

Clinical Case

A 76-year-old man presents to clinic with his wife, who is concerned about his memory. Over the past 2 years, she has found him to be increasingly forgetful and repetitive. He complains that he frequently misplaces items around the house and has left the stove on after cooking twice in the past year. On two occasions, he has gotten lost while driving home from the post office and store.

E. Finger (✉)
Clinical Neurological Sciences, University of Western Ontario,
268 Grosvenor Street, Suite D0-224, London, ON, Canada N6A 4V2
e-mail: elizabeth.finger@lhsc.on.ca

J.G. Burneo et al. (eds.), *Neurology: An Evidence-Based Approach*,
DOI 10.1007/978-0-387-88555-1_8, © Springer Science+Business Media, LLC 2012

Clinical Case Questions

What is the incidence across age groups of Alzheimer's disease?
What is the prevalence across age groups of Alzheimer's disease?
What is the risk of Alzheimer's disease for individuals with one or two copies of the
    APOE ε4 allele?

Search Strategy

Ovid MEDLINE database was searched from 1950 to December 12, 2008. Medical
subject heading (MeSH) terms "incidence or prevalence" and "Alzheimer's disease"
were searched and combined using the Boolean "AND." After limiting the retrieval
to English and human, a final set of 683 citations were obtained. From this set, ten
articles using community-based samples with large sample sizes were selected for
review. EMBASE, PubMed, and the Cochrane Library databases were also searched
implementing the same strategy of MeSH terms and keywords. No additional relevant
articles were detected.

Results

Incidence

Based on a meta-analysis from 1998 of 23 community-based studies of the incidence of dementia and Alzheimer's disease in Europe, Japan, China, and the USA
and two subsequent community-based studies in the USA, aging is associated with
an increased incidence of Alzheimer's disease (see Table 8.1) [1]. In addition to age,
lower levels of education are associated with an increased risk of developing
Alzheimer's disease, with an estimated relative risk reduction of 0.91 (CI: 0.86–
0.97) per year of education [2]. This effect of education has been attributed to greater
cognitive reserve, and not reduction in the neuropathologic changes of Alzheimer's
disease [4].

Prevalence

Prevalence rates in the USA based on the aging, demographics, and memory study
cohort were recently estimated at 2.32% (1.26–3.37) for individuals aged 71–79,
18% (13.5–22.7) for individuals aged 80–89, and 30% (18.6–40.8) for those ≥90
years of age [5]. A meta-analysis of 20 studies of the prevalence of AD in Caucasians,
excluding the East Boston Study as an outlier, reported the higher prevalence rates
for AD (combined mild, moderate or severe): 65–69 years: 1.1–1.9, 70–74 years:
2.3–3.9, 75–79 years: 4.8–8.2, 80–84 years: 9.8–16.3, 85–89 years: 19.4–31.9,
90–94 years: 36.4–58.7 [6]. A pooled analysis of 11 European population-based

Table 8.1 Incidence of Alzheimer's disease by age per 1,000 Person-years

Age	Meta-analysis (European – US) [1]	ACT cohort [2]	Rochester Epidemiology Project [3]
65–69	2.5–6.1	3.53	1.03
70–74	5.2–11.1	5.88	3.15
75–79	10.7–20.1	9.36	9.89
80–84	22.1–38.4	29.63	19.44
85–90	46.1–74.5	46.38	32.49
+90	144.8	61.01	46.55–56.77

studies of individuals >65 years of age also demonstrated increasing prevalence of Alzheimer's disease with age, with somewhat lower prevalence estimates of 1.8–4.3% of individuals ages 75–79 and 6.3–14.2% of those aged 80–90 [7].

Risk of Alzheimer's Disease and APOE ε4 Status

Several studies have consistently found an increased risk of Alzheimer's disease for individuals carrying one or two APOE ε4 alleles compared to noncarriers. Based on these studies, the relative risk of carrying a single ε4 allele is 1.3–4.77 times higher than noncarriers while the relative risk of two copies ranges from 6.2 to 8.5 times above that of noncarriers [2, 8, 9] (Table 8.1).

Clinical Bottom Lines

The incidence and prevalence rates of Alzheimer's disease increase with age.
Greater years of education are associated with a modest reduction in the risk of developing clinical Alzheimer's dementia.
Heterozygous and homozygous carriers of the APOE ε4 allele have an increased risk of developing Alzheimer's compared to noncarriers.

Diagnosis

Clinical Questions

How accurate are the diagnostic criteria for Alzheimer's disease?
Which neuropsychological tests are best for diagnosing Alzheimer's disease?
What is the role of neuroimaging in diagnosing Alzheimer's disease? Which neuroimaging study is best?
What is the role of CSF biomarkers in the diagnosis of Alzheimer's disease?
Should patients be screened for Alzheimer's disease-associated genetic polymorphisms and mutations?

Table 8.2 NINCDS-ADRDA core criteria for Alzheimer's disease [10]

I. Probable Alzheimer's disease:
   a. Dementia established by clinical examination and documented by the MMSE, Blessed dementia scale or similar exam and confirmed by neuropsychological tests
   b. Deficits in two or more areas of cognition
   c. Progressive worsening of memory and other cognitive functions
   d. Onset between ages 40 and 90, most often after age 65
   e. Absence of systemic disorders or other brain diseases that could account for the dementia

II. Possible Alzheimer's disease
   a. Dementia syndrome, in the absence of other neurologic, psychiatric, or systemic disorders sufficient to cause dementia, and in the presence of variations in onset, in the presentation, or in clinical course
   b. Presence of second systemic or brain disorder sufficient to produce dementia, which is not considered to be the cause of dementia and
   c. A single, gradually progressive severe cognitive deficits identified in the absence of other identifiable causes

III. Definite Alzheimer's disease
   a. The clinical criteria for probable Alzheimer's disease and
   b. Histopathologic evidence obtained from a biopsy or autopsy

Search Strategy

Ovid MEDLINE database was searched from 1950 to December 28, 2008. MeSH terms "Alzheimer's disease" and "diagnostic criteria" were searched and combined using the Boolean "AND." After limiting the retrieval to English and human a final set of 371 citations was obtained. Additional searches combining the terms "Alzheimer's disease," "diagnosis," and "neuroimaging" limited to English language and human studies resulted in 199 articles; "Alzheimer's disease," "biomarkers," and "diagnosis" yielded 371 citations, and a search using "Alzheimer's disease" and "genetic testing" yielded 354 results. From these, studies were selected for review based on the sample size, clinical relevance of control groups, and practical clinical availability of tests or analytic methods. Studies evaluating the additive benefit of specific diagnostic tests beyond routine clinical diagnostic accuracy were given preference. EMBASE, PubMed, and the Cochrane Library databases were also searched implementing the same strategy of MeSH terms and keywords. No additional relevant articles were detected.

Results

Clinical Criteria

Based on autopsy series of patients with various types of dementia, the NINCDS-ARDRA criteria (see Table 8.2) have a sensitivity of 66–93% and a specificity of 23–70% for diagnosing Alzheimer's disease [11–13]. The DSM-III, IIIR, and IV have also been commonly used. Available evidence on the PPV of the DSM-IIIR for probable dementia of the Alzheimer type and Alzheimer's dementia is high (89–100%) but the negative predictive value is low, ranging from 33 to 63% [14].

Neuropsychology

Cognitive Screening Tests

Mini-Mental Status Exam

Overall, the mini-mental status exam (MMSE) was most effective at ruling out dementia in community or primary care settings, where the prevalence of dementia was low. The MMSE was not useful in these settings to rule in dementia, as the majority of persons (60%) below the cutoff would be false positives [15]. In specialist settings where the prevalence of dementia is significantly higher, at best the MMSE may be modestly useful in ruling in dementia. MMSE scores vary significantly according to education, and thus accuracy of the test is lower in persons with low education [15, 16].

Montreal Cognitive Assessment

While early impressions of the Montreal cognitive assessment (MoCA) suggest a high sensitivity but low specificity [17, 18], to date there is insufficient evidence regarding the sensitivity and specificity to distinguish between normal aging nor among dementia subtypes.

Neuropsychological Testing

While patients with AD may exhibit short-term memory deficits, executive functioning impairment, and anomia, delayed recall tests are the best predictors/discriminators of patients with AD vs. normal controls (see Table 8.3).

NeuroImaging

MRI-regular clinical scan: In addition to the role of CT and MRI in ruling out non-neurodegenerative causes of cognitive impairment, including mass lesions or normal pressure hydrocephalus, MRI demonstrates additive benefit above comprehensive clinical diagnosis (clinical diagnosis + neuropsychological testing) for distinguishing dementias (Alzheimer's disease, frontotemporal dementia (FTD), and LBD pooled) from VaD [31]. Medial temporal lobe atrophy has been associated with AD and with 2–7 times increased risk of progression of MCI to AD [32–34]. FDG-PET: A recent study with autopsy confirmation comparing sensitivity of PET to clinical

Table 8.3 Sensitivity and specificity of diagnostic tests in Alzheimer's disease

Modality	Diagnostic tool	Sensitivity (%)	Specificity (%)	References
Clinical criteria	NINDS-CRADA	66–93	23–70	[11–13]
Neuropsychology	MMSE (average cutoff score of 23–24)	80	81	[15]
	Delayed Recall (various paradigms)	87–96	84–87	[19–21]
NeuroImaging	MRI with Medial Temporal Lobe Atrophy Measures	92	94	[22]
	FDG-PET	74–86	74–86	[23, 24]
	SPECT	71–90	76	[25]
	PIB-PET	100	?	[26, 27]
CSF Biomarkers	Reduced a-beta and/or elevated tau	61–95	80–83	[28, 29]
Genetics	APOε4 (+clinical assessment)	84	64	[30]

diagnosis of Alzheimer's at initial presentation found that PET was superior to that of the initial clinical evaluation while PET and clinical evaluation were comparable approximately 4 years later [23]. SPECT: SPECT does not appear more accurate than clinical criteria for diagnosing Alzheimer's disease; however, it may be more specific than the criteria (91% vs. 70%) for distinguishing between AD and non-AD dementias [25].

PIB-PET: While small studies PIB-PET have demonstrated a 100% sensitivity for patients with clinical diagnosis of Alzheimer's disease [26, 27], significant PIB binding in Lewy body disease and healthy controls limit the current role of PIB-PET to distinguish between these disorders and Alzheimer's disease [27, 35]. While lower PIB binding has been reported in clinically probable FTD vs. Alzheimer's disease [27], up to 20–30% of clinically diagnosed FTD patients showed PIB+ [36, 37]. Thus, further studies of the sensitivity and specificity of PIB-PET with autopsy confirmed diagnosis are required.

Biomarkers

Alzheimer's disease has been associated with low levels of CSF a-beta and high levels of CSF tau proteins [38]. At present, biomarkers are not recommended in the routine evaluation for Alzheimer's disease given insufficient evidence of additive diagnostic accuracy above other clinical measures [19].

Genetics

The ε4 allele of the apolipoprotein E is the most common genotype associated with Alzheimer's disease to date. However, whether APOε4 genotype shows an additive benefit above comprehensive clinical diagnostic accuracy is not determined. North

American and recent European practice guidelines do not recommend routine testing of APOE genotype in patients with suspected dementia [19, 39]. The prevalence of identifiable mutations in amyloid precursor protein (APP), presenilin 1 and 2 is <5% in all Alzheimer's patients, though is significantly higher in early-onset familial patients (approximately 20%) [40, 41], and up to 50% in autosomal dominant familial forms [42]. At present, genetic screening for these mutations is only recommended in the setting genetic counseling and a clear autosomal dominant familial pattern of inheritance [39].

Clinical Bottom Lines

For the most commonly used diagnostic criteria, NINCDS-ARDA criteria lack sensitivity.

The MMSE may be useful as a screening tool for identifying patients in the community or primary care setting who may require further assessment.

Routine clinical CT or MRI should be performed in all patients with suspected Alzheimer's disease to rule out non-neurodegenerative etiologies.

PET imaging may improve clinical diagnostic accuracy of AD at initial presentation. SPECT imaging may be helpful in distinguishing between Alzheimer's disease and non-Alzheimer's disease dementias.

Visualization of in vivo amyloid using PIB-PET is promising new technique; however, further validation is required.

Routine use of CSF biomarkers for the diagnosis of Alzheimer's disease is not supported given insufficient evidence for an additive value above routine clinical measures.

At present, routine genetic testing is not recommended for patients with suspected Alzheimer's disease or dementia.

Tables 8.2 and 8.3.

Treatment

Clinical Questions

What is the evidence for efficacy of cholinesterase inhibitors (CHEIs) in Alzheimer's disease? Are there significant differences among the CHEIs?

What is the evidence for the use of memantine in Alzheimer's disease?

What are the proven benefits and risks associated with atypical neuroleptics for agitation and confusion in Alzheimer's disease?

Is there a role for antioxidant, anti-inflammatory, or statin therapy for Alzheimer's disease?

Search Strategy

The Cochrane database was searched with the terms "Alzheimer's disease" and "treatment." Limiting results to publications from 2003 to February 16, 2009 produced 475 articles. Additional searches for articles published in 2008 and 2009 were conducted in Medline and Pubmed. 21 articles were selected for review based on design (randomized, double-blind, placebo-controlled trials, and meta-analysis).

Results

Cholinesterase Inhibitors

A Cochrane systematic review (literature search in June 2005) of CHEIs (pooled analysis of donepezil, galantamine, and rivastigmine) in mild, moderate, and severe AD included ten randomized, controlled, blinded trials of at least 6 months duration [43] (see Table 8.4). Modest improvements were found in cognitive outcomes and general clinical impression. Modest benefits on various scales of activities of daily living and behavior were also reported. Higher rate of adverse events and withdrawal were observed in the CHEI groups (29% vs. 18% in placebo). More frequent adverse events associated with CHEI treatment were nausea, vomiting, abdominal pain, diarrhea, headache, insomnia, and dizziness. One head-to-head study was included which compared donepezil to rivastigmine and demonstrated no difference in cognitive outcomes, activities of daily living or behavioral measures at 2 years. Fewer side effects were observed with donepezil compared to rivastigmine OR 0.64 (95% CI 0.5–0.8).

Donepezil

A Cochrane systematic review of 15 unconfounded, double-blind, randomized controlled trials of donepezil vs. placebo in patients with mild, moderate, or severe AD was reviewed [45]. Modest improvements in cognition and several scales of activities of daily living were found (see Table 8.4). Withdrawal rates were highest at the 10 mg/day dose (24% vs. 20% placebo), though not significantly higher at 5 mg/day (18% drug and 18% placebo). A separate 12-week randomized placebo-controlled trial assessed the efficacy of donepezil 10 mg/day vs. placebo in 272 patients with AD and agitation [46]. No significant differences on Cohen-Mansfield Agitation Inventory, neuropsychiatric inventory (NPI), NPI-Caregiver Distress Scale, or Clinician's Global Impression of Change were found.

Table 8.4 Cochrane review and meta-analysis results: effects of cholinesterase inhibitors and memantine in Alzheimer's disease

Drug	Effect dose and duration	Clinical scales
Cholinesterase inhibitors (pooled analysis of donepezil, galantamine, and rivastigmine) [43]	Donepezil 10 mg/day; galantamine 12–24 mg/day divided bid; rivastigmine 8.5–12 mg/day divided bid >= 6 months	ADAS-Cog: −2.7/70 points (95% CI −3.0 to −2.3) MMSE: +1.37/30 points (95% CI 1.13–1.61) PDS: 2.40 (95% CI 1.55–3.37) DAD: 4.39 (95% CI 1.96–6.81) NPI: -2.44/120 points (95% CI −4.12 to −0.76) CBIC: OR 1.84 (95% CI 1.47–2.3)
Memantine [44]	20 mg/day for 6 months	SIB: 2.97/100 points (95% CI 1.68–4.26) ADCS-ADL: 1.27/54 points (95% CI 0.44–2.09) NPI: 2.76/144 points (95% CI 0.88–4.63) ADAS-Cog: 0.99/70 points (95% CI 0.21–1.78)

ADAS-Cog Alzheimer's Disease Assessment Scale maximum score (most impaired) is 70 points
SIB Severe Impairment Battery: Maximum score = 100 points indicates no impairment
MMSE Mini-mental Status Exam, maximum score 30 points indicates no impairment
ADCS-ADL Alzheimer's Disease Cooperative Study activities of daily living inventory for moderate to severe dementia. Maximum score of 54 indicates no impairment
NPI Neuropsychiatric Inventory: Score range from 12 to 120, with 120 indicating severe impairment
PDS Progressive Deterioration Scale. Maximum score of 100 indicates no impairment
DAD Disability Assessment for Dementia scale: Maximum score of 100 indicates no impairment
CBIC Clinician's Interview-Based Impression of Change scale. Scored from 1–7, with score of 4 = patient's baseline. Higher scores indicate worsening, lower scores indicate improvement

Galantamine

A Cochrane systematic review assessed randomized, double-blind, parallel group trials with treatment duration of >4 weeks in mild to moderate probable AD for a total of 6,805 subjects [47]. For doses greater than 8 mg/day, significant improvement or stabilization of global scale ratings and modest improvement in cognitive measures were found (see Table 8.4). Extended release formulations of 16–24 mg QD had similar efficacy and side effect profile as bid dosing. Side effects frequency was summarized to be similar to other CHEI, with the best optimization of efficacy and side effects at 16 mg/day [OR adverse side effects at 16 mg vs. placebo 2.79 (CI 1.7–5.3)].

Rivastigmine

A Cochrane systematic review of double-blind, randomized, placebo-controlled trials in parallel groups for greater than 2 weeks included seven trials [48]. Compared to placebo, doses of 6–12 mg/day were associated with an improvement in cognition and activities of daily living. Adverse effects of nausea, vomiting, diarrhea, headache, syncope, abdominal pain, and dizziness were reported in 23% of patients receiving rivastigmine vs. 8% receiving placebo.

Memantine

A Cochrane systematic review of blinded, parallel group, placebo-controlled, randomized trials of memantine in patients with dementia was reviewed [44]. Memantine was associated with a slightly lower incidence of agitation, especially in moderate to severe Alzheimer's disease (12% on memantine vs. 18% on placebo). There was no significant difference in adverse event rates between memantine and placebo groups, and the dropout rate was lower in memantine groups (20.3% on memantine vs. 27.9% on placebo). Subsequent recent studies of memantine in mild to moderate AD have shown mixed results. A recent randomized, double-blind placebo-controlled trial of 6 weeks of memantine (20 mg/day) in mild to moderate Alzheimer's disease did not show any significant effects on outcome measures of ADAS-cog or CIBIC-plus, NPI, MMSE, or ADCS-ADLs [49]. A second study of memantine (20 mg/day) for 24 weeks in mild to moderate Alzheimer's disease showed improvement at weeks 12 and 18 on the ADAS-cog and CIBIC-plus score but not at 24 weeks [50]. A recent meta-analysis of randomized, placebo-controlled, double-blinded studies of memantine for 4 weeks or greater in patients with probable Alzheimer's disease and outcome ratings on the NPI included five studies (three of which were included in the Cochrane review above). Patients mean MMSE scores ranged from 7.9 to 17.3 [51]. A modest improvement in mean NPI scores was reported in the pooled analysis (−1.99/144 points; 95% CI 0.08 to −3.91). Retrospective studies of combination treatment with memantine and CHEIs suggest a benefit in ADLs, cognition, and time to nursing home placement [52, 53]. Shorter duration placebo-controlled studies of memantine added to stable dosing of a CHEI indicate combination therapy is safe, but have shown mixed results as to whether combination therapy improves cognition, ADLs or behavior [49, 54, 55].

Neuroleptics

A Cochrane systematic review for randomized, double-blind, placebo-controlled, parallel group studies of atypical antipsychotic (olanzapine, quetiapine, risperidone, clozapine, and aripiprazole) treatment for Alzheimer's disease for at least 6 weeks, with validated measures of aggression or psychosis included 16 studies [56]. Risperidone, at doses between 0.5 and 2 mg/day, was associated with a modest improvement in behavioral ratings [NPI or BEHAVE-AD: SMD 0.17–0.29 (95% CI 0.05–0.51)]. Aggression ratings on risperidone (1–2 mg/day) were also improved [Cohen-Mansfield Agitation Inventory: MD −0.84 to −1.50 (95% CI −0.4 to −2.05)]. Risperidone was associated with a higher rate of adverse events at 1 mg (11.5% vs. 9 % on placebo) and 2 mg doses (41% vs. 27% on placebo). Patients treated with risperidone showed significantly more extrapyramidal symptoms, upper respiratory tract infections, urinary tract infections, falls, and cerebrovascular events (3% on risperidone vs. 1% on placebo). Olanzapine 5–10 mg/day was associated with a modest benefit in aggression [NPI-NH aggression MD: −0.77 (95% CI −1.44 to −0.1)] but also a higher dropout rate due to adverse effects (11% on olanzapine vs. 4% placebo). Aripiprazole: One 10-week study demonstrated an improvement in psychosis but adverse effects of somnolence. Quetiapine (50–100 mg/day) was associated with a worse performance on the severe impairment battery. A separate meta-analysis of mortality data from published and unpublished studies demonstrated a small but significant increase in mortality in patients with dementia, 87% of whom had Alzheimer's disease, treated with atypical neuroleptic mediations (OR 1.54; 95% CI 1.06–2.23) [57]. There were no significant differences in risk for specific drugs (olanzapine, risperidone, quetiapine, or aripiprazole), disease severity, sample selection, or diagnosis.

A recent prospective, placebo-controlled withdrawal study of continuation of neuroleptic medications in patients with Alzheimer's disease for 12 months found that continuation of antipsychotic medications was associated with a significant increased risk of death compared to placebo with 24-month survival of 41% of patients on antipsychotic medication vs. 71% on placebo [58]. Phase 1 results from the Clinical Antipsychotic Trials of Intervention Effectiveness – Alzheimer's Disease (CATIE-AD) study of masked, flexible dosing of risperidone (0.5 or 1 mg), olanzapine (2.5 or 5 mg), quetiapine (25 or 50 mg), vs. placebo for an average of 7 weeks found small improvements for risperidone on total NPI score [difference in least mean squares −8.2 (95% CI −13 to −2.4)], clinical global impression of change (−0.7; 95% CI −1.1 to −0.3), and brief psychiatric rating scale hostile suspiciousness factor (Mean difference 2.9 points, SE 1.1) [59]. No significant differences from placebo were found for cognition, functioning, care needs, or quality of life for risperidone or quetiapine, but olanzapine, was associated with a worsening in these measures.

A separate multicentered, double-blind, placebo-controlled trial examined the effects of olanzapine (mean doses 5.5 mg/day), quetiapine (56.5/day), risperidone (1 mg/day), or placebo on time to medication discontinuation and CGIC scores at 12 weeks [60]. Overall, duration to discontinuation rates of the neuroleptics was not different than placebo, with 77 to 85% of patients discontinuing treatment or placebo for lack of efficacy or for adverse events. Parkinsonism occurred in 12% of patients on olanzapine or risperidone compared to 2% on quetiapine and 1% on placebo. No significant differences were observed for clinical global impression scores at 12 weeks. Higher rates of sedation (15–24%) occurred in neuroleptic groups compared to placebo (5%). Confusion and mental status changes were more common with olanzapine (18%) and risperidone (11%) than placebo (5%).

Antioxidants

NSAIDS

A majority of studies of NSAIDS in Alzheimer's disease have failed to show clinically significant effects on disease progression, progression from MCI to AD, and most show an increased risk of adverse events with NSAIDS: rofecoxib or naproxen [61, 62], celecoxib [63], indomethacin [64], and aspirin [65].

Vitamin E

A Cochrane systematic review [66] found one randomized, placebo-controlled study of vitamin E in patients with probable AD [67] and one study of the effects of vitamin E on progression rates from amnestic MCI to probable AD [68]. In patients with moderate AD, vitamin E was associated with reduced frequency of patients reaching an endpoint of progression in CDR scores from 2.0 to 3.0. There was also a significant increase in falls in patients receiving vitamin E compared to placebo (16% vs. 5%) [67]. There was no significant difference in the rates of progression from amnestic MCI to probable AD between vitamin E and placebo-treated patients [68]. Due to the availability of only one sufficiently controlled trial in AD and one in MCI, the Cochrane review concludes that the replication of these studies is required before vitamin E should be prescribed for patients with AD [66]. A meta-analysis of vitamin E supplementation suggests a slight increase in mortality associated with high-dose vitamin E supplementation: pooled all-cause mortality risk difference in high-dosage vitamin E trials (>400 IU/day) was 39 per 10,000 persons (95% CI, 3 to 74 per 10,000 persons; $p=0.035$) [66, 69].

Statins

Recent studies have suggested a role of statins and beta-amyloid processing, but human studies of an association between statins, development of Alzheimer's disease and beta-amyloid deposition show mixed results [70, 71]. Population studies of risk of development of AD suggest reduced risk with statin use [72], but earlier meta-analysis did not find an association between statin use and development of AD [73]. Some pilot randomized studies have reported potential benefits of statin therapy in patients with AD on cognitive and functional outcomes [74], but further larger scale, placebo-controlled trials of statins are required (Table 8.4).

Clinical Bottom Lines

All three CHEIs (donepezil, galantamine, rivastigmine) show modest benefit in patients with Alzheimer's disease on measures of cognition, activities of daily living, and behavior, with similar side effect profiles.

Recent studies of memantine show a very small improvement in measures of cognition, behavior, activities of daily living and agitation in patients with moderate to severe Alzheimer's disease, with no significant side effects. At present, there is not sufficient evidence to recommend memantine in patients with mild Alzheimer's disease.

Because of increased risk of cerebrovascular events, death, and other serious adverse events, the use of neuroleptic medications for agitation and confusion in Alzheimer's disease should be used only as a last resort after other behavioral interventions have been tried. Treatment with these medications requires a review with caregivers of the potential risks, careful monitoring, and frequent attempts at discontinuation.

At present, there is insufficient evidence to support the use of nonsteroidal anti-inflammatory medications or vitamin E in Alzheimer's disease.

Prognosis

Clinical Question

What is the average survival time for a patient diagnosed with Alzheimer's disease from time of symptom onset and from time of diagnosis?

Search Strategy

Ovid MEDLINE database was searched from 1950 to November 28, 2008. MeSH terms "Alzheimer disease" and "prognosis" were searched and combined using the Boolean "AND" limiting results to English and human, resulting in 504 references. Additional articles were found by tracking references to these articles. No additional articles were found in Cochrane reviews or EMBASE. Five studies were selected for detailed review based on sample size, incident diagnosis of Alzheimer's disease, and reported statistics on survival estimates.

Results

Estimates of the average survival time for patients with Alzheimer's disease are affected by age and gender, with reduced survival times for advanced age at symptom onset or diagnosis (see Table 8.5), and reduced survival times for men compared to women [75–77, 79]. For a patient aged 65 years of age at diagnosis, there is an approximate 17-year reduction in expected remaining lifespan compared to controls, 3–5 years less for those diagnosed at age 70–75, and at age 90 the reduction in remaining life span is approximately 2 years compared to controls [76–78].

Table 8.5 Estimated survival time from symptom onset and time of diagnosis in patients with probable Alzheimer's disease

Age	Median survival in years from symptom onset (SD) [75]	Median survival in years from initial diagnosis [76–78]
<75 years	8.9 (4.5)	6–9.9
75–84 years	6.13 (3.3)	4.9–6.9
>=85 years	4.38 (2.46)	3.2–4.4

Clinical Bottom Lines

With advanced age of onset, the median expected remaining survival decreases for patients with Alzheimer's disease. In younger patients (age 65), there is a dramatic difference in life expectancy compared with controls (Table 8.5).

Frontotemporal Dementia

Introduction

Frontotemporal dementia (FTD), or frontotemporal lobar dementia (FTLD) describes a group of neurodegenerative disorders classically characterized by the mid-life onset of gradually progressive changes in behavior and/or language, and which share a predilection for neurodegeneration of the frontal and or temporal lobes. Several clinical variants of FTD have been recognized, including behavioral variant FTD (bv-FTD), primary progressive aphasia (PPA), and semantic dementia (also called temporal variant FTD (tv-FTD)). In bv-FTD, patients present with striking behavioral changes which can include loss of appropriate social conduct, neglect of personal hygiene, development of obsessions and compulsions, emotional blunting, distractibility, and inattention. Typically, patients lack insight into these behavioral and personality changes. In PPA, language is the predominant feature, with gradually progressive difficulties in expressive speech as in a progressive nonfluent aphasia. In semantic dementia, patients present with loss of knowledge of the meaning of words, with generally preserved fluency. Patients with combined symptoms of FTD and motor neuron disease are increasingly recognized. Several genetic mutations are associated with FTD, including mutations in the genes for tau, progranulin, CHMP2B, and valosin-containing protein. Neuropathologically, FTD is characterized by atrophy of the frontal and or temporal lobes, with gliosis, neuronal loss, and microvaculation. Several protein inclusions have been identified in patients, most commonly TDP-43 inclusions associated with ubiquitin, followed by intraneuronal tau inclusions termed Pick bodies. Recent cases have also been reported with ubiquitin + FUS + pathology and other neurofilament inclusions.

Epidemiology

Clinical Case

A 65-year-old man presents with 5–6 years of gradually progressive changes in his behavior, including increased jocularity, impulsive spending, poor hygiene, and deficits in attention and concentration. There is no known family history of FTD, though limited information is available for his father who died at age 40 of a myocardial infarction. Based on his presentation, neurocognitive tests, and an MRI demonstrating atrophy of the frontal lobes, a diagnosis of FTD is made.

Clinical Questions

What is the incidence of FTD?
What is the prevalence of FTD?
If my family member has FTD, what is my chance of getting the disease?

Search Strategy

Ovid MEDLINE database was searched from 1950 to November 21, 2008. MeSH terms "incidence or prevalence" and "frontotemporal dementia or frontotemporal lobar degeneration or Pick's disease" were searched and combined using the Boolean "AND." After limiting the retrieval to English and human, a final set of 99 citations were obtained. From this set, six articles were reviewed: two incidence studies, two prevalence studies, and two studies of risk in first-degree relatives. EMBASE, PubMed, and the Cochrane Library databases were also searched implementing the same strategy of MeSH terms and keywords. No additional relevant articles were detected.

Results

Incidence

One recent study was reviewed which screened databases of specialized early onset dementia, memory and Huntington's disease clinics to ascertain cases of patients <65 years of age at time on symptom onset in Cambridgeshire, England [80]. This study reported an incidence of 3.5 cases per 100,000 person years (95% CI 2.0–5.7) in persons age 45–65 years of age. This estimate is consistent with a smaller, earlier study of the incidence of FTD in Rochester, Minnesota which estimated an incidence of 4.1 per 100,000 person years age 40–69 [81].

Table 8.6 Neary core criteria core diagnostic features for FTD and semantic dementia and progressive nonfluent aphasia subtypes

I.   FTD
  a. Insidious onset and gradual progression
  b. Early decline in social interpersonal conduct
  c. Early impairment in regulation of personal conduct
  d. Early emotional blunting
  e. Early loss of insight
II. Progressive nonfluent aphasia
  f. Insidious onset and gradual progression
  g. Nonfluent spontaneous speech with at least one of the following: agrammatism, phonemic paraphasias, anomia
III. Semantic dementia
  h. Insidious onset and gradual progression
  i. Language disorder characterized by
    • Progressive, fluent, empty spontaneous speech
    • Loss of word meaning, manifest by impaired naming and comprehension
    • Semantic paraphasias and/or
  j. Perceptual disorder characterized by
    • Prosopagnosia: impaired recognition of identity of familiar faces and/or
    • Associative agnosia: impaired recognition of object identity
  k. Preserved perceptual matching and drawing reproductions
  l. Preserved single word repetition
  m. Preserved ability to read aloud and write to dictation orthographically regular words

Prevalence

Two retrospective studies conducted in the Netherlands and in England assessed the community-based prevalence of FTD via ascertainment of cases from area clinics, physicians, hospitals, and nursing homes and a review of medical records from area medical centers specializing in dementia [82, 83]. Results from these two studies suggest the prevalence of FTD ranges from 9.6 to 15/100,000 in younger onset patients (<65 years of age and 60–69 years of age, respectively). Two additional studies using outreach screening of older community members indicate that prevalence rates among older age groups are higher than initially presumed (see Table 8.6).

Risk of dementia in family members: Two studies of the relative risk of dementia in first-degree relatives using the family history method were reviewed [84, 85]. The relative risk of developing any form of dementia varied significantly between the studies, from no increased risk to a twofold increase in risk (from 11% risk of dementia before age 80 in relatives of controls, vs. a 22% risk of dementia in first-degree relatives of FTD). Based on these studies, the relative risk of a first-degree relative developing FTD ranged from 3.5 to 10 times higher than that of the general population. These estimates may be low, as other studies have reported that 38% had a history of a first-degree relative with dementia, and 13% of FTD patients show an autosomal dominant pattern of inheritance. The highest hereditability rates were found for FTD-ALS, followed by fv-FTD, while semantic dementia was associated with the lowest rate of hereditability [86]. The differences in these estimates likely stem from differences in the control populations used to estimate control incidence rates, limitations of the family history method for case ascertainment, and from inclusion of differing numbers of patients with each FTD subtype.

Clinical Bottom Lines

Based on the best evidence to date, the incidence of FTD is estimated to be at least 3.5–4.1 per 100,000 person years.

Based on the best evidence to date, the prevalence of FTD is estimated to be 9.4–15/100,000 persons.

First-degree family members of patients with FTD have a 3.5- to 10-fold increased risk of developing FTD.

Diagnosis

Clinical Questions

How sensitive and specific are the clinical criteria for frontotemporal dementia?

Are neuropsychological tests are useful in distinguishing FTD from AD?

Are neuroimaging techniques useful in the diagnosis of FTD and distinction from AD and other neuropsychiatric diseases?

Are there any biomarkers or genetic tests that can be ordered to confirm the diagnosis of FTD?

Search Strategy

Ovid MEDLINE database was searched from 1950 to October 14, 2008. MeSH terms "frontotemporal dementia or frontotemporal lobar degeneration or Pick's disease" and "diagnostic criteria" were searched and combined using the Boolean "AND." After limiting the retrieval to English and human a final set of 77 citations were obtained. A second search of the terms "frontotemporal dementia or frontotemporal lobar degeneration or Pick's disease" and "MRI or SPECT" resulted in 384 articles. A third search using the terms "frontotemporal dementia or frontotemporal lobar degeneration or Pick's disease" and "biomarkers or biochemical markers" yielded 64 articles. Studies were selected that specifically addressed the most difficult diagnostic distinctions between FTD, Alzheimer's, and other neuropsychiatric disorders at patients' initial presentation. Studies with neuropathologic diagnostic confirmation and using diagnostic methodologies widely available were given preference. From this set, six articles were reviewed. EMBASE, PubMed, and the Cochrane Library databases were also searched implementing the same strategy of MeSH terms and keywords. No additional relevant articles were detected.

Results

Clinical Criteria

The Neary criteria [87] are the most common criteria used in current FTD clinical practice and research (see Table 8.6). The sensitivity and specificity of the Neary criteria were recently evaluated in a retrospective assessment of patients referred to a specialized clinic for the evaluation of possible FTD [88]. Note the high pretest prevalence of this sample (47%) was due to prior evaluations by neurologists and psychiatrists which did reveal alternate diagnosis.

Neuropsychological Assessment

The frontal behavourial inventory (FBI), a caregiver interviewer of symptoms of FTD, has been demonstrated to distinguish FTD from AD and controls (see Table 8.7). In the Mendez et al. study described above, the utility of two neuropsychological batteries, the Consortium to Establish a Registry in Alzheimer's disease and the frontal assessment battery, were assessed in patients with possible FTD. The results suggest that initial composite neuropsychological scores on these batteries did not discriminate between FTD and non-FTD patients, although progressive worsening over time was significant in patients with FTD [88]. In a meta-analysis of published neuropsychological studies of patients diagnosed with FTD (all subtypes combined) or Alzheimer's disease found patients with FTD performed significantly worse on several tests of language, while patients with Alzheimer's disease showed poorer performance on memory tests [96]. While the meta-analysis did not find differences between the two groups in performance on executive function tasks, prior work has suggested grouping of tv- and fv-FTD patients may obscure differences in neuropsychological test results [97]. In a smaller study comparing tv-FTD, fv-FTD, AD patients and controls on standard neuropsychological tests, patients with tv-FTD showed deficits in semantic memory (Palms and Pyramids) but better performance on attention and executive tests than patients with AD or fv-FTD while patients with fv-FTD showed greater deficits in attention and executive functioning domain scores (Test of Everyday Attention, Wisconsin Card Sort Task) than patients with AD or tv-FTD [97].

Neuroimaging

MRI

Possible FTD (see Table 8.7). FTD vs. AD: Comparison of visual inspection ratings of regional atrophy on initial presenting T1 MRI scans of patients with biopsy or autopsy confirmed FTD found a specificity of only 60% vs. patients with Alzheimer's [91].

Table 8.7 Sensitivity and specificity of diagnostic tests in frontotemporal dementia

Modality	Diagnostic tool	Sensitivity (%)	Specificity (%)	References
Clinical criteria	Neary criteria	30[a]	100	[88]
Neuropsychology	Frontal behavioral inventory	70–97	85–95	[89, 90]
NeuroImaging	MRI: frontotemporal atrophy in possible FTD (pretest probability of FTD 47%)	64	70	[88]
	MRI: frontal lobe atrophy in FTD vs. controls	76	74	[91]
	PET cortical and hippocampal ratings in FTD vs. AD	98	94	[92]
	SPECT FTD vs. AD (combined reduced frontal and preserved parietal CBF)	80	81	[93]
CSF Biomarkers	Reduced a-beta and/or elevated tau to discriminate AD from FTD	79–90	64–97	[94, 95]

[a]At initial assessment

PET

A recent study evaluating the diagnostic benefit of FDG-PET scanning in autopsy-confirmed patients with FTD or AD [92] found PET resulted in an inappropriate change of diagnosis or increased confidence in the correct diagnosis in 42% of cases, had no effect on clinical impression in 42% of cases, and inappropriately changed the diagnosis in 11.5%.

SPECT: FTD vs. AD (see Table 8.7).

Possible FTD: One study in patients with possible FTD found the sensitivity of reduced frontotemporal blood flow on SPECT/PET combined was 90.5% with a specificity of 74.6%, giving a PPV of 76.0% and negative predictive value of 89.8% [88].

CSF Biomarkers

While several studies have demonstrated that an elevated Tau/AB42 ratio can discriminate between patients with FTD and AD, this has not been shown to improve clinical diagnostic accuracy [94].

Genetics

Studies of the two most common genetic mutations associated with FTD, tau and progranulin show lower rates for sporadic FTD, and significantly higher rates for familial forms. Estimates of the prevalence of tau mutations in sporadic cases of

FTD range from 0 to 3.6% [83, 98]. Recent studies of the prevalence of progranulin mutations in sporadic FTD may be somewhat higher, ranging from 0 to 30%, but further studies are required [99–101]. Thus, genetic screening of individuals without a family history of FTD is not currently recommended [98]. In patients with an autosomal dominant pattern of FTD, prevalence rates of tau mutations increases from 9 to 32% [83, 98]. A higher prevalence of progranulin mutations is also suggested (range 17–28% [99, 101]). Referral to a genetic counselor prior to consideration of screening for familial forms of FTD-associated mutations, including tau and progranulin mutations, is recommended.

Clinical Bottom Lines

The Neary criteria commonly used for a diagnosis of FTD show high specificity but lower sensitivities indicate these criteria may miss early cases of FTD.

Neuropsychological tests of language, memory, and executive functioning help to discriminate between patients with tv-FTD, fv-FTD, and Alzheimer's disease.

Patterns of frontal lobe atrophy on MRI or frontal lobe hypometabolism on PET and SPECT may aid in the diagnosis of FTD.

At present, there is insufficient evidence for the use of biomarkers in the routine clinical evaluation of patients with possible FTD.

At present, genetic screening is not recommended for sporadic cases of FTD. For patients with a significant family history, referral to a genetic counselor is appropriate.

As yet there is no single test with adequate sensitivity and specificity for antemortem diagnosis of FTD. The best available evidence suggests that diagnostic accuracy is maximized by combined clinical assessment, including neuropsychological tests of memory, language, and executive functioning along with MRI and/or PET or SPECT scanning.

Tables 8.6 and 8.7.

Treatment

Clinical Question

Are there any treatments proven to be effective in the management of behavioral problems in patients with FTD?

Search Strategy

Ovid MEDLINE database was searched from 1950 to October 14, 2008. MeSH terms "frontotemporal dementia or frontotemporal lobar degeneration or Pick's disease" and "treatment" were searched and combined using the Boolean "AND." After limiting the retrieval to English and human a final set of 132 citations were obtained. Of these citations, 20 were treatment studies in FTD, including seven case reports and case series, seven open label studies, one randomized open label study, two randomized controlled trials, and three randomized placebo-controlled trials. EMBASE, PubMed, and the Cochrane Library databases were also searched implementing the same strategy of MeSH terms and keywords. One additional Cochrane review article was found which reviewed two articles, one of which was relevant to patients with FTD. Based on the small number of studies available, we reviewed the five published treatment trials employing at least a randomization arm.

Results

Serotonergic Medications

Paroxetine

Two randomized controlled trials evaluated the effect of paroxetine on neuropsychiatric symptoms in patients with FTD. One double-blind, placebo-controlled crossover design study ($n = 10$ total) found no effects of paroxetine (2 weeks titration followed by 40 mg for 4 weeks) on neuropsychiatric deficits as measured by caregiver interviews using the NPI or the Cambridge behavioral inventory [102]. A second randomized controlled trial comparing patients with FTD ($n = 8$ per group) receiving paroxetine (10 mg/day for 2 weeks, then 20 mg/day for 14 months) or piracetam (1,200 mg/day) found improvements in behavioral measures, including the BEHAVE-AD (baseline score -2.5 ± 0.2 compared to piracetam group $+13.08 \pm 2.12$) and the NPI (drop -8.25 ± 1.6 in paroxetine vs. $+5 \pm 1.0$ in piracetam group) [103]. Using these figures, we calculate an estimated effect size of $d = 0.6$ of paroxetine vs. piracetam for NPI, and $d = 0.8$ for the BEHAVE-AD (though note the piracetam group showed a significant worsening in this rating over time). Several open-label studies of SSRIs, including paroxetine, fluvoxamine, and sertraline, have reported improvement in behaviors of patients with FTD [104–106].

Trazadone

One randomized double-blind placebo-controlled crossover design trial has examined the efficacy of trazadone on neuropsychiatric symptoms in $n = 26$ patients with FTD [107]. Patients receiving trazadone 150 mg in the first 6 weeks demonstrated a significant improvement in NPI scores ($p < 0.03$) compared to the placebo group (mean drop in NPI score 26 points vs. 8 points). Improvements were strongest for subitems of irritability, agitation, depression, and eating disorders. Insufficient data was reported to calculate effect sizes. Side effects occurred in 11 patients during the trazadone phase, though were generally reported as mild and included fatigue, dizziness, hypotension, and cold extremities. Three patients in the placebo phase reported fatigue and dizziness.

Cholinesterase Inhibitors

Compared to control groups, there has been no evidence of improvement in language score ratings in patients with FTD treated with either galantamine [108] nor in cognitive scores in patients treated with donepezil [109]. The study of galantamine did not find medication effects on FBI and CGIS ratings of neuropsychiatric symptoms and behaviors.

Methylphenidate

A randomized, double-blind, placebo-controlled crossover study examined cognitive effects of a single dose of 40 mg of methylphenidate in patient with FTD [110]. Cognitive effects were examined using the CANTAB cognitive battery, Tower of London test, and the Cambridge gambling task. Significant medication effects were reported only for the Cambridge gambling task, indicating that methylphenidate reduced risk-taking bets in patients with FTD. Though an interesting result with potential relevance for the treatment of FTD, limitations include limited treatment duration, lack of ecological behavioral indices, and noncorrection for multiple comparisons.

Clinical Bottom Lines

There are few published studies of treatment trials in patients with FTD, and fewer double-blind, randomized, placebo-controlled trials.
Of published trials, sample sizes remain small, and thus conclusions are preliminary and require further study and replication.
While SSRIs are one of the most commonly prescribed medications for FTD and have been associated with reduced aggression and improved behaviors in open-label studies, controlled randomized trials using SSRIs have show mixed results. Thus, further study of the efficacy of SSRIs in FTD is warranted.
Results from one randomized, controlled trial suggest trazadone may be helpful in reducing common neuropsychiatric symptoms in FTD, including irritability and agitation.
Current studies suggest CHEIs are not beneficial in FTD.
To date, there have been no published randomized, placebo-controlled trials of memantine or atypical neuroleptic medications in patients with FTD.

Prognosis

Clinical Questions

What is the average survival for patients with FTD from time of first symptoms? From time of diagnosis?
Are there differences in prognosis between FTD subtypes?

Search Strategy

Ovid MEDLINE database was searched from 1950 to November 28, 2008. MeSH terms "frontotemporal dementia or frontotemporal lobar degeneration or Pick's disease" and "mortality" were searched and combined using the Boolean "AND" limiting results to English and human. Two articles that were not relevant to the topic were found. A second search with the terms "survival or progression" yielded 122 articles. From these, six relevant articles identified. One additional article was found by searching citations from these six articles. No additional articles were found in Cochrane reviews, with searches for mortality, survival or progression. Based on sample size, autopsy confirmation, separation of FTD subtypes, and the statistical approach, two of the six studies were selected for detailed review.

Results

Average Survival

Based on two retrospective, longitudinal studies together evaluating survival in 248 patients with FTD, mean survival estimates based on retrospective assessment of first symptom onset ranges from 6 to 8.7 years, while mean survival from time of diagnosis is 3 years [111].

Prognosis Across FTD Subtypes

These studies indicate that the subset of patients with FTD plus motor neuron disease have a significantly shorter survival than other subtypes (see Table 8.8) [111, 112]. There is growing evidence that patients with underlying tau positive pathology have a longer survival than patients with tau negative pathology, even when FTD-MND cases are excluded from the tau negative group (see Table 8.8). Results are inconclusive as to whether patients with semantic dementia or progressive nonfluent aphasia subtypes have a longer survival time than patients with bv-FTD.

Clinical Bottom Lines

Patients with FTD have a mean survival of approximately 7 years from time of first symptom onset.

Patients with FTD (behavioral variant, SD, or PNFA) who have underlying tau positive inclusions may survive on average 4 years longer than patients with tau negative pathology.

Table 8.8.

Table 8.8 Mean survival from symptom onset and time of diagnosis in FTD and subtypes

	Mean survival from symptom onset (SD)		Mean survival from diagnosis (SD)	
	Hodges et al. [111]	Roberson et al. [112]	Hodges et al. [111]	Roberson et al. [112]
Whole group	6.0	8.7	3.0	3.0
fvFTD	8.2 (0.8)	8.7 (1.2)	4.7 (0.6)	3 (0.5)
Semantic dementia	6.9 (1.2)	11.9 (0.2)	4.0 (1.1)	5.3 (0.4)
Progressive nonfluent aphasia	10.6 (1.8)	9.4 (2.4)	5.5 (1.1)	4.2 (1.1)
FTD-MND	2.4 (0.4)[a]	4.9 (1.6)[b]	1.3 (0.3)[a]	1.4 (0.2)[b]
Tau+	9 (95% CI: 8.1–9.9)		10.2 (5.0)	
Tau−	5.0 (95% CI: 3.9–6.1)		5.6 (0.3)	

[a]Based on autopsy
[b]Based on neurologic symptoms

Dementia with Lewy Bodies

Introduction

Dementia with Lewy Bodies (DLB) is a neurodegenerative disorder classically featuring progressive cognitive impairment, parkinsonism, visual hallucinations, and fluctuations in attention and confusion. On neuropathologic examination, cytoplasmic inclusions of alpha-synuclein aggregates termed Lewy bodies are found in the brainstem and often in limbic and neocortical regions. Lewy bodies can also be found in 22–75% of patients with neuropathologic changes associated with Alzheimer's disease [113–115]. Thus, current consensus criteria suggest that DLB is the cause of dementia when Lewy bodies are present in regions beyond the brainstem and absent, low, or intermediate levels of Alzheimer's pathologic changes are found [116].

Epidemiology

Clinical Case

A 70-year-old woman presents with 2 years of gradually progressive difficulties with short-term memory and with tasks, such as managing her financial accounts and cooking. Her family is struck by the fluctuations they have observed; on some days, she seems quite well, and on other days she is quite confused. They are worried that recently she has begun to "see" children in her home when no one else is there. On exam she has features of mild parkinsonism, and a diagnosis of DLB disease is made.

Clinical Questions

What is the prevalence of DLB?
What are the risk factors associated with DLB?

Search Strategy

Ovid MEDLINE database was searched from 1950 to December 21, 2008. MeSH terms "incidence or prevalence" and "DLB or Lewy body disease or diffuse Lewy bodies" were searched and combined using the Boolean "AND." After limiting the retrieval to English and human, a final set of 93 citations were obtained. From this set, two population-based prevalence studies with an emphasis on DLB and four articles related to genetic risk factors were selected for review. EMBASE, PubMed, and the Cochrane Library databases were also searched implementing the same strategy of MeSH terms and keywords. No additional relevant articles were detected.

Results

Prevalence

There are few prevalence studies of DLB and none with prevalence rates stratified according to age. Based on available data, using the 1996 consensus criteria [117], the prevalence of DLB in adults aged 65 years and older ranges between 0.4 and 11% [118–120].

Risk Factors

Few studies assessing risk factors for DLB are available to date. While a few families have been identified with mutations in the alpha-synuclein gene [121], this is not found in most patients with DLB [122]. Two recent reports have highlighted a possible association with a mutation in a gene for glucocerebrocidase with a frequency of 3.5–23% in patients with DLB compared to 0.4% of controls [123, 124].

A familial pattern and association with mutations in alpha-synuclein has been described in a small number of families world-wide; however, most patients with DLB are not associated with this mutation.

Clinical Bottom Lines

There are few studies of the incidence and prevalence of Lewy body disease in population-based samples and none available using the current consensus criteria.

Prior estimates of the prevalence of DLB based on the 1995 consensus criteria range from 0.4 to 11%, and likely underestimate the true prevalence of the disorder due to low sensitivity of the older criteria.

Diagnosis

Clinical Questions

What are the diagnostic criteria and supportive tests required for a diagnosis of probable DLB?
How can DLB be distinguished from other neurodegenerative disorders?

Search Strategy

The terms "Lewy body disease or DLB" and "diagnosis" were combined with the Boolean "AND" and searched in Medline, yielding 452 articles. Additional searches in Medline and Pubmed were conducted combining the terms "Lewy body" and "biomarkers" and "Lewy body" and "gene." Additional references cited in the revised clinical criteria for DLB [116] were reviewed. From these searches, 48 articles were selected for detailed review based on relevance, sample size, and availability of autopsy-confirmed diagnosis.

Results

Clinical Criteria

The clinical criteria for DLB were revised in 2006 (see Table 8.9). In addition to the core features, a diagnosis of DLB is made if dementia precedes or is concurrent with the development of parkinsonism. Use of the revised clinical criteria has been reported to increase the number of patients with diagnosis of probable DLB by 25% compared to prior criteria [125]. One cited difficulty with the old core criteria was accurate clinical assessment of fluctuations in cognition and attention. To address this issue, a study of 70 patients evaluated discrimination between DLB and AD with the Mayo fluctuations scale [126]. Endorsement by caregivers of three out of four items from the scale (see Table 8.10) was found in 63% of DLB vs. 12% of AD patients, with PPV of 80% for DLB vs. AD and NPV of 70%.

Neuropsychology

The central neurocognitive features of DLB include deficits in attention, executive function, visuospatial abilities, and memory. Multiple studies have shown that when

Table 8.9 Revised criteria for clinical diagnosis of dementia with Lewy bodies [116]

1. *Central feature* (essential for a diagnosis of possible or probable DLB)
   Dementia defined as progressive cognitive decline of sufficient magnitude to interfere with normal social or occupational function.
   Prominent or persistent memory impairment may not necessarily occur in the early stages but is usually evident with progression.
   Deficits on tests of attention, executive function, and visuospatial ability may be especially prominent.

2. *Core* features (two core features are sufficient for a diagnosis of probable DLB, one for possible DLB)
   Fluctuating cognition with pronounced variations in attention and alertness
   Recurrent visual hallucinations that are typically well formed and detailed
   Spontaneous features of parkinsonism

3. *Suggestive features* (If one or more of these is present in the presence of one or more core features, a diagnosis of probable DLB can be made. In the absence of any core features, one or more suggestive features are sufficient for possible DLB. Probable DLB should not be diagnosed on the basis of suggestive features alone.)
   REM sleep behavior disorder
   Severe neuroleptic sensitivity
   Low dopamine transporter uptake in basal ganglia demonstrated by SPECT or PET imaging

4. *Supportive features* (commonly present but not proven to have diagnostic specificity)
   Repeated falls and syncope
   Transient, unexplained loss of consciousness
   Severe autonomic dysfunction, e.g., orthostatic hypotension, urinary incontinence
   Hallucinations in other modalities
   Systematized delusions
   Depression
   Relative preservation of medial temporal lobe structures on CT/MRI scan
   Generalized low uptake on SPECT/PET perfusion scan with reduced occipital activity
   Abnormal (low uptake) MIBG myocardial scintigraphy
   Prominent slow wave activity on EEG with temporal lobe transient sharp waves

Table 8.10 Discriminant Items from Mayo Fluctuations scale [126]

1. Are there times when the patient's flow of ideas seem disorganized, unclear, or not logical?
2. How often is the patient drowsy and lethargic during the day, despite getting enough sleep the night before?
   (a) All the time or several times a day   (b) Once a day or less
3. How much time does the patient spend sleeping during the day (before 7:00 p.m.)? (a) 2 h or more   (b) Less than 2 h
4. Does the patient stare into space for long periods of time?

compared to patients with Alzheimer's disease, patients with DLB show relatively worse performance on tasks of visuospatial perception and construction and attention, and relatively better performance on tasks of memory and naming [127–130].

Table 8.11 Sensitivity and specificity of diagnostic tests in Lewy body dementia

Modality	Diagnostic tool	Sensitivity (%)	Specificity (%)	References
Clinical criteria	McKeith 1996 criteria	18–83	71–95	[131, 132]
Neuropsychology	Mayo Fluctuations Scale (for DLB vs. AD)	PPV 80	NPV 70	[15]
	Trails A, Boston Naming Test, AVLT % Retention, and Rey-Osterrieth Complex Figure Copy to distinguish DLB from AD	83	91	[133]
NeuroImaging	DAT-SPECT	78	90	[134]
	FP-CIT/SPECT	100	83	[135]
	FDG-PET for DLB vs. AD	90	80	[136]
	Cardiac MIBG (discriminate DLB from AD)	99–100	87–100	[137–139]
CSF biomarkers	Reduced a-beta and/or elevated tau to discriminate AD from FTD	79–90	64–97	[94, 95]

Imaging

DAT-SPECT

Several neuroimaging modalities are included as supporting evidence in the 2006 consensus criteria for DLB (see Table 8.11).

SPECT

Occipital hypoperfusion on SPECT blood flow imaging is observed in DLB compared to patients with AD or normal controls [140]. However, a recent study of patients with DLB diagnosed by I-FP-CIT/ SPECT imaging reported occipital hypoperfusion only in 28% of DLB vs. 31% of patients with a non-DLB dementia [141].

PET

FDG-PET has been used to show patterns of reduced occipital metabolism in patients with DLB compared with patients with AD [142–144].

Cardiac MIBG

A pattern of reduced heart-to-mediastinum (H/M) uptake ratio of MIBG scintigraphy which examines postganglionic cardiac sympathetic innervation has been associated with DLB and Parkinson's disease [137, 145]. Recent studies suggest excellent discrimination between DLB and AD. A recent small study also suggests a reduced H/M MIBG ratio may help to distinguish DLB from FTD [146].

MRI

Volumetric assessment of occipital lobes has not been shown to discriminate between DLB and AD [147]. Other single studies have suggested that decreased putamen/whole brain volume ratios [148], or midbrain, hypothalamus and SI, atrophy in DLB plus sparing of temporal/parietal cortex may distinguish DLB from AD [149], but further validation studies are required.

EEG

The revised consensus criteria list prominent slow wave activity on EEG with transient temporal sharp waves as supportive features of DLB [116]. While this has been reported in some studies [150–152], other studies of visual inspection of EEG in clinical or autopsy confirmed DLB have failed to find significant EEG differences between patients with DLB and AD [153, 154]. Various quantitative EEG measure have been recently associated with DLB in comparison to AD [155–157], but further validation is required.

Biomarkers

The revised consensus criteria for DLB do not include CSF biomarkers as a supportive feature [116]. Patients with DLB tend to show lower CSF tau levels than patients with AD [158]; however, beta-amyloid 42 and tau levels are often overlapping in patients with DLB and AD [38, 159], and thus use of these markers at present is inferior to other diagnostic tests [160]. Recent studies of CSF-alpha-synuclein [161] and other a-beta peptide ratios have shown promise [162] but to date there has been a lack of sufficient evidence to support an additive diagnostic benefit [163].

Genetics

While DLB has been considered a sporadic disease, a small number of familial cases have been identified [164, 165]. Study of these familial cases has associated triplication of the alpha-synuclein gene with DLB and PD [121]. However, this appears to be a rare mutation in a general sample of patients with DLB [166]. Current consensus guidelines do not recommend genetic testing in suspected DLB.

Clinical Bottom Lines

Clinical Criteria

Prior clinical consensus criteria for DLB showed low sensitivity. Validation with autopsy confirmed studies is required to determine the sensitivity and specificity of the revised criteria and supporting features.

Neuropsychology

Overall, patients with DLB perform worse on visual perception, construction, and attention tasks while patients with AD perform worse on memory and naming tasks.

NeuroImaging

FP-SPECT appears to show good discrimination between patients with DLB and AD or controls, but not with patients with PD or PD + D. PET shows promise but further studies are required to determine whether it provides an additive diagnostic benefit.

Cardiac MIBG heart-to-mediastinal uptake ratios appear to be sensitive and specific for distinguishing DLB from AD.

Biomarkers

At present, there is insufficient evidence of additive diagnostic benefit to recommend CSF biomarker evaluation in patients with suspected DLB.

Genetics

At present, no genetic testing is recommended for patients with suspected DLB. Tables 8.9–8.11.

Treatment

Clinical Questions

What treatments are effective for management of hallucinations in DLB?
What treatments are effective for management of parkinsonism in DLB?
Are any treatments effective in improving cognitive deficits in DLB?

Search Strategy

A search in Medline of terms "diffuse Lewy body" or "Lewy body disease" and "treatment" combined with the Boolean "AND" yielded 272 results. An additional search of these terms in the Cochrane database resulted in two articles. From these, 15 articles were selected for detailed review.

Results

Management of Hallucinations: Neuroleptic Medications

Quetiapine

Open label studies of quetiapine in DLB suggested efficacy in reducing hallucinations and aggression [167]. A double-blind, randomized, placebo-controlled parallel group trial of quetiapine (mean 120 mg/day) for 10 weeks, including patients with DLB plus psychosis or agitation ($n=23$) measured efficacy via the brief psychiatric rating scale and unified PD rating scale and found no significant differences between placebo and quetiapine groups [168].

Olanzapine

A post-hoc analysis of a prospective, blinded, randomized placebo-controlled trial of olanzapine (5 mg, 10 mg or 15 mg) in patients with dementia assessed effects in a subset of participants meeting criteria for DLB ($n=29$) and found improvements in delusions, hallucinations or NPI-NH scores at 5 or 10 mg, but no differences compared to the placebo group at 15 mg [169]. No significant differences were found on the MMSE or on evaluation of parkinsonian symptoms between olanzapine and placebo groups. In an open label study of olanzapine (mean dose 4.21–7.32 mg/day) with $n=4$ patients with DLB, significant improvements in hallucinations and aggression were reported, as well as improvements in NPI, BEHAVE, and RSS scores [170]. Approximately 30% of patients with DLB experienced somnolence or postural instability and 17% developed postural hypotension.

Risperidone

No published, controlled trials of risperidone in DLB were found. While some early cases series were favorable [171], others included reported of severe extrapyramidal side effects in patients with DLB treated with this medication, which have been attributed to the D2 antagonistic properties of risperidone [172].

Clozapine

Several randomized, controlled trials and a meta-analysis have found clozapine to be effective in the treatment of hallucinations and psychosis in Parkinson's disease [173]. In patients with DLB, case reports of the effectiveness and tolerability of clozapine have been mixed [174, 175]. There are no randomized, controlled trials of clozapine in DLB to date.

Management of Parkinsonism

Two open label studies measuring acute response to levadopa reported positive motor responses (at least 20% improvement in UPDRS ratings) in 13.8–50% of patients with DLB and some measure of improvement in 36–75% of patients after 6 months treatment studies [176, 177]. Approximately 10% of patients developed acute worsening of hallucinations or confusion following initiation of levadopa therapy which resolved upon discontinuation [177].

Treatment of Cognitive Deficits

Cholinesterase Inhibitors

A Cochrane review from 2003 of the use of CHEIs found only one randomized, blind, placebo-controlled trial of rivastigmine in DLB ($n = 120$, mean dose 9.4 mg/day for 20 weeks) [178]. Based on the McKeith et al. [178] study, the review found no significant effects on the NPI, MMSE, or the clinicians global change scale in the intention to treat analysis. In the observed cases only analysis, a 6 point improvement was found on the NPI at 20 weeks in the treated group compared to placebo. Significantly higher rates of nausea (37%), vomiting (25%), anorexia (19%), and somnolence (9%) were reported for the rivastigmine group. Follow up analysis of this study reported significant improvements in cognition using the COGDRAS but not in other cognitive measures [179]. A meta-analysis of CHEIs in DLB [180] which also included case reports and open label studies of donepezil and rivastigmine found preliminary evidence supporting modest efficacy of both drugs on cognitive and behavioral measures. Subsequent open label studies of galantamine and donepezil in patients with DLB have reported improvements in the NPI but lesser or nonsignificant effects on cognitive measures [181, 182]. Reported rates of adverse effects, including nausea, anorexia, and vomiting, were consistent with prior studies. A review of the cardiovascular safety of rivastigmine in DLB based on the McKeith et al. [178] study found a mean 1.5–2 bpm slowing of heart rate, with no clinically significant ECG changes or bradycardia, and no increase in adverse vascular events or syncope [183].

Clinical Bottom Lines

The atypical neuroleptic medications olanzapine and quetiapine may decrease delusions and hallucinations in DLB. Due to frequent side effects, including extrapyramidal symptoms and sedation, these medications should be used at the lowest effective dose and discontinued as soon as possible. Controlled trials of clozapine are needed in patients with DLB to determine its efficacy and tolerability in the management of psychosis and hallucinations.

Cholinesterase Inhibitors

Available evidence suggests donepezil, galantamine, and rivastigmine are associated with a modest improvement in some cognitive and behavioral outcome measures in DLB. Long-term efficacy of these medications in DLB is not known.

Open label studies of levodopa for parkinsonism in DLB suggest a subset of patients respond favorably, though levodopa may increase confusion or hallucinations.

Prognosis

Clinical Questions

What is the expected survival for patients diagnosed with DLB from symptom onset?

Search Strategy

In Medline, the terms "Lewy body" and "prognosis or survival or mortality" were searched resulting in 99 references. The same terms were searched in EMBASE, producing 192 articles. Of these, seven articles were judged to be original research articles relevant to the topic. One study was selected for detailed review which included a prospective clinical cohort with autopsy confirmed diagnosis.

Results

Based on a longitudinal prospective study with autopsy confirmation, including $n = 63$ confirmed cases of DLB with a mean age of onset at 70 years, the median survival from time of symptom onset was 7.28 years (95% CI 5.7–8.8) [184]. Median time to nursing home placement was 6.1 years (95% CI 4.1–7.8). These figures suggest a slightly more rapid decline compared to patients with Alzheimer's disease in the same study, who had a mean age 75 years at disease onset and median survival of 8.5 years (95% CI 7.8–9.1). These findings were consistent with autopsy-based series suggesting shorter survival times in patients with DLB relative to AD [185, 186].

Clinical Bottom Line

Based on one prospective cohort of patients with definite DLB, an estimated time from symptom onset to nursing home placement is 6 years and survival time is approximately 7.3 years.

Vascular Dementia

Introduction

Vascular dementia is diagnosed when dementia arises from cerebrovascular disease. Included in this category are patients with poststroke dementia, multiple lacunar or subcortical infarctions, CADASIL, cerebral amyloid angiopathy and hemorrhages, and severe white matter changes that are thought to be ischemic in etiology. Vascular cognitive impairment is used to denote patients with cognitive deficits arising from these forms of cerebrovascular disease, who do not meet the criteria for dementia. Vascular dementia can occur alone or in combination with Alzheimer's disease, and is often quoted as the second most common cause of dementia.

Epidemiology

Clinical Case

An 82-year-old man with a history of hypertension and diabetes presents with 5 years of increasing confusion and memory problems. His family reports that the decline began 5 years ago when he presented with right side visual deficits and was diagnosed with a stroke. Since then, he has had four additional spells, including transient visual loss, transient aphasia with mild residual word finding deficits, and transient left body numbness. His MRI demonstrates a chronic left occipital cortex infarction with significant white matter changes and microhemorrhages (Fig. 8.1). Based on his evaluation, he is diagnosed with vascular dementia.

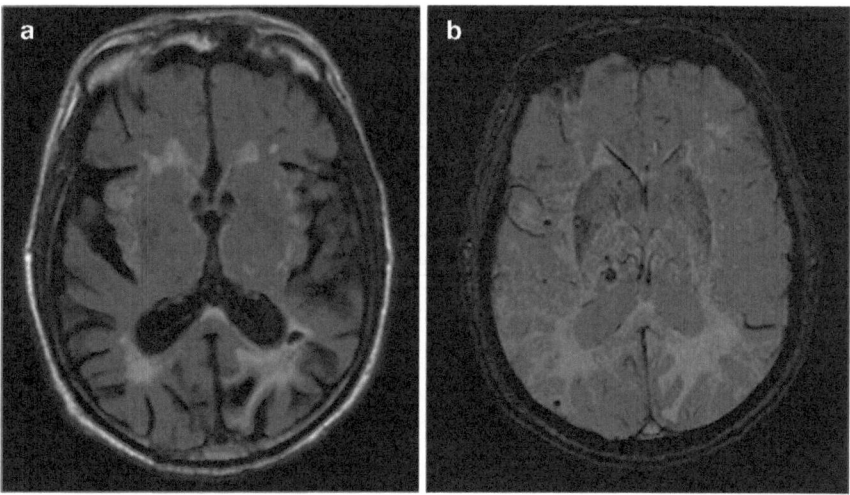

Fig. 8.1 Axial FLAIR image (**a**) demonstrating large vessel ischemic stroke, lacunar infarctions and white matter disease and (**b**) susceptibility weighted image demonstrating multiple microhemorrhages in a 72-year-old man with a clinical diagnosis of vascular dementia

Clinical Questions

What is the incidence of vascular dementia?
What is the prevalence of vascular dementia?
What are proven risk factors for the development of vascular dementia?

Search Strategy

Ovid MEDLINE database was searched from 1950 to December 10, 2008. MeSH terms "incidence or prevalence" and "vascular dementia or vascular cognitive impairment" were searched and combined using the Boolean "AND." After limiting the retrieval to English and human, a final set of 241 citations were obtained. A second search combining the terms "vascular dementia or vascular cognitive impairment" and "risk factors" limited to human and English produced 409 citations. From this set, three population-based studies were selected for detailed review based on sample size and report of age-stratified rates. An additional six population-based studies of risk factors were reviewed. PubMed and the Cochrane Library databases were also searched implementing the same strategy of MeSH terms and keywords. No additional relevant articles were detected.

Table 8.12 Incidence rates of vascular dementia by age per 1,000 (rate among survivors-estimated rate including deaths)

| Age, y | Canadian Health and Aging Study[a] | | Pitea River Study[b] |
	Women	Men	All
65–69	0.67–1.36	1.18–2.23	0.94
70–74	0.72–1.14	3.07–4.61	1.75
75–79	3.84–7.04	3.52–6.63	3.71
80–84	5.25–7.25	5.26–7.01	5.26
>85	6.78–9.28	6.64–8.28	6.74

[a]Herbert et al. [187]
[b]Andreason et al. [188]

Results

Incidence

Based on the findings from the Canadian Health and Aging Study and the Pitea River Valley Study in Sweden, aging is associated with an increasing incidence of vascular dementia (see Table 8.12) [187, 188]. Despite use of two different clinical criteria for diagnosis (ICD-10 and NINDS-AIREN) and different forms of case ascertainment, these two large population-based studies report highly concordant estimates of incidence rates.

Prevalence

Prevalence rates of vascular dementia as estimated by a pooled examination of 11 studies from across Europe using DSM-III-R, NINCDS-AIREN, CAMDEX, ICD-10, or Hachinski Ischemia Scores as criteria for a clinical diagnosis of vascular dementia report an increasing prevalence with aging, peaking at approximately 4–5% in elderly 90 years of age and older [7]. In an autopsy series of patients with dementia, 30–41% were found to have pure AD at autopsy, 16–38% had AD with cerebral infarcts, 5% showed mixed AD and VaD pathologic changes, while 10–12% had "pure" VaD [189, 190].

Associated Risk Factors

Age has been repeatedly identified as a risk factor for the development of vascular dementia [187]. The presence of 1 or 2 APOE ε4 alleles was also associated with an increased risk, OR 2.34 (1.29–4.15) [187]. Heart disease and associated vascular risk factors of hypertension and diabetes have been repeatedly associated with a higher risk of developing vascular cognitive impairment and vascular dementia,

Age	Women (%)	Men (%)
65–69	0.1	0.5
70–74	0.6	0.8
75–79	0.9	1.9
80–84	2.3	2.4
85–89	3.5	2.4
90+	5.8	3.6

Table 8.13 Prevalence rates of vascular dementia by age from Lobo et al. [7]

with OR ranging from 1.62 to 3.3 for diabetes [187, 191–193] and 1.02 to 11.8 for hypertension [187, 194–196].

Clinical Bottom Lines

Aging is associated increasing incidence and prevalence of vascular dementia.
Cerebral infarctions are commonly seen in patients with Alzheimer's disease while "pure" vascular dementia is less common.
Cardiovascular risk factors of hypertension and diabetes are associated with an increased risk of developing vascular cognitive impairment and vascular dementia.
The presence of the APOE ε4 allele is associated with increased risk of developing vascular dementia.

Tables 8.12 and 8.13.

Diagnosis

Clinical Questions

How sensitive and specific are clinical criteria for the diagnosis of vascular dementia?
What tests are useful to diagnose vascular dementia and distinguish it from Alzheimer's disease?

Search Strategy

Medline was searched from 2000 to February 27, 2009 using the terms "vascular dementia" and "diagnosis." Limiting results to human studies in English, 425 articles were retrieved. From these, 12 articles were selected for detailed review with preference given to studies with autopsy confirmation of diagnosis and evidence of an additive diagnostic benefit to standard clinical evaluation.

Table 8.14 NINDS-AIREN Clinical Criteria for Vascular Dementia (Roman et al. [197])

I. Criteria for clinical diagnosis of probable vascular dementia include all of the following:
  • Dementia is defined by cognitive decline from a previously higher level of functioning and manifested by impairment of memory and two or more cognitive domains
  • Evidence of cerebrovascular disease by focal signs on neurological examination consistent with stroke
  • Evidence of relevant cerebrovascular disease by brain imaging, including multiple large vessel infarcts or a single strategically placed infarct as well as multiple basal ganglia and white matter lacunae or extensive periventricular white matter lesions or combinations thereof
II. Clinical features consistent with the diagnosis of probable vascular dementia include the following:
  • Early presence of gait disturbance
  • History of unsteadiness and frequent, unprovoked falls
  • Early urinary frequency, urgency, and other urinary symptoms not explained by urologic disease
  • Pseudobulbar palsy
  • Personality and mood changes, abulia, depression, emotional incontinence, or other subcortical deficits, including psychomotor retardation and abnormal executive function.

Results

Clinical Criteria

Several criteria for the diagnosis of vascular dementia have been developed and used over the past several years, including DSM-IV, Hachinski Ischemic Score, ICD-10, ADDTC, and the NINDS-AIREN criteria (see Table 8.14). An autopsy validated comparison of the sensitivity and specificity of several of the major clinical criteria for vascular dementia found sensitivities ranging from 0.2 to 0.7 for possible and probable vascular dementia with specificities ranging from 0.78 to 0.94 [198]. A significant range was also found in the ability of the criteria to distinguish mixed etiologies with 9–40% of mixed vascular dementia and AD cases diagnosed as pure vascular dementia. Reports of a stepwise decline vs. a more gradually progressive course are not necessarily discriminative as vascular dementia without significant AD pathology may show a pattern of gradual progression of deficits [199].

Diagnostic Tests

Neuropsychology

In patients with a history of stroke or TIA, clinical diagnosis of vascular dementia has been associated with a profile of impairment in abstraction, mental flexibility, information processing speed and working memory relative to controls [200]. A similar pattern has been reported in patients with subcortical vascular dementia who showed more impairment on semantic memory, executive/attention functioning, and visuospatial and perceptual skills, while patients with AD show greater impairments in episodic memory [201]. Significant associations have been found between increasing white matter hyperintensities over time and cognitive impairment [202] and between impairment on executive function tests and degree of cerebrovascular white matter changes on CT [203]. A recent study of neuropsychological profiles in patients with autopsy confirmed diagnosis of vascular dementia or AD found that those with AD generally demonstrated more severe deficits in episodic memory compared to executive functioning, while patients with vascular dementia showed a mild predominance of executive function deficits compared to verbal memory performance [199].

NeuroImaging

CT or MRI brain imaging is a part of the routine assessment of patients with suspected vascular dementia to confirm the location of strokes or the presence silent infarcts, leukoaraiosis (white matter hyperintensities on FLAIR), or microhemorrhages. Lack of sufficient radiologic evidence of cerebrovascular disease has been cited as the most important factor in distinguishing vascular dementia from AD [197]. The NINDS-AIREN criteria for vascular dementia include radiographic findings associated with vascular dementia (see Table 8.14) but emphasize that no radiologic findings are pathognomomic for the disorder, and thus diagnosis requires an appropriate history of dementia in association with cerebrovascular disease. In addition to other diseases causing white matter hyperintensities, moderate to severe white matter hyperintensities may be found in 9–22% of noncognitively impaired elderly [204].

PET: A pattern of reduced temporo-parietal metabolism in the presence of leukoaraiosis has been suggested to correlate with AD while a pattern of preserved temporal–parietal metabolism in this setting may suggest vascular dementia [205]. While subsequent studies suggest PET may discriminate between clinically diagnosed vascular dementia and AD [206, 207], no evidence is available to support an additive diagnostic benefit of this test at present.

Biomarkers

CSF amyloid and tau ratios may discriminate between clinical AD and vascular dementia [208–210], but an additive diagnostic value has not yet been demonstrated. Tables 8.14 and 8.15.

Clinical Bottom Lines

Clinical Criteria

Currently used clinical criteria overall show low sensitivity and high specificity for the diagnosis of vascular dementia.

Table 8.15 Brain imaging lesions associated with vascular dementia in NINDS-AIREN criteria (Roman et al. [197])

I. Topography
   Radiologic lesions associated with dementia include ANY of the following or combinations thereof:
   1. Large-vessel strokes in the following territories:
      - Bilateral anterior cerebral artery
      - Posterior cerebral artery, including paramedian thalamic infarctions, inferior medial temporal lobe lesions
      - Association areas: parietotemporal, temporo-occipital territories
      - Watershed carotid territories
   2. Small-vessel disease:
      - Basal ganglia and frontal white matter lacunes
      - Extensive periventricular white matter lesions
      - Bilateral thalamic lesions
II. Severity
   In addition to the above, relevant radiologic lesions associated with dementia include:
   - Large vessel lesions of the dominant hemisphere
   - Bilateral large-vessel hemispheric strokes
   - Leukoencephalopathy involving at least one-fourth of the total white matter

Neuropsychology

A profile of slow processing speed with impaired executive and attentional performance supports a diagnosis of pure vascular dementia while greater impairment in episodic memory suggests concomitant Alzheimer's disease.

Neuroimaging

Brain imaging with MRI or CT is essential for the diagnosis of vascular dementia to confirm the presence of significant cerebrovascular disease.

Further studies with autopsy confirmation are required to determine whether PET adds to clinical diagnostic discrimination between VaD, AD, and mixed VaD/AD.

Treatment

Clinical Questions

What treatments are effective in improving cognitive and function in patients with vascular dementia?

Are any treatments effective and preventing or slowing the progression of vascular dementia?

Search Strategy

The terms "vascular dementia" and "treatment" were entered into the Cochrane database and combined with the Boolean "AND" to search for articles from 1950 to March 4, 2009. After limiting results to human studies and English, 42 articles were retrieved. Entering the same search terms into Medline resulted in 515 articles. From these, 11 articles were selected for detailed review with preference given to meta-analysis and randomized, blind, placebo-controlled trials in patients with vascular dementia.

Results

Cognitive Enhancers

Cholinesterase Inhibitors

A recent meta-analysis examined the efficacy and adverse effects of donepezil, galantamine, and rivastigmine in patients with vascular dementia (including large and small vessel subtypes) [211]. The pooled analysis demonstrated modest cognitive benefit in patients treated with CHEI, with a mean improvement on the ADAS-Cog of ~2 points/100 points; however, significant improvements in global functioning or activities of daily living were not found. Increased rates of adverse side effects, including nausea, emesis, diarrhea, and anorexia, were more common in the CHEI group ranging from 6.4 to 16.6% vs. 3.6 to 10.2% in placebo groups. Since the meta-analysis, an additional randomized, placebo-controlled trial of donepezil (10 mg) for 18 weeks in patients <70 years of age with genetic or biopsy confirmed diagnosis of CADASIL was reported [212]. The study found no significant differences between donepezil and placebo groups on the primary outcome measure, the vascular ADAS-Cog, nor on the ADAS-Cog or MMSE, though improvements were found for secondary outcome tests of executive functioning (Trails test and EXIT-25).

Memantine

The Kavirajan and Schneider meta-analysis also assessed efficacy and adverse effects of memantine in patients with vascular dementia, including controlled trials of patients with large or small vessel disease [211]. Based on two randomized, blind, placebo-controlled trials of 20 mg of memantine for 28 weeks, the meta-analysis demonstrated a mean improvement on the ADAS-Cog of −1.86 points (95% CI −2.79 to −0.94). Significant effects on global measures and functioning were not found. Rates of adverse effects were not significantly different between memantine and placebo groups.

Secondary Stroke Prevention

Antihypertensive Medications

Data from population studies suggest treatment with antihypertensive medications reduces the risk of vascular dementia [213]. A Cochrane systematic review from 2006 included three randomized, placebo-controlled trials (Syst-Eur, SCOPE, SHEP, $n=12,091$ patients, mean age 72.8 years) of antihypertensive treatment which measured cognitive outcomes and incidence of dementia at 5 years [214]. In the pooled analysis, no significant difference was found in incidence of dementia for treated vs. placebo groups (OR 0.89, 95% CI 0.69–1.16), nor in cognitive measures (MMSE). Interpretation of these results has been limited by the observations that high numbers (up to 84%) of patients in the placebo group were also treated with antihypertensive medications during the course of the trial, and differential dropout rates in placebo and treatment groups may have confounded results [214].

Statins

Treatment with statins has been associated with reduced rates of ischemic stroke and a slightly higher occurrence of hemorrhage stroke in patients with a history of stroke or TIA [215]. Population cohort studies have not found a reduced risk of vascular dementia in patients taking statins [216]. A controlled, randomized trial of pravastatin in elderly individuals with risk factors for vascular disease did not find any effect on cognitive function or white matter lesions [217, 218]. Further controlled trials in younger patients and longitudinal follow up are required to determine whether statins reduce the incidence or severity of vascular dementia.

Aspirin

In population studies, aspirin use has not been associated with reduced risk of vascular dementia [219]. A Cochrane review from 2000 found one controlled study of aspirin and cognitive measures in patients with vascular dementia which suggested a modest benefit of treatment [220, 221], but further studies are required.

Clinical Bottom Lines

While CHEIs are associated with modest improvement in cognitive outcome measures, the side effects of these agents may outweigh potential benefits in patients with pure vascular dementia.

There is not significant evidence supporting use of memantine in patients with vascular dementia.

Antihypertensive, statin, and antiplatelet treatments have been associated with reduced risk of recurrent strokes. However, direct evidence for effects on incidence or progression of vascular dementia is lacking.

Prognosis

Clinical Question

What is the prognosis for patients diagnosed with vascular dementia?

Search Strategy

The terms "vascular dementia" and "survival or prognosis" were combined with the Boolean "AND" and entered in Medline searching from 1950 to March 6, 2009, resulting in 115 citations. From these, four relevant articles were selected for detailed review.

Results

In the prospective, longitudinal cardiovascular health cognition study, estimated median survival from dementia onset to death was 3.9 years for those with vascular dementia (mean age 78 years at onset), compared to 7.1 years for AD, 5.4 years for AD+vascular dementia, and 11.0 years for matched controls with normal cognition [222]. Similar estimates of median survival of 3.3 years from onset of vascular dementia were found by the Canadian Study of Health and aging and the Rochester Epidemiology Project [223, 224]. The leading causes of death in patients with vascular dementia are cerebrovascular events, cardiovascular events, and respiratory diseases [222, 223, 225].

Clinical Bottom Lines

The median survival for patients with vascular dementia is estimated at 3.3–3.9 years from time of disease onset – a shorter median survival than patients with Alzheimer's disease. The majority of patients with vascular dementia die from cerebrovascular or cardiovascular events.

References

1. Jorm AF, Jolley D. The incidence of dementia: a meta-analysis. Neurology. 1998;51:728–33.
2. Kukull WA, Higdon R, Bowen JD, McCormick WC, Teri L, Schellenberg GD, et al. Dementia and Alzheimer disease incidence: a prospective cohort study. Arch Neurol. 2002;59:1737–46.
3. Edland SD, Rocca WA, Petersen RC, Cha RH, Kokmen E. Dementia and Alzheimer disease incidence rates do not vary by sex in Rochester, Minn. Arch Neurol. 2002;59:1589–93.
4. Mortimer JA, Snowdon DA, Markesbery WR. Head circumference, education and risk of dementia: findings from the Nun Study. J Clin Exp Neuropsychol. 2003;25:671–9.
5. Plassman BL, Langa KM, Fisher GG, Heeringa SG, Weir DR, Ofstedal MB, et al. Prevalence of dementia in the United States: the aging, demographics, and memory study. Neuroepidemiology. 2007;29:125–32.
6. Hy LX, Keller DM. Prevalence of AD among whites: a summary by levels of severity. Neurology. 2000;55:198–204.
7. Lobo A, Launer LJ, Fratiglioni L, Andersen K, Di Carlo A, Breteler MM, et al. Prevalence of dementia and major subtypes in Europe: A collaborative study of population-based cohorts. Neurologic Diseases in the Elderly Research Group. Neurology. 2000;54:S4–9.
8. Breitner JC, Wyse BW, Anthony JC, Welsh-Bohmer KA, Steffens DC, Norton MC, et al. APOE-epsilon4 count predicts age when prevalence of AD increases, then declines: the Cache County Study. Neurology. 1999;53:321–31.
9. Slooter AJ, Cruts M, Kalmijn S, Hofman A, Breteler MM, Van Broeckhoven C, et al. Risk estimates of dementia by apolipoprotein E genotypes from a population-based incidence study: the Rotterdam Study. Arch Neurol. 1998;55:964–8.
10. McKhann G, Drachman D, Folstein M, Katzman R, Price D, Stadlan EM. Clinical diagnosis of Alzheimer's disease: report of the NINCDS-ADRDA Work Group under the auspices of Department of Health and Human Services Task Force on Alzheimer's Disease. Neurology. 1984;34:939–44.
11. Holmes C, Cairns N, Lantos P, Mann A. Validity of current clinical criteria for Alzheimer's disease, vascular dementia and dementia with Lewy bodies. Br J Psychiatry. 1999;174:45–50.
12. Kazee AM, Eskin TA, Lapham LW, Gabriel KR, McDaniel KD, Hamill RW. Clinicopathologic correlates in Alzheimer disease: assessment of clinical and pathologic diagnostic criteria. Alzheimer Dis Assoc Disord. 1993;7:152–64.
13. Varma AR, Snowden JS, Lloyd JJ, Talbot PR, Mann DM, Neary D. Evaluation of the NINCDS-ADRDA criteria in the differentiation of Alzheimer's disease and frontotemporal dementia. J Neurol Neurosurg Psychiatry. 1999;66:184–8.
14. Nagy Z, Esiri MM, Hindley NJ, Joachim C, Morris JH, King EM, et al. Accuracy of clinical operational diagnostic criteria for Alzheimer's disease in relation to different pathological diagnostic protocols. Dement Geriatr Cogn Disord. 1998;9:219–26.
15. Mitchell AJ. A meta-analysis of the accuracy of the mini-mental state examination in the detection of dementia and mild cognitive impairment. J Psychiatr Res. 2009;43:411–31.
16. Narasimhalu K, Lee J, Auchus AP, Chen CP. Improving detection of dementia in Asian patients with low education: combining the Mini-Mental State Examination and the Informant Questionnaire on Cognitive Decline in the Elderly. Dement Geriatr Cogn Disord. 2008;25:17–22.
17. Luis CA, Keegan AP, Mullan M. Cross validation of the Montreal Cognitive Assessment in community dwelling older adults residing in the Southeastern US. Int J Geriatr Psychiatry. 2009;24:197–201.
18. Smith T, Gildeh N, Holmes C. The Montreal Cognitive Assessment: validity and utility in a memory clinic setting. Can J Psychiatry. 2007;52:329–32.
19. Knopman DS, DeKosky ST, Cummings JL, Chui H, Corey-Bloom J, Relkin N, et al. Practice parameter: diagnosis of dementia (an evidence-based review). Report of the Quality Standards Subcommittee of the American Academy of Neurology. Neurology. 2001;56:1143–53.

20. Welsh K, Butters N, Hughes J, Mohs R, Heyman A. Detection of abnormal memory decline in mild cases of Alzheimer's disease using CERAD neuropsychological measures. Arch Neurol. 1991;48:278–81.
21. Cahn DA, Salmon DP, Butters N, Wiederholt WC, Corey-Bloom J, Edelstein SL, et al. Detection of dementia of the Alzheimer type in a population-based sample: neuropsychological test performance. J Int Neuropsychol Soc. 1995;1:252–60.
22. Wahlund LO, Julin P, Johansson SE, Scheltens P. Visual rating and volumetry of the medial temporal lobe on magnetic resonance imaging in dementia: a comparative study. J Neurol Neurosurg Psychiatry. 2000;69:630–5.
23. Jagust W, Reed B, Mungas D, Ellis W, Decarli C. What does fluorodeoxyglucose PET imaging add to a clinical diagnosis of dementia? Neurology. 2007;69:871–7.
24. Patwardhan MB, McCrory DC, Matchar DB, Samsa GP, Rutschmann OT. Alzheimer disease: operating characteristics of PET–a meta-analysis. Radiology. 2004;231:73–80.
25. Dougall NJ, Bruggink S, Ebmeier KP. Systematic review of the diagnostic accuracy of 99mTc-HMPAO-SPECT in dementia. Am J Geriatr Psychiatry. 2004;12:554–70.
26. Klunk WE, Engler H, Nordberg A, Wang Y, Blomqvist G, Holt DP, et al. Imaging brain amyloid in Alzheimer's disease with Pittsburgh Compound-B. Ann Neurol. 2004;55:306–19.
27. Rowe CC, Ng S, Ackermann U, Gong SJ, Pike K, Savage G, et al. Imaging beta-amyloid burden in aging and dementia. Neurology. 2007;68:1718–25.
28. Hansson O, Zetterberg H, Buchhave P, Londos E, Blennow K, Minthon L. Association between CSF biomarkers and incipient Alzheimer's disease in patients with mild cognitive impairment: a follow-up study. Lancet Neurol. 2006;5:228–34.
29. Herukka SK, Hallikainen M, Soininen H, Pirttila T. CSF Abeta42 and tau or phosphorylated tau and prediction of progressive mild cognitive impairment. Neurology. 2005;64:1294–7.
30. Mayeux R, Saunders AM, Shea S, Mirra S, Evans D, Roses AD, et al. Utility of the apolipoprotein E genotype in the diagnosis of Alzheimer's disease. Alzheimer's Disease Centers Consortium on Apolipoprotein E and Alzheimer's Disease. N Engl J Med. 1998;338:506–11.
31. Hentschel F, Kreis M, Damian M, Krumm B, Frolich L. The clinical utility of structural neuroimaging with MRI for diagnosis and differential diagnosis of dementia: a memory clinic study. Int J Geriatr Psychiatry. 2005;20:645–50.
32. DeCarli C, Frisoni GB, Clark CM, Harvey D, Grundman M, Petersen RC, et al. Qualitative estimates of medial temporal atrophy as a predictor of progression from mild cognitive impairment to dementia. Arch Neurol. 2007;64:108–15.
33. Geroldi C, Rossi R, Calvagna C, Testa C, Bresciani L, Binetti G, et al. Medial temporal atrophy but not memory deficit predicts progression to dementia in patients with mild cognitive impairment. J Neurol Neurosurg Psychiatry. 2006;77:1219–22.
34. Korf ES, Wahlund LO, Visser PJ, Scheltens P. Medial temporal lobe atrophy on MRI predicts dementia in patients with mild cognitive impairment. Neurology. 2004;63:94–100.
35. Aizenstein HJ, Nebes RD, Saxton JA, Price JC, Mathis CA, Tsopelas ND, et al. Frequent amyloid deposition without significant cognitive impairment among the elderly. Arch Neurol. 2008;65:1509–17.
36. Engler H, Santillo AF, Wang SX, Lindau M, Savitcheva I, Nordberg A, et al. In vivo amyloid imaging with PET in frontotemporal dementia. Eur J Nucl Med Mol Imaging. 2008;35:100–6.
37. Rabinovici GD, Furst AJ, O'Neil JP, Racine CA, Mormino EC, Baker SL, et al. 11 C-PIB PET imaging in Alzheimer disease and frontotemporal lobar degeneration. Neurology. 2007;68: 1205–12.
38. Andreasen N, Minthon L, Davidsson P, Vanmechelen E, Vanderstichele H, Winblad B, et al. Evaluation of CSF-tau and CSF-Abeta42 as diagnostic markers for Alzheimer disease in clinical practice. Arch Neurol. 2001;58:373–9.
39. Waldemar G, Dubois B, Emre M, Georges J, McKeith IG, Rossor M, et al. Recommendations for the diagnosis and management of Alzheimer's disease and other disorders associated with dementia: EFNS guideline. Eur J Neurol. 2007;14:e1–26.

40. Cruts M, van Duijn CM, Backhovens H, Van den Broeck M, Wehnert A, Serneels S, et al. Estimation of the genetic contribution of presenilin-1 and −2 mutations in a population-based study of presenile Alzheimer disease. Hum Mol Genet. 1998;7:43–51.

41. Kamimura K, Tanahashi H, Yamanaka H, Takahashi K, Asada T, Tabira T. Familial Alzheimer's disease genes in Japanese. J Neurol Sci. 1998;160:76–81.

42. Janssen JC, Beck JA, Campbell TA, et al. Early onset familial Alzheimer's disease: mutation frequency in 31 families. Neurology. 2003;60:235–9.

43. Birks J. Cholinesterase inhibitors for Alzheimer's disease. Cochrane Database Syst Rev. 2006:CD005593.

44. McShane R, Areosa Sastre A, Minakaran N. Memantine for dementia. Cochrane Database Syst Rev. 2006:CD003154.

45. Birks J, Harvey RJ. Donepezil for dementia due to Alzheimer's disease. Cochrane Database Syst Rev. 2006:CD001190.

46. Howard RJ, Juszczak E, Ballard CG, Bentham P, Brown RG, Bullock R, et al. Donepezil for the treatment of agitation in Alzheimer's disease. N Engl J Med. 2007;357:1382–92.

47. Loy C, Schneider L. Galantamine for Alzheimer's disease and mild cognitive impairment. Cochrane Database Syst Rev. 2006:CD001747.

48. Birks J, Grimley Evans J, Iakovidou V, Tsolaki M. Rivastigmine for Alzheimer's disease. Cochrane Database Syst Rev. 2000:CD001191.

49. Porsteinsson AP, Grossberg GT, Mintzer J, Olin JT. Memantine treatment in patients with mild to moderate Alzheimer's disease already receiving a cholinesterase inhibitor: a randomized, double-blind, placebo-controlled trial. Curr Alzheimer Res. 2008;5:83–9.

50. Bakchine S, Loft H. Memantine treatment in patients with mild to moderate Alzheimer's disease: results of a randomised, double-blind, placebo-controlled 6-month study. J Alzheimers Dis. 2008;13:97–107.

51. Maidment ID, Fox CG, Boustani M, Rodriguez J, Brown RC, Katona CL. Efficacy of memantine on behavioral and psychological symptoms related to dementia: a systematic meta-analysis. Ann Pharmacother. 2008;42:32–8.

52. Atri A, Shaughnessy LW, Locascio JJ, Growdon JH. Long-term course and effectiveness of combination therapy in Alzheimer disease. Alzheimer Dis Assoc Disord. 2008;22:209–21.

53. Lopez OL, Becker JT, Wahed AS, Saxton J, Sweet RAD, Wolk DA, et al. Memantine augments the effects of cholinesterase inhibition in the treatment of Alzheimer's disease. J Neurol Neurosurg Psychiatry. 2009. doi:10.1136/jnnp. 2008.158964.

54. Cummings JL, Schneider E, Tariot PN, Graham SM. Behavioral effects of memantine in Alzheimer disease patients receiving donepezil treatment. Neurology. 2006;67:57–63.

55. Feldman HH, Schmitt FA, Olin JT. Activities of daily living in moderate-to-severe Alzheimer disease: an analysis of the treatment effects of memantine in patients receiving stable donepezil treatment. Alzheimer Dis Assoc Disord. 2006;20:263–8.

56. Ballard CG, Waite J, Birks J. Atypical antipsychotics for aggression and psychosis in Alzheimer's disease. Cochrane Database Syst Rev. 2009:CD003476.

57. Schneider LS, Dagerman KS, Insel P. Risk of death with atypical antipsychotic drug treatment for dementia: meta-analysis of randomized placebo-controlled trials. JAMA. 2005;294:1934–43.

58. Ballard C, Hanney ML, Theodoulou M, Douglas S, McShane R, Kossakowski K, et al. The dementia antipsychotic withdrawal trial (DART-AD): long-term follow-up of a randomised placebo-controlled trial. Lancet Neurol. 2009;8:151–7.

59. Sultzer DL, Davis SM, Tariot PN, Dagerman KS, Lebowitz BD, Lyketsos CG, et al. Clinical symptom responses to atypical antipsychotic medications in Alzheimer's disease: phase 1 outcomes from the CATIE-AD effectiveness trial. Am J Psychiatry. 2008;165:844–54.

60. Schneider LS, Tariot PN, Dagerman KS, Davis SM, Hsiao JK, Ismail MS, et al. Effectiveness of atypical antipsychotic drugs in patients with Alzheimer's disease. N Engl J Med. 2006;355:1525–38.

61. Aisen PS, Schafer KA, Grundman M, Pfeiffer E, Sano M, Davis KL, et al. Effects of rofecoxib or naproxen vs placebo on Alzheimer disease progression: a randomized controlled trial. JAMA. 2003;289:2819–26.

62. Reines SA, Block GA, Morris JC, Liu G, Nessly ML, Lines CR, et al. Rofecoxib: no effect on Alzheimer's disease in a 1-year, randomized, blinded, controlled study. Neurology. 2004;62:66–71.
63. Soininen H, West C, Robbins J, Niculescu L. Long-term efficacy and safety of celecoxib in Alzheimer's disease. Dement Geriatr Cogn Disord. 2007;23:8–21.
64. de Jong D, Jansen R, Hoefnagels W, Jellesma-Eggenkamp M, Verbeek M, Borm G, et al. No effect of one-year treatment with indomethacin on Alzheimer's disease progression: a randomized controlled trial. PLoS ONE. 2008;3:e1475.
65. Bentham P, Gray R, Sellwood E, Hills R, Crome P, Raftery J. Aspirin in Alzheimer's disease (AD2000): a randomised open-label trial. Lancet Neurol. 2008;7:41–9.
66. Isaac MG, Quinn R, Tabet N. Vitamin E for Alzheimer's disease and mild cognitive impairment. Cochrane Database Syst Rev. 2008:CD002854.
67. Sano M, Ernesto C, Thomas RG, Klauber MR, Schafer K, Grundman M, et al. A controlled trial of selegiline, alpha-tocopherol, or both as treatment for Alzheimer's disease. The Alzheimer's Disease Cooperative Study. N Engl J Med. 1997;336:1216–22.
68. Petersen RC, Thomas RG, Grundman M, Bennett D, Doody R, Ferris S, et al. Vitamin E and donepezil for the treatment of mild cognitive impairment. N Engl J Med. 2005;352:2379–88.
69. Miller 3rd ER, Pastor-Barriuso R, Dalal D, Riemersma RA, Appel LJ, Guallar E. Meta-analysis: high-dosage vitamin E supplementation may increase all-cause mortality. Ann Intern Med. 2005;142:37–46.
70. Arvanitakis Z, Grodstein F, Bienias JL, Schneider JA, Wilson RS, Kelly JF, et al. Relation of NSAIDs to incident AD, change in cognitive function, and AD pathology. Neurology. 2008;70:2219–25.
71. Li G, Larson EB, Sonnen JA, Shofer JB, Petrie EC, Schantz A, et al. Statin therapy is associated with reduced neuropathologic changes of Alzheimer disease. Neurology. 2007;69:878–85.
72. Haag MD, Hofman A, Koudstaal PJ, Stricker BH, Breteler MM. Statins are associated with a reduced risk of Alzheimer disease regardless of lipophilicity. The Rotterdam Study. J Neurol Neurosurg Psychiatry. 2009;80:13–7.
73. Zhou B, Teramukai S, Fukushima M. Prevention and treatment of dementia or Alzheimer's disease by statins: a meta-analysis. Dement Geriatr Cogn Disord. 2007;23:194–201.
74. Sparks DL, Sabbagh MN, Connor DJ, Lopez J, Launer LJ, Browne P, et al. Atorvastatin for the treatment of mild to moderate Alzheimer disease: preliminary results. Arch Neurol. 2005;62:753–7.
75. Ganguli M, Dodge HH, Shen C, Pandav RS, DeKosky ST. Alzheimer disease and mortality: a 15-year epidemiological study. Arch Neurol. 2005;62:779–84.
76. Brookmeyer R, Corrada MM, Curriero FC, Kawas C. Survival following a diagnosis of Alzheimer disease. Arch Neurol. 2002;59:1764–7.
77. Larson EB, Shadlen MF, Wang L, McCormick WC, Bowen JD, Teri L, et al. Survival after initial diagnosis of Alzheimer disease. Ann Intern Med. 2004;140:501–9.
78. Helzner EP, Scarmeas N, Cosentino S, Tang MX, Schupf N, Stern Y. Survival in Alzheimer disease: a multiethnic, population-based study of incident cases. Neurology. 2008;71:1489–95.
79. Helmer C, Joly P, Letenneur L, Commenges D, Dartigues JF. Mortality with dementia: results from a French prospective community-based cohort. Am J Epidemiol. 2001;154:642–8.
80. Mercy L, Hodges JR, Dawson K, Barker RA, Brayne C. Incidence of early-onset dementias in Cambridgeshire, United Kingdom. Neurology. 2008;71:1496–9.
81. Knopman DS, Petersen RC, Edland SD, Cha RH, Rocca WA. The incidence of frontotemporal lobar degeneration in Rochester, Minnesota, 1990 through 1994. Neurology. 2004;62:506–8.
82. Ratnavalli E, Brayne C, Dawson K, Hodges JR. The prevalence of frontotemporal dementia. Neurology. 2002;58:1615–21.
83. Rosso SM, Donker Kaat L, Baks T, Joosse M, de Koning I, Pijnenburg Y, et al. Frontotemporal dementia in The Netherlands: patient characteristics and prevalence estimates from a population-based study. Brain. 2003;126:2016–22.

84. Grasbeck A, Horstmann V, Nilsson K, Sjobeck M, Sjostrom H, Gustafson L. Dementia in first-degree relatives of patients with frontotemporal dementia. A family history study. Dement Geriatr Cogn Disord. 2005;19:145–53.

85. Stevens M, van Duijn CM, Kamphorst W, de Knijff P, Heutink P, van Gool WA, et al. Familial aggregation in frontotemporal dementia. Neurology. 1998;50:1541–5.

86. Goldman JS, Farmer JM, Wood EM, Johnson JK, Boxer A, Neuhaus J, et al. Comparison of family histories in FTLD subtypes and related tauopathies. Neurology. 2005;65:1817–9.

87. Neary D, Snowden JS, Gustafson L, Passant U, Stuss D, Black S, et al. Frontotemporal lobar degeneration: a consensus on clinical diagnostic criteria. Neurology. 1998;51:1546–54.

88. Mendez MF, Shapira JS, McMurtray A, Licht E, Miller BL. Accuracy of the clinical evaluation for frontotemporal dementia. Arch Neurol. 2007;64:830–5.

89. Blair M, Kertesz A, Davis-Faroque N, Hsiung GY, Black SE, Bouchard RW, et al. Behavioural measures in frontotemporal lobar dementia and other dementias: the utility of the frontal behavioural inventory and the neuropsychiatric inventory in a national cohort study. Dement Geriatr Cogn Disord. 2007;23:406–15.

90. Milan G, Lamenza F, Iavarone A, Galeone F, Lore E, de Falco C, et al. Frontal Behavioural Inventory in the differential diagnosis of dementia. Acta Neurol Scand. 2008;117:260–5.

91. Likeman M, Anderson VM, Stevens JM, Waldman AD, Godbolt AK, Frost C, et al. Visual assessment of atrophy on magnetic resonance imaging in the diagnosis of pathologically confirmed young-onset dementias. Arch Neurol. 2005;62:1410–5.

92. Foster NL, Heidebrink JL, Clark CM, Jagust WJ, Arnold SE, Barbas NR, et al. FDG-PET improves accuracy in distinguishing frontotemporal dementia and Alzheimer's disease. Brain. 2007;130:2616–35.

93. McNeill R, Sare GM, Manoharan M, Testa HJ, Mann DMA, Neary D, et al. Accuracy of single-photon emission computed tomography in differentiating frontotemporal dementia from Alzheimer's disease. J Neurol Neurosurg Psychiatry. 2007;78:350–5.

94. Bian H, Van Swieten JC, Leight S, Massimo L, Wood E, Forman M, et al. CSF biomarkers in frontotemporal lobar degeneration with known pathology. Neurology. 2008;70:1827–35.

95. Kapaki E, Paraskevas GP, Papageorgious SG, Bonakis A, Kalfakis N, Zalonis I, et al. Diagnostic value of CSF biomarker profile in frontotemporal lobar degeneration. Alzheimer Dis Assoc Disord. 2008;22:47–53.

96. Hutchinson AD, Mathias JL. Neuropsychological deficits in frontotemporal dementia and Alzheimer's disease: a meta-analytic review. J Neurol Neurosurg Psychiatry. 2007;78:917–28.

97. Perry RJ, Hodges JR. Differentiating frontal and temporal variant frontotemporal dementia from Alzheimer's disease. Neurology. 2000;54:2277–84.

98. Houlden H, Baker M, Adamson J, Grover A, Waring S, Dickson D, et al. Frequency of tau mutations in three series of non-Alzheimer's degenerative dementia. Ann Neurol. 1999;46:243–8.

99. Benussi L, Ghidoni R, Pegoiani E, Moretti DV, Zanetti O, Binetti G. Progranulin Leu271LeufsX10 is one of the most common FTLD and CBS associated mutations worldwide. Neurobiol Dis. 2009;33:379–85.

100. Kruger J, Kaivorinne AL, Udd B, Majamaa K, Remes AM. Low prevalence of progranulin mutations in Finnish patients with frontotemporal lobar degeneration. Eur J Neurol. 2009;16:27–30.

101. Pickering-Brown SM, Rollinson S, Du Plessis D, Morrison KE, Varma A, Richardson AM, et al. Frequency and clinical characteristics of progranulin mutation carriers in the Manchester frontotemporal lobar degeneration cohort: comparison with patients with MAPT and no known mutations. Brain. 2008;131:721–31.

102. Deakin JB, Rahman S, Nestor PJ, Hodges JR, Sahakian BJ. Paroxetine does not improve symptoms and impairs cognition in frontotemporal dementia: a double-blind randomized controlled trial. Psychopharmacology (Berl). 2004;172:400–8.

103. Moretti R, Torre P, Antonello RM, Cazzato G, Bava A. Frontotemporal dementia: paroxetine as a possible treatment of behavior symptoms. A randomized, controlled, open 14-month study. Eur Neurol. 2003;49:13–9.

104. Ikeda M, Shigenobu K, Fukuhara R, Hokoishi K, Maki N, Nebu A, et al. Efficacy of fluvoxamine as a treatment for behavioral symptoms in frontotemporal lobar degeneration patients. Dement Geriatr Cogn Disord. 2004;17:117–21.

105. Mendez MF, Shapira JS, Miller BL. Stereotypical movements and frontotemporal dementia. Mov Disord. 2005;20:742–5.

106. Swartz JR, Miller BL, Lesser IM, Darby AL. Frontotemporal dementia: treatment response to serotonin selective reuptake inhibitors. J Clin Psychiatry. 1997;58:212–6.

107. Lebert F, Stekke W, Hasenbroekx C, Pasquier F. Frontotemporal dementia: a randomised, controlled trial with trazodone. Dement Geriatr Cogn Disord. 2004;17:355–9.

108. Kertesz A, Morlog D, Light M, Blair M, Davidson W, Jesso S, et al. Galantamine in fronto-temporal dementia and primary progressive aphasia. Dement Geriatr Cogn Disord. 2008;25:178–85.

109. Mendez MF, Shapira JS, McMurtray A, Licht E. Preliminary findings: behavioral worsening on donepezil in patients with frontotemporal dementia. Am J Geriatr Psychiatry. 2007;15:84–7.

110. Rahman S, Robbins TW, Hodges JR, Mehta MA, Nestor PJ, Clark L, et al. Methylphenidate ('Ritalin') can ameliorate abnormal risk-taking behavior in the frontal variant of frontotem-poral dementia. Neuropsychopharmacology. 2006;31:651–8.

111. Hodges JR, Davies R, Xuereb J, Kril J, Halliday G. Survival in frontotemporal dementia. Neurology. 2003;61:349–54.

112. Roberson ED, Hesse JH, Rose KD, Slama H, Johnson JK, Yaffe K, et al. Frontotemporal dementia progresses to death faster than Alzheimer disease. Neurology. 2005;65:719–25.

113. Bergeron C, Pollanen M. Lewy bodies in Alzheimer disease–one or two diseases? Alzheimer Dis Assoc Disord. 1989;3:197–204.

114. Gibb WR, Lees AJ. Prevalence of Lewy bodies in Alzheimer's disease. Ann Neurol. 1989;26:691–3.

115. Iseki E. Dementia with Lewy bodies: reclassification of pathological subtypes and boundary with Parkinson's disease or Alzheimer's disease. Neuropathology. 2004;24:72–8.

116. McKeith IG. Consensus guidelines for the clinical and pathologic diagnosis of dementia with Lewy bodies (DLB): report of the Consortium on DLB International Workshop. J Alzheimers Dis. 2006;9:417–23.

117. McKeith IG, Galasko D, Kosaka K, Perry EK, Dickson DW, Hansen LA, et al. Consensus guidelines for the clinical and pathologic diagnosis of dementia with Lewy bodies (DLB): report of the consortium on DLB international workshop. Neurology. 1996;47:1113–24.

118. Jhoo JH, Kim KW, Huh Y, Lee SB, Park JH, Lee JJ, et al. Prevalence of dementia and its subtypes in an elderly urban korean population: results from the Korean Longitudinal Study on Health And Aging (KLoSHA). Dement Geriatr Cogn Disord. 2008;26:270–6.

119. Rahkonen T, Eloniemi-Sulkava U, Rissanen S, Vatanen A, Viramo P, Sulkava R. Dementia with Lewy bodies according to the consensus criteria in a general population aged 75 years or older. J Neurol Neurosurg Psychiatry. 2003;74:720–4.

120. Stevens T, Livingston G, Kitchen G, Manela M, Walker Z, Katona C. Islington study of dementia subtypes in the community. Br J Psychiatry. 2002;180:270–6.

121. Singleton AB, Farrer M, Johnson J, Singleton A, Hague S, Kachergus J, et al. Alpha-Synuclein locus triplication causes Parkinson's disease. Science. 2003;302:841.

122. Lockhart PJ, Kachergus J, Lincoln S, Hulihan M, Bisceglio G, Thomas N, et al. Multiplication of the alpha-synuclein gene is not a common disease mechanism in Lewy body disease. J Mol Neurosci. 2004;24:337–42.

123. Goker-Alpan O, Giasson BI, Eblan MJ, Nguyen J, Hurtig HI, Lee VM, et al. Glucocerebrosidase mutations are an important risk factor for Lewy body disorders. Neurology. 2006;67:908–10.

124. Mata IF, Samii A, Schneer SH, Roberts JW, Griffith A, Leis BC, et al. Glucocerebrosidase gene mutations: a risk factor for Lewy body disorders. Arch Neurol. 2008;65:379–82.

125. Aarsland D, Rongve A, Nore SP, Skogseth R, Skulstad S, Ehrt U, et al. Frequency and case identification of dementia with Lewy bodies using the revised consensus criteria. Dement Geriatr Cogn Disord. 2008;26:445–52.

126. Ferman TJ, Smith GE, Boeve BF, Ivnik RJ, Petersen RC, Knopman D, et al. DLB fluctuations: specific features that reliably differentiate DLB from AD and normal aging. Neurology. 2004;62:181–7.

127. Calderon J, Perry RJ, Erzinclioglu SW, Berrios GE, Dening TR, Hodges JR. Perception, attention, and working memory are disproportionately impaired in dementia with Lewy bodies compared with Alzheimer's disease. J Neurol Neurosurg Psychiatry. 2001;70:157–64.

128. Crowell TA, Luis CA, Cox DE, Mullan M. Neuropsychological comparison of Alzheimer's disease and dementia with lewy bodies. Dement Geriatr Cogn Disord. 2007;23:120–5.

129. Mori E, Shimomura T, Fujimori M, Hirono N, Imamura T, Hashimoto M, et al. Visuoperceptual impairment in dementia with Lewy bodies. Arch Neurol. 2000;57:489–93.

130. Tiraboschi P, Salmon DP, Hansen LA, Hofstetter RC, Thal LJ, Corey-Bloom J. What best differentiates Lewy body from Alzheimer's disease in early-stage dementia? Brain. 2006;129:729–35.

131. Litvan I, MacIntyre A, Goetz CG, Wenning GK, Jellinger K, Verny M, et al. Accuracy of the clinical diagnoses of Lewy body disease, Parkinson disease, and dementia with Lewy bodies: a clinicopathologic study. Arch Neurol. 1998;55:969–78.

132. McKeith IG, Ballard CG, Perry RH, Ince PG, O'Brien JT, Neill D, et al. Prospective validation of consensus criteria for the diagnosis of dementia with Lewy bodies. Neurology. 2000;54:1050–8.

133. Ferman TJ, Smith GE, Boeve BF, Graff-Radford NR, Lucas JA, Knopman DS, et al. Neuropsychological differentiation of dementia with Lewy bodies from normal aging and Alzheimer's disease. Clin Neuropsychol. 2006;20:623–36.

134. McKeith I, O'Brien J, Walker Z, Tatsch K, Booij J, Darcourt J, et al. Sensitivity and specificity of dopamine transporter imaging with [123] I-FP-CIT SPECT in dementia with Lewy bodies: a phase III, multicentre study. Lancet Neurol. 2007;6:305–13.

135. Walker Z, Costa DC, Walker RWH, Shaw K, Gacinovic S, Stevens T, et al. Differentiation of dementia with Lewy bodies from Alzheimer's disease using a dopaminergic presynaptic ligand. J Neurol Neurosurg Psychiatry. 2002;73:134–40.

136. Minoshima S, Foster NL, Sima AA, Frey KA, Albin RL, Kuhl DE. Alzheimer's disease versus dementia with Lewy bodies: cerebral metabolic distinction with autopsy confirmation. Ann Neurol. 2001;50:358–65.

137. Yoshita M, Taki J, Yamada M. A clinical role for [(123)I]MIBG myocardial scintigraphy in the distinction between dementia of the Alzheimer's-type and dementia with Lewy bodies. J Neurol Neurosurg Psychiatry. 2001;71:583–8.

138. Estorch M, Camacho V, Paredes P, Rivera E, Rodriguez-Revuelto A, Flotats A, et al. Cardiac (123)I-metaiodobenzylguanidine imaging allows early identification of dementia with Lewy bodies during life. Eur J Nucl Med Mol Imaging. 2008;35:1636–41.

139. Hanyu H, Shimizu S, Hirao K, Kanetaka H, Iwamoto T, Chikamori T, et al. Comparative value of brain perfusion SPECT and [(123)I]MIBG myocardial scintigraphy in distinguishing between dementia with Lewy bodies and Alzheimer's disease. Eur J Nucl Med Mol Imaging. 2006;33:248–53.

140. Colloby SJ, Fenwick JD, Williams ED, Paling SM, Lobotesis K, Ballard C, et al. A comparison of (99 m)Tc-HMPAO SPET changes in dementia with Lewy bodies and Alzheimer's disease using statistical parametric mapping. Eur J Nucl Med Mol Imaging. 2002;29:615–22.

141. Kemp PM, Hoffmann SA, Tossici-Bolt L, Fleming JS, Holmes C. Limitations of the HMPAO SPECT appearances of occipital lobe perfusion in the differential diagnosis of dementia with Lewy bodies. Nucl Med Commun. 2007;28:451–6.

142. Albin RL, Minoshima S, D'Amato CJ, Frey KA, Kuhl DA, Sima AA. Fluoro-deoxyglucose positron emission tomography in diffuse Lewy body disease. Neurology. 1996;47:462–6.

143. Gilman S, Koeppe RA, Little R, An H, Junck L, Giordani B, et al. Differentiation of Alzheimer's disease from dementia with Lewy bodies utilizing positron emission tomography

with [18 F]fluorodeoxyglucose and neuropsychological testing. Exp Neurol. 2005;191 Suppl 1:S95–103.

144. Ishii K, Soma T, Kono AK, Sofue K, Miyamoto N, Yoshikawa T, et al. Comparison of regional brain volume and glucose metabolism between patients with mild dementia with lewy bodies and those with mild Alzheimer's disease. J Nucl Med. 2007;48:704–11.

145. Taki J, Yoshita M, Yamada M, Tonami N. Significance of 123I-MIBG scintigraphy as a pathophysiological indicator in the assessment of Parkinson's disease and related disorders: it can be a specific marker for Lewy body disease. Ann Nucl Med. 2004;18:453–61.

146. Novellino F, Bagnato A, Salsone M, Cascini GL, Nicoletti G, Arabia G, et al. Myocardial (123)I-MIBG scintigraphy for differentiation of Lewy Bodies Disease from FTD. Neurobiol Aging. 2009;31(11):1903–11.

147. Middelkoop HA, van der Flier WM, Burton EJ, Lloyd AJ, Paling S, Barber R, et al. Dementia with Lewy bodies and AD are not associated with occipital lobe atrophy on MRI. Neurology. 2001;57:2117–20.

148. Cousins DA, Burton EJ, Burn D, Gholkar A, McKeith IG, O'Brien JT. Atrophy of the putamen in dementia with Lewy bodies but not Alzheimer's disease: an MRI study. Neurology. 2003;61:1191–5.

149. Whitwell JL, Weigand SD, Shiung MM, Boeve BF, Ferman TJ, Smith GE, et al. Focal atrophy in dementia with Lewy bodies on MRI: a distinct pattern from Alzheimer's disease. Brain. 2007;130:708–19.

150. Briel RC, McKeith IG, Barker WA, Hewitt Y, Perry RH, Ince PG, et al. EEG findings in dementia with Lewy bodies and Alzheimer's disease. J Neurol Neurosurg Psychiatry. 1999;66:401–3.

151. Crystal HA, Dickson DW, Lizardi JE, Davies P, Wolfson LI. Antemortem diagnosis of diffuse Lewy body disease. Neurology. 1990;40:1523–8.

152. Doran M, Larner AJ. EEG findings in dementia with Lewy bodies causing diagnostic confusion with sporadic Creutzfeldt-Jakob disease. Eur J Neurol. 2004;11:838–41.

153. Barber PA, Varma AR, Lloyd JJ, Haworth B, Snowden JS, Neary D. The electroencephalogram in dementia with Lewy bodies. Acta Neurol Scand. 2000;101:53–6.

154. Londos E, Passant U, Brun A, Rosen I, Risberg J, Gustafson L. Regional cerebral blood flow and EEG in clinically diagnosed dementia with Lewy bodies and Alzheimer's disease. Arch Gerontol Geriatr. 2003;36:231–45.

155. Andersson M, Hansson O, Minthon L, Rosen I, Londos E. Electroencephalogram variability in dementia with lewy bodies, Alzheimer's disease and controls. Dement Geriatr Cogn Disord. 2008;26:284–90.

156. Bonanni L, Thomas A, Tiraboschi P, Perfetti B, Varanese S, Onofrj M. EEG comparisons in early Alzheimer's disease, dementia with Lewy bodies and Parkinson's disease with dementia patients with a 2-year follow-up. Brain. 2008;131:690–705.

157. Roks G, Korf ES, van der Flier WM, Scheltens P, Stam CJ. The use of EEG in the diagnosis of dementia with Lewy bodies. J Neurol Neurosurg Psychiatry. 2008;79:377–80.

158. Bibl M, Mollenhauer B, Esselmann H, Lewczuk P, Trenkwalder C, Brechlin P, et al. CSF diagnosis of Alzheimer's disease and dementia with Lewy bodies. J Neural Transm. 2006;113:1771–8.

159. Mollenhauer B, Cepek L, Bibl M, Wiltfang J, Schulz-Schaeffer WJ, Ciesielczyk B, et al. Tau protein, Abeta42 and S-100B protein in cerebrospinal fluid of patients with dementia with Lewy bodies. Dement Geriatr Cogn Disord. 2005;19:164–70.

160. Wada-Isoe K, Kitayama M, Nakaso K, Nakashima K. Diagnostic markers for diagnosing dementia with Lewy bodies: CSF and MIBG cardiac scintigraphy study. J Neurol Sci. 2007;260:33–7.

161. Mollenhauer B, Cullen V, Kahn I, Krastins B, Outeiro TF, Pepivani I, et al. Direct quantification of CSF alpha-synuclein by ELISA and first cross-sectional study in patients with neurodegeneration. Exp Neurol. 2008;213:315–25.

162. Bibl M, Mollenhauer B, Esselmann H, Lewczuk P, Klafki HW, Sparbier K, et al. CSF amyloid-beta-peptides in Alzheimer's disease, dementia with Lewy bodies and Parkinson's disease dementia. Brain. 2006;129:1177–87.

163. Ohrfelt A, Grognet P, Andreasen N, Wallin A, Vanmechelen E, Blennow K, et al. Cerebrospinal fluid alpha-synuclein in neurodegenerative disorders – a marker of synapse loss? Neurosci Lett. 2009;450:332–5.

164. Gwinn-Hardy K, Singleton AA. Familial Lewy body diseases. J Geriatr Psychiatry Neurol. 2002;15:217–23.

165. Tsuang DW, DiGiacomo L, Bird TD. Familial occurrence of dementia with Lewy bodies. Am J Geriatr Psychiatry. 2004;12:179–88.

166. Johnson J, Hague SM, Hanson M, Gibson A, Wilson KE, Evans EW, et al. SNCA multiplication is not a common cause of Parkinson disease or dementia with Lewy bodies. Neurology. 2004;63:554–6.

167. Takahashi H, Yoshida K, Sugita T, Higuchi H, Shimizu T. Quetiapine treatment of psychotic symptoms and aggressive behavior in patients with dementia with Lewy bodies: a case series. Prog Neuropsychopharmacol Biol Psychiatry. 2003;27:549–53.

168. Kurlan R, Cummings J, Raman R, Thal L. Quetiapine for agitation or psychosis in patients with dementia and parkinsonism. Neurology. 2007;68:1356–63.

169. Cummings JL, Street J, Masterman D, Clark WS. Efficacy of olanzapine in the treatment of psychosis in dementia with lewy bodies. Dement Geriatr Cogn Disord. 2002;13:67–73.

170. Moretti R, Torre P, Antonello RM, Cazzato G, Griggio S, Bava A. Olanzapine as a treatment of neuropsychiatric disorders of Alzheimer's disease and other dementias: a 24-month follow-up of 68 patients. Am J Alzheimers Dis Other Demen. 2003;18:205–14.

171. Allen RL, Walker Z, D'Ath PJ, Katona CL. Risperidone for psychotic and behavioural symptoms in Lewy body dementia. Lancet. 1995;346:185.

172. McKeith IG, Ballard CG, Harrison RW. Neuroleptic sensitivity to risperidone in Lewy body dementia. Lancet. 1995;346:699.

173. Frieling H, Hillemacher T, Ziegenbein M, Neundorfer B, Bleich S. Treating dopamimetic psychosis in Parkinson's disease: structured review and meta-analysis. Eur Neuropsychopharmacol. 2007;17:165–71.

174. Burke WJ, Pfeiffer RF, McComb RD. Neuroleptic sensitivity to clozapine in dementia with Lewy bodies. J Neuropsychiatry Clin Neurosci. 1998;10:227–9.

175. Chacko RC, Hurley RA, Jankovic J. Clozapine use in diffuse Lewy body disease. J Neuropsychiatry Clin Neurosci. 1993;5:206–8.

176. Bonelli SB, Ransmayr G, Steffelbauer M, Lukas T, Lampl C, Deibl M. L-dopa responsiveness in dementia with Lewy bodies, Parkinson disease with and without dementia. Neurology. 2004;63:376–8.

177. Molloy S, McKeith IG, O'Brien JT, Burn DJ. The role of levodopa in the management of dementia with Lewy bodies. J Neurol Neurosurg Psychiatry. 2005;76:1200–3.

178. McKeith I, Del Ser T, Spano P, Emre M, Wesnes K, Anand R, et al. Efficacy of rivastigmine in dementia with Lewy bodies: a randomised, double-blind, placebo-controlled international study. Lancet. 2000;356:2031–6.

179. Wesnes KA, McKeith IG, Ferrara R, Emre M, Del Ser T, Spano PF, et al. Effects of rivastigmine on cognitive function in dementia with lewy bodies: a randomised placebo-controlled international study using the cognitive drug research computerised assessment system. Dement Geriatr Cogn Disord. 2002;13:183–92.

180. Simard M, van Reekum R. The acetylcholinesterase inhibitors for treatment of cognitive and behavioral symptoms in dementia with Lewy bodies. J Neuropsychiatry Clin Neurosci. 2004;16:409–25.

181. Edwards K, Royall D, Hershey L, Lichter D, Hake A, Farlow M, et al. Efficacy and safety of galantamine in patients with dementia with Lewy bodies: a 24-week open-label study. Dement Geriatr Cogn Disord. 2007;23:401–5.

182. Mori S, Mori E, Iseki E, Kosaka K. Efficacy and safety of donepezil in patients with dementia with Lewy bodies: preliminary findings from an open-label study. Psychiatry Clin Neurosci. 2006;60:190–5.

183. Ballard C, Lane R, Barone P, Ferrara R, Tekin S. Cardiac safety of rivastigmine in Lewy body and Parkinson's disease dementias. Int J Clin Pract. 2006;60:639–45.

184. Williams MM, Xiong C, Morris JC, Galvin JE. Survival and mortality differences between dementia with Lewy bodies vs. Alzheimer disease. Neurology. 2006;67:1935–41.

185. Jellinger KA, Wenning GK, Seppi K. Predictors of survival in dementia with lewy bodies and Parkinson dementia. Neurodegener Dis. 2007;4:428–30.

186. Olichney JM, Galasko D, Salmon DP, Hofstetter CR, Hansen LA, Katzman R, et al. Cognitive decline is faster in Lewy body variant than in Alzheimer's disease. Neurology. 1998;51:351–7.

187. Hebert R, Lindsay J, Verreault R, Rockwood K, Hill G, Dubois MF. Vascular dementia: incidence and risk factors in the Canadian study of health and aging. Stroke. 2000;31:1487–93.

188. Andreasen N, Blennow K, Sjodin C, Winblad B, Svardsudd K. Prevalence and incidence of clinically diagnosed memory impairments in a geographically defined general population in Sweden. The Pitea Dementia Project. Neuroepidemiology. 1999;18:144–55.

189. Jellinger KA, Attems J. Neuropathological evaluation of mixed dementia. J Neurol Sci. 2007;257:80–7.

190. Schneider JA, Arvanitakis Z, Bang W, Bennett DA. Mixed brain pathologies account for most dementia cases in community-dwelling older persons. Neurology. 2007;69:2197–204.

191. Hayden KM, Zandi PP, Lyketsos CG, Khachaturian AS, Bastian LA, Charoonruk G, et al. Vascular risk factors for incident Alzheimer disease and vascular dementia: the Cache County study. Alzheimer Dis Assoc Disord. 2006;20:93–100.

192. MacKnight C, Rockwood K, Awalt E, McDowell I. Diabetes mellitus and the risk of dementia, Alzheimer's disease and vascular cognitive impairment in the Canadian Study of Health and Aging. Dement Geriatr Cogn Disord. 2002;14:77–83.

193. Xu WL, Qiu CX, Wahlin A, Winblad B, Fratiglioni L. Diabetes mellitus and risk of dementia in the Kungsholmen project: a 6-year follow-up study. Neurology. 2004;63:1181–6.

194. Launer LJ, Ross GW, Petrovitch H, Masaki K, Foley D, White LR, et al. Midlife blood pressure and dementia: the Honolulu-Asia aging study. Neurobiol Aging. 2000;21:49–55.

195. Posner HB, Tang MX, Luchsinger J, Lantigua R, Stern Y, Mayeux R. The relationship of hypertension in the elderly to AD, vascular dementia, and cognitive function. Neurology. 2002;58:1175–81.

196. Yoshitake T, Kiyohara Y, Kato I, Ohmura T, Iwamoto H, Nakayama K, et al. Incidence and risk factors of vascular dementia and Alzheimer's disease in a defined elderly Japanese population: the Hisayama Study. Neurology. 1995;45:1161–8.

197. Roman GC, Tatemichi TK, Erkinjuntti T, Cummings JL, Masdeu JC, Garcia JH, et al. Vascular dementia: diagnostic criteria for research studies. Report of the NINDS-AIREN International Workshop. Neurology. 1993;43:250–60.

198. Gold G, Bouras C, Canuto A, Bergallo MF, Herrmann FR, Hof PR, et al. Clinicopathological validation study of four sets of clinical criteria for vascular dementia. Am J Psychiatry. 2002;159:82–7.

199. Reed BR, Mungas DM, Kramer JH, Ellis W, Vinters HV, Zarow C, et al. Profiles of neuropsychological impairment in autopsy-defined Alzheimer's disease and cerebrovascular disease. Brain. 2007;130:731–9.

200. Sachdev PS, Brodaty H, Valenzuela MJ, Lorentz L, Looi JC, Wen W, et al. The neuropsychological profile of vascular cognitive impairment in stroke and TIA patients. Neurology. 2004;62:912–9.

201. Graham NL, Emery T, Hodges JR. Distinctive cognitive profiles in Alzheimer's disease and subcortical vascular dementia. J Neurol Neurosurg Psychiatry. 2004;75:61–71.

202. Longstreth Jr WT, Arnold AM, Beauchamp Jr NJ, Manolio TA, Lefkowitz D, Jungreis C, et al. Incidence, manifestations, and predictors of worsening white matter on serial cranial

magnetic resonance imaging in the elderly: the Cardiovascular Health Study. Stroke. 2005;36:56–61.

203. Price CC, Jefferson AL, Merino JG, Heilman KM, Libon DJ. Subcortical vascular dementia: integrating neuropsychological and neuroradiologic data. Neurology. 2005;65:376–82.

204. Hunt AL, Orrison WW, Yeo RA, Haaland KY, Rhyne RL, Garry PJ, et al. Clinical significance of MRI white matter lesions in the elderly. Neurology. 1989;39:1470–4.

205. Mendez MF, Ottowitz W, Brown CV, Cummings JL, Perryman KM, Mandelkern MA. Dementia with leukoaraiosis: clinical differentiation by temporoparietal hypometabolism on (18)FDG-PET imaging. Dement Geriatr Cogn Disord. 1999;10:518–25.

206. Kerrouche N, Herholz K, Mielke R, Holthoff V, Baron JC. 18FDG PET in vascular dementia: differentiation from Alzheimer's disease using voxel-based multivariate analysis. J Cereb Blood Flow Metab. 2006;26:1213–21.

207. Nagata K, Maruya H, Yuya H, Terashi H, Mito Y, Kato H, et al. Can PET data differentiate Alzheimer's disease from vascular dementia? Ann NY Acad Sci. 2000;903:252–61.

208. de Jong D, Jansen RW, Kremer BP, Verbeek MM. Cerebrospinal fluid amyloid beta42/phosphorylated tau ratio discriminates between Alzheimer's disease and vascular dementia. J Gerontol A Biol Sci Med Sci. 2006;61:755–8.

209. Paraskevas GP, Kapaki E, Papageorgiou SG, Kalfakis N, Andreadou E, Zalonis I, et al. CSF biomarker profile and diagnostic value in vascular dementia. Eur J Neurol. 2009;16: 205–11.

210. Stefani A, Bernardini S, Panella M, Pierantozzi M, Nuccetelli M, Koch G, et al. AD with subcortical white matter lesions and vascular dementia: CSF markers for differential diagnosis. J Neurol Sci. 2005;237:83–8.

211. Kavirajan H, Schneider LS. Efficacy and adverse effects of cholinesterase inhibitors and memantine in vascular dementia: a meta-analysis of randomised controlled trials. Lancet Neurol. 2007;6:782–92.

212. Dichgans M, Markus HS, Salloway S, Verkkoniemi A, Moline M, Wang Q, et al. Donepezil in patients with subcortical vascular cognitive impairment: a randomised double-blind trial in CADASIL. Lancet Neurol. 2008;7:310–8.

213. in't Veld BA, Ruitenberg A, Hofman A, Stricker BH, Breteler MM. Antihypertensive drugs and incidence of dementia: the Rotterdam Study. Neurobiol Aging. 2001;22:407–412.

214. McGuinness B, Todd S, Passmore P, Bullock R. The effects of blood pressure lowering on development of cognitive impairment and dementia in patients without apparent prior cerebrovascular disease. Cochrane Database Syst Rev. 2006:CD004034.

215. Amarenco P, Bogousslavsky J, Callahan 3rd A, Goldstein LB, Hennerici M, Rudolph AE, et al. High-dose atorvastatin after stroke or transient ischemic attack. N Engl J Med. 2006;355:549–59.

216. Rea TD, Breitner JC, Psaty BM, Fitzpatrick AL, Lopez OL, Newman AB, et al. Statin use and the risk of incident dementia: the Cardiovascular Health Study. Arch Neurol. 2005;62:1047–51.

217. Shepherd J, Blauw GJ, Murphy MB, Bollen EL, Buckley BM, Cobbe SM, et al. Pravastatin in elderly individuals at risk of vascular disease (PROSPER): a randomised controlled trial. Lancet. 2002;360:1623–30.

218. ten Dam VH, van den Heuvel DM, van Buchem MA, Westendorp RG, Bollen EL, Ford I, et al. Effect of pravastatin on cerebral infarcts and white matter lesions. Neurology. 2005;64:1807–9.

219. Szekely CA, Breitner JC, Fitzpatrick AL, Rea TD, Psaty BM, Kuller LH, et al. NSAID use and dementia risk in the Cardiovascular Health Study: role of APOE and NSAID type. Neurology. 2008;70:17–24.

220. Meyer JS, Rogers RL, McClintic K, Mortel KF, Lotfi J. Randomized clinical trial of daily aspirin therapy in multi-infarct dementia. A pilot study. J Am Geriatr Soc. 1989;37:549–55.

221. Williams PS, Rands G, Orrel M, Spector A. Aspirin for vascular dementia. Cochrane Database Syst Rev. 2000:CD001296.

222. Fitzpatrick AL, Kuller LH, Lopez OL, Kawas CH, Jagust W. Survival following dementia onset: Alzheimer's disease and vascular dementia. J Neurol Sci. 2005;229–230:43–9.
223. Knopman DS, Rocca WA, Cha RH, Edland SD, Kokmen E. Survival study of vascular dementia in Rochester, Minnesota. Arch Neurol. 2003;60:85–90.
224. Wolfson C, Wolfson DB, Asgharian M, M'Lan CE, Ostbye T, Rockwood K, et al. A reevaluation of the duration of survival after the onset of dementia. N Engl J Med. 2001;344:1111–6.
225. Brunnstrom HR, Englund EM. Cause of death in patients with dementia disorders. Eur J Neurol. 2009;16(4):488–92.

Chapter 9
Neuromuscular Disorders

Brian A. Crum, Devon I. Rubin, Elliot L. Dimberg, and Brent P. Goodman

Keywords Amyotrophic lateral sclerosis • Riluzole • Diabetic peripheral neuropathy • Alpha lipoic acid • Inclusion body myositis • Muscle biopsy • Intravenous immunoglobulin • Myasthenia gravis • Mycophenolate • Thymectomy • Single-fiber electromyography • Acetylcholine receptor antibodies

Amyotrophic Lateral Sclerosis

Amyotrophic lateral sclerosis (ALS) is classically defined as a progressive disorder of both upper and lower motor neurons leading to progressive skeletal muscle weakness and death in an average of 3 years from symptom onset. The disease typically begins asymmetrically in a hand or foot or sometimes in the bulbar segment with dysarthria (less commonly dysphagia at onset). Lower motor neuron signs include atrophy, fasciculations, weakness, and neurogenic abnormalities on electromyography (EMG) (fibrillation and fasciculation potentials, reduced numbers of large motor units). Upper motor neuron signs include hyperreflexia, spasticity, Babinski signs, and spastic dysarthria (with or without pseudobulbar affect). The mixture of these signs in multiple segments of the body (bulbar, cervical, thoracic, lumbosacral) defines the degree of certainty of the diagnosis based on El Escorial criteria.

The incidence of the disease is near 2/100,000 per year. A study from Olmsted county, Minnesota, showed no increasing incidence in the disease [1], though other studies have found this to be true perhaps due to the aging population as the incidence of the disease does increase with age, at least to the age of 85 [2].

B.A. Crum (✉)
Neurology Department, Mayo Clinic, 200 First Street, SW, Rochester, MN 55905, USA
e-mail: crum.brian@mayo.edu

J.G. Burneo et al. (eds.), *Neurology: An Evidence-Based Approach*,
DOI 10.1007/978-0-387-88555-1_9, © Springer Science+Business Media, LLC 2012

Prognosis

The prognosis in ALS is grim. The average life expectancy is around 3 years from symptom onset and 2 years from diagnosis. There are, however, exceptions to this on both ends of the spectrum. Patients are often interested to know if they will be more on the rapid or slow track following diagnosis. This helps with planning and with the overall acceptance of the condition.

Clinical Case Example

A 58-year-old man who presented with dysarthria, then dysphagia beginning 6 months ago, was just diagnosed with ALS. He is beginning to have some mild right hand and arm weakness and some mild spasticity with gait. He inquires as to whether he is more likely to have a faster progression of disease.

Clinical Question

In a newly diagnosed patient with ALS, what factors predict a slower or faster course?

Search Strategy

PubMed Clinical Queries were used. Prognosis articles for ALS topics were searched. Limits were applied to this as "Human" and "English language." This yielded 284 articles. These were reviewed from most recent onward. The most recent article that addressed this question with suitable methodology (population-based as opposed to specialty clinic-based) was selected. Cochrane database was also searched, though no additional articles were found.

Prognosis Study

Zoccolella et al. [3] reviewed the factors that were predictors of prognosis in ALS patients. These cases were derived from a population-based registry of ALS patients in Southern Italy who were diagnosed in 1998 or 1999. One hundred and thirty new cases were identified and most were followed in the local ALS clinics. The features of these patients matched generally well with the expected demographics and initial symptoms in large ALS populations. The main outcome measure was time from diagnosis to death or mechanical ventilation. A secondary measure was time from symptom onset to death or mechanical ventilation. Variables considered included age, gender, time from first symptoms of ALS diagnosis, localization of symptoms at onset, El Escorial category at entry, riluzole, use, percutaneous endoscopic gastrostomy (PEG) and noninvasive ventilation (NIV), UMN sign predominance, and management by ALS clinic.

Median survival from symptom onset was 27.5 months and from diagnosis 15.7 months. Riluzole was prescribed in 58%, and a minority of patients had PEG, NIV, or tracheostomy. Multivariate analysis showed that advanced age (over 45, especially over 75) and bulbar or generalized onset were the main factors that predicted poorer prognosis – meaning a shorter time from symptom onset or diagnosis to death or mechanical ventilation. Factors that did not seem to predict survival included gender, time to diagnosis, or care in multidisciplinary ALS clinics. There was a borderline-significant longer survival time for those with predominant UMN involvement. The median survival time from onset in those under 45 was 39.3 months, those with spinal onset 34.2 months, and those with UMN predominance 45.2 months. This was a sound study with solid enrollment and follow-up.

Mandrioli et al. [4] performed a study in ALS patients in an Italian province with diagnoses between 1989 and 1998 using a variety of methods of ascertainment. Time to death (from symptom onset) was the outcome measure (or time to study end). Factors, including gender, age, form of ALS, area of residence in the province, and type of work, were analyzed. The median survival in the 123 patients was 29 months. Features that predicted faster progression included age of 75, bulbar or upper limb involvement at onset, residence in mountainous areas, and agricultural work. Those less than 60 years of age and with lower limb symptoms at onset had the slowest progression. Multivariate analysis was not done.

Clinical Bottom Lines

1. Average survival in ALS is about 2–2.5 years from time of symptom onset.
2. Factors that predict slower progression include younger age (less than 45 and perhaps even less than 60) and lack of bulbar onset of symptoms.
3. Younger patients, those with lower limb onset, and those with UMN predominate signs at onset tend to have slower progression.

Summary

Two population-based studies outlined the factors predictive of a worse outcome (i.e., shorter survival) in ALS patients. The methodology was sound, though there was not a detailed account (in the first study) of how complete ascertainment was reached, only that "several sources of information" were used to identify ALS patients. There was no comment regarding the inclusion or exclusion of familial ALS cases. In the second study, no multivariate analysis was done as it was felt that there would not be enough power (patient numbers) to make meaningful conclusions. The follow-up was at least 5 years in the first study and only 1 year in the second study; this could have reduced the ability to draw conclusions regarding survival, especially in the second study. The studies' conclusions are consistent with other prognosis studies that have been published and help to provide information to counsel patients.

Treatment

ALS is a rapidly progressive disease which leads to skeletal muscle weakness, dysarthria, dysphagia, and respiratory insufficiency. Treatment of the disease, thus, is multifactorial. As no cure exists, much of the treatment is management of these eventual complications of the disease. Rehabilitation medicine is important for issues of mobility, transferring, pain, and upper extremity use. Speech therapists assist with communicative devices. Speech and occupational therapists assist in the evaluation and treatment of dysphagia – from initial changes in types of food eaten to eventual placement of a feeding tube (PEG) if desired by a patient. Respiratory insufficiency is initially treated with NIV in the form of a BiPAP or CPAP with the eventual decision for or against mechanical ventilation. Treatment also encompasses the spiritual and emotional needs of the patient and the family/caregivers and ultimately, many need the services of a hospice team.

Pharmacological treatment of ALS boils down to symptomatic treatment of complications (such as tricyclic antidepressants for sialorrhea) and disease-modifying therapies. Of the latter, many medications and supplements have been studied with only riluzole being found to be effective, though only modestly so. Randomized, double-blind, placebo trials are ongoing of multiple therapies in ALS with the hope (and expectation) that there will be more positive results.

Clinical Question

In patients with ALS, does treatment with riluzole lead to increased survival?

Search Strategy

In PubMed, the following search string was used: "ALS and riluzole and survival." This was limited to English language, humans, and randomized, controlled studies. This yielded nine articles, including the original riluzole study of 1994. In addition, a search of the Cochrane database using the search "ALS and riluzole" yielded a review on this topic which discussed three randomized, controlled studies of riluzole in treatment of ALS.

Treatment Studies

Bensimon et al. [5] conducted a randomized, double-blinded, controlled study in the use of riluzole (50 mg twice a day) in patients with ALS. Patients were 20–75 with probably or definite ALS. Patients were excluded if they had symptoms of the disease for more than 5 years, had a vital capacity below 60% predicted, or had dementia. Patients were stratified into limb or bulbar onset disease and were followed for the main outcome measure of tracheostomy-free survival at 12 months.

A total of 155 patients were studied. At 12 months, 74% of the riluzole-treated patients were alive and 58% of the placebo-treated patients were alive. Overall survival was 449 days in the placebo group and 532 in the riluzole group. This improvement in survival was more pronounced in the bulbar onset group, whereas it was not clearly statistically significant in the limb onset group. The slope of the decline of functional scores was also slowed in the riluzole group.

Patients tolerated riluzole well with the main adverse affects leading to medication stoppage being increasing asthenia, nausea, stiffness, and elevation of liver enzymes (AST or ALT). No serious adverse events were noted related to the medication.

In the Cochrane review [6], a pooled analysis of three randomized, controlled studies was performed and the overall length of survival in treated versus placebo groups was 14.8 months compared to 11.8 months; a 3-month increase in survival.

Clinical Bottom Lines

1. Riluzole prolongs ventilator-free survival by about 3 months and increases the likelihood of surviving 1 year by 40%.
2. The largest benefit was seen in the bulbar onset ALS patients.
3. Riluzole was tolerated well, though liver enzymes need to be monitored and patients need to be questioned about increasing asthenia and stiffness.

Summary

The initial randomized, controlled study of riluzole in ALS was methodologically sound study. Several issues, though, must be raised. First, 24 patients were enrolled who originally did not meet inclusion/exclusion criteria in their entirety, though post-hoc analysis showed that they did not influence the final results. There was a high dropout rate in the riluzole-treated group (25%) – this may have actually diluted the treatment effect. Patients were also on average 2.3 years into their disease (from symptom onset), which may indicate a later stage of the disease. Today, it takes about 1 year to secure a diagnosis of ALS, therefore whether treatment at an earlier stage would be more beneficial is not known.

Diabetic Peripheral Neuropathy

Introduction

Distal symmetric polyneuropathy is the most common peripheral neuromuscular disorder encountered in neurologic practice. Although numerous etiologies may be associated with distal symmetric polyneuropathy, the cause is unknown in approximately 40–70% of cases, despite extensive evaluations [7–9]. The evaluation of patients with symptoms of neuropathy includes assessment for general medical diseases, endocrine disorders, vitamin deficiencies, and autoimmune disorders. Diabetes is the most commonly identified acquired cause of peripheral neuropathy, and therefore screening for impaired glucose metabolism or diabetes is a necessary component of a neuropathy evaluation. When identified, treatment of diabetic peripheral neuropathy can be challenging and focuses on prevention of progression and treatment of symptoms. This section provides an evidence-based review of several topics related to the diagnosis and treatment of diabetic peripheral neuropathy.

Diagnosis

Introduction

Peripheral neuropathy is a common manifestation of diabetes. Approximately 45–60% of patients with diabetes develop manifestations of peripheral neuropathy. The most common symptoms are distal, symmetric sensory loss, or paresthesias, often associated with pain. Although neuropathy often occurs well after the development and diagnosis of diabetes, in some instances neuropathic symptoms may occur early in the course of the disease or even begin prior to the development of impaired glucose metabolism. In these cases, what may be initially considered as "idiopathic" or "cryptogenic" peripheral neuropathy may actually be an early diabetic neuropathy. The presence of neuropathic symptoms prior to the development of diabetes in some patients suggests that the mechanisms involved in the development of diabetic peripheral neuropathy are likely more than directly related to the length and degree of hyperglycemia. However, poor glycemic control increases the risk of complications of diabetes, such as retinopathy or cardiovascular disease, and therefore optimal management of hyperglycemia with intensive glycemic control is necessary to reduce diabetic complications. Therefore, optimal screening is necessary to identify the earliest stages of diabetes in patients presenting with peripheral neuropathy. Several tests are used to screen for impaired glucose metabolism, including fasting serum glucose and the 2-h oral glucose tolerance test (OGTT). Recently, the American Diabetes Association (ADA) revised the criteria for the diagnosis of impaired glucose tolerance (IGT) and diabetes mellitus, lowering the threshold for levels of glucose considered to be abnormal [10]. In order to optimize the diagnosis and management of patients presenting with early diabetic peripheral neuropathy, the treating physician must select the most useful test to identify impaired glucose metabolism.

Clinical Case Example

A 62-year-old right-handed male presents with a 6-month history of numbness, tingling, and pain in both of his feet. The symptoms began gradually and have slowly spread to his ankles. His examination demonstrates distal sensory loss to pinprick, vibration, and proprioception to his ankles and absent Achilles reflexes. Electrodiagnostic testing demonstrates findings compatible with a distal sensorimotor peripheral neuropathy. As part of the evaluation for etiologies of the neuropathy, screening for diabetes is considered. The physician is considering whether a fasting serum glucose or a 2-h OGTT would be preferable to screen for diabetes as part of the patient's neuropathy evaluation.

Clinical Question

Is a 2-h OGTT more useful than fasting plasma glucose as a screen for impaired glucose tolerance or early diabetes in the evaluation of peripheral neuropathy?

Search Strategy

Ovid MEDLINE database was searched for the time period of January 1990 to May, Week 3, 2009. Medical Subject Heading (MeSH) term "diabetes" combined with the Boolean "AND" "neuropathy" yielded 7,331 articles. Similarly, a search for the term "glucose tolerance test" combined with the Boolean "AND" "fasting glucose" yielded 1,172 articles. Combining these two searches yielded eight citations. From this set, three articles specifically addressed neuropathy. Two articles were selected, one by Singleton et al. [11] and one by Hoffman-Snyder et al. [12] as they represented the only studies which specifically compared the utility of fasting glucose and the glucose tolerance testing in patients presenting with neuropathy. PubMed and the Cochrane Library databases were also searched implementing the same strategy of MeSH terms and keywords. No additional relevant articles were detected.

DM Screening

Two recent studies addressed the value of the OGTT in the evaluation of patients with diabetes. Singleton et al. prospectively evaluated 107 sequential patients with idiopathic peripheral neuropathy to identify the presence of impaired fasting glucose

Table 9.1 Comparison of the frequency of abnormal glucose metabolism in patients with idiopathic peripheral neuropathy

Study	Number of subjects	Impaired glucose tolerance	Diabetes mellitus
Novella et al. [14]	48	13 (27%)	11 (23%)
Singleton et al. [11]	72	36 (50%)	13 (18%)
Sumner et al. [15]	73	26 (36%)	15 (20%)
Hoffman-Snyder et al. [12]	100	38 (38%)	24 (24%)

(IFG) or IGT using 1997 ADA criteria. Fasting plasma glucose was assessed in 105 of 107 patients and the 2-h OGTT was only performed in 72 of 107 patients. The OGTT was not performed at the same institution in all patients; some patients had the study performed by their primary care physician at different locations. The method of performance of the OGTT was not described. Of the 72 patients in whom both fasting glucose test and 2-h OGTT were performed, 34 (50%) had evidence of IGT on OGTT (defined by 2-h glucose of ≥140 but <200), but not with fasting glucose. Only three (4%) patients were found to have impaired fasting glucose without IGT on OGTT. The mean age and body mass index (BMI) were similar among the patients with IGT, diabetes, and those with normal tests of glucose metabolism. Patients with diabetes and neuropathy were found to be significantly more likely to have a family history of diabetes than those with IGT or normal glucose testing.

In a second study, Hoffman-Snyder et al. retrospectively reviewed 100 consecutive patients with symptoms of peripheral neuropathy over a 24-month period. All patients underwent a fasting glucose level as well as a 2-h OGTT with a 75-g oral D-glucose (dextrose) load, both performed at a single institution. Revised 2003 ADA criteria were used to classify patients with "impaired fasting glucose" (plasma glucose >100 and <126 mg/dL), "IGT" (2-h glucose >140 and <200 mg/dL), or "new onset diabetes" (fasting plasma glucose >126 mg/dL or 2-h glucose >200 mg/dL) [12]. Of the 100 patients, 39% of patients had abnormal fasting plasma glucose metabolism, whereas 62% had abnormal glucose metabolism when assessed with the OGTT. Using the 2003 ADA criteria, the frequency of identifying abnormal glucose metabolism in chronic idiopathic neuropathy by the 2-h OGTT was significantly higher using the OGTT than fasting plasma glucose levels (p 0.001, 95% confidence interval (CI) 10–35%). The study compared the prevalence of undiagnosed glucose metabolism in patients presenting with neuropathy (62%) with previously published, age-matched prevalence rates (33%) in the general population, and found a nearly twofold higher rate in the neuropathy patients [13]. The study additionally characterized the neuropathy into three subtypes (sensorimotor, pure sensory, and small fiber) and found that abnormal glucose metabolism rates were similar among the three subtypes.

A comparison of the frequency of abnormal glucose metabolism in these studies with several other published studies (that did not directly compare fasting plasma glucose with the OGTT is shown in Table 9.1.

Clinical Bottom Lines

1. Using the 2003 ADA criteria for determining abnormal fasting glucose metabolism in patients presenting with distal symmetric peripheral neuropathy of unknown etiology, the 2-h OGTT is a more sensitive measure of abnormal glucose metabolism than fasting plasma glucose.
2. Up to 62% of patients with peripheral neuropathy may have evidence of IGT or diabetes using the 2-h OGTT.

Summary

Each of these studies had several methodological limitations. The study by Singleton et al. prospectively identified the prevalence of IGT in patients with peripheral neuropathy using older (1997) ADA criteria, and their findings indicated that the OGTT was more sensitive than the fasting serum glucose. However, not all patients were administered both tests of glucose metabolism, the tests were not administered at the same institution, and no mention was made regarding the uniformity of the method of performance of the OGTT.

The study by Hoffman-Snyder et al. was retrospective in nature and the inclusion criteria required that the patients had undergone a 2-h OGTT. Four hundred and sixty two patients were screened and excluded from the study for a variety of reasons. However, there was no mention of how many were excluded because the 2-h OGTT was not performed. Therefore, the 100 consecutive patients in whom the 2-h OGTT was performed may have demonstrated features (such as a high BMI) that led the investigators to perform the test and may have skewed the data toward a higher prevalence rate.

Both studies compared the prevalence of undiagnosed abnormal fasting glucose metabolism in the neuropathy patients studied with the prevalence reported in an age-matched population, and control groups were not directly studied. Thus, comparison of the prevalence of abnormal fasting glucose in neuropathy patients to the population can only be made indirectly. When comparing the prevalence rates with the published rates for the general population in cross-sectional studies, factors such as BMI were not controlled for, limiting direct comparison to published population results.

Treatment

Introduction

Treatment of diabetic peripheral neuropathy focuses on two aspects. First, methods are utilized to attempt to slow the progression of the neuropathy. To that extent, optimizing control of the diabetes is frequently considered to have an effect at halting or improving the neuropathy. Second, symptomatic reduction of the neuropathic features, such as pain or paresthesias, is usually the mainstay of treatment. Many different classes of pharmacologic therapies, such as anticonvulsant and antidepressant medications, have been used to reduce neuropathic pain in diabetic neuropathy [16]. Alternative treatments and nutritional supplements, such as alpha-lipoic acid (ALA), have also been used for symptomatic relief [17]. ALA's mechanisms of action may include anti-inflammatory, antioxidant, cytoprotective, and neuroprotective effects, which may favorably influence the underlying pathophysiology of neuropathy and relieve neuropathic pain.

Clinical Case Scenario

A 62-year-old right-handed male with a 3-year history of poorly controlled diabetes presents with a 2-year history of symmetric numbness and burning, stabbing pain in both of his feet. The symptoms began gradually and have slowly spread to his ankles. His examination demonstrates distal sensory loss to pinprick, vibration, and proprioception to his ankles and absent Achilles reflexes. He has previously been prescribed anticonvulsant and antidepressant medications, which had no significant effect in reducing his neuropathic pain. He questions what can be done to stop the progression of his neuropathy and whether there are any alternative medications that can be used to reduce his foot pain.

Clinical Questions

1. Does tight glycemic control in DM prevent peripheral neuropathic complications in diabetic neuropathy?
2. Is ALA effective in treating painful peripheral neuropathy?

Search Strategy

Does tight glycemic control in DM prevent peripheral neuropathic complications in diabetic neuropathy?

Ovid MEDLINE database was searched for the time period of 1994 to May, Week 2, 2009. MeSH term "diabetes" was combined with the Boolean "AND" neuropathy with a yield of 7,326 articles. Similarly, a search for the term "intensive" combined with the Boolean "AND" "therapy" yielded 119 articles. Combining these two searches yielded 30 articles. After limiting the retrieval to English and human, 28 citations were identified. From this set, only three articles specifically addressed neuropathy, two of which were review articles on diabetic neuropathy. An article by the Diabetes Control and Complications Trial Research Group was selected as it represented the only study which specifically evaluated the effect of diabetes therapy on neuropathy [18]. PubMed and the Cochrane Library databases were also searched implementing the same strategy of MeSH terms and keywords. No additional relevant articles were detected.

Is ALA effective in treating painful peripheral neuropathy?

Ovid MEDLINE database was searched for the time period 1966 to May, Week 2, 2009. MEDLINE was searched using MeSH term "thioctic acid" and using text word "alpha-lipoic acid." These searches were combined using the Boolean "OR." In the same manner, MEDLINE was searched using MeSH term "diabetic neuropathies." These two searches were combined using the Boolean "AND." Results were limited to English language and human subjects. Further limits were applied utilizing search filters or strategies for therapy – emphasizing relevance – to locate randomized clinical trials (RCTs). The yield was nine articles. The same terms were searched in the PubMed and Cochrane Library databases, but no additional relevant articles were located. From the set of nine articles, a single, recent, relevant RCT of oral ALA and a relevant systematic review of intravenous ALA were located [19]. The RCT was selected as the best available evidence to answer the clinical question.

The Effect of Glycemic Control in DM in Preventing Peripheral Neuropathic Complications

The Diabetes Control and Complications Trial Research Group performed a prospective, multicenter RCT of 1,441 patients with type 1 diabetes comparing intensive diabetic therapy with three or more daily insulin injections or continuous subcutaneous insulin infusion with conventional therapy of one or two daily insulin injections. Although the major study outcome was the prevention or slowing the progression of diabetic retinopathy, a secondary outcome, and the focus of this publication, was the development and progression of clinically significant peripheral neuropathy. All patients had insulin-dependent diabetes; patients with diabetic neuropathy were not excluded at entry unless the patient or investigator believed that the symptoms were severe enough to warrant treatment. Subjects were divided into a primary prevention group and a secondary intervention group. Patients were randomly assigned by cohort and clinical center to receive either conventional therapy or intensive therapy for diabetes. No additional information regarding the method of randomization was available.

Patients were followed to assess the effect of the diabetes therapy on the development of clinical neuropathy, diagnosed by history or physical examination features along with nerve conduction study or autonomic testing abnormalities. Neurologic examination was performed by neurologists masked to treatment assignment. The primary neurologic end point was defined as the development of "confirmed clinical neuropathy" (abnormal neurologic examination and either abnormal nerve conduction studies or autonomic testing). Secondary neurologic end points included clinical (without electrophysiologic) neuropathy and subclinical neuropathy. Statistical analysis to compare variables among the groups were performed, and the percentage risk reduction of intensive therapy compared with conventional therapy was calculated.

A total of 1,422 patients completed the study to the end point. The baseline demographic characteristics between the two cohorts were similar although confirmed clinical neuropathy at baseline was 3.5% of the primary prevention cohort and 9.4% of the secondary intervention cohort ($p=0.04$). The data from these patients was excluded in the final analysis of the effect of therapy on the development of neuropathy. Subjects were followed for a mean of 6.5 years (range 3.5–9 years). At 5 years follow-up, the subjects in the primary prevention cohort had a 71% (95% CI 34–87%) risk reduction in developing confirmed clinical neuropathy with intensive therapy compared to conventional therapy. In the secondary intervention cohort, patients who were treated with intensive therapy had a 64% risk reduction in the development of neuropathy (95% CI, 45–76%) [18].

Follow-up of 84 patients who had confirmed clinical neuropathy at baseline found that 42% of those in the intensive therapy group, compared to 56% in the conventional group, continued to meet the criteria for confirmed clinical neuropathy based on clinical symptoms. Therefore, 58% of intensive therapy and 44% of conventional therapy groups had resolution of clinical features of neuropathy. Electrophysiologic findings did not improve, even with improved clinical symptoms.

There have been no large randomized trials that have specifically looked at the effect of tight glycemic control on the development or progression of peripheral neuropathy in patients with type 2 diabetes.

The Utility of Alpha-Lipoic Acid in Treating Painful Peripheral Neuropathy

The Symptomatic Diabetic Neuropathy (SYDNEY) 2 was a four-arm, parallel-group, randomized, double-blinded, placebo-controlled, multicenter trial of three oral doses of ALA (600 mg, 1,200 mg, and 1,800 mg) in patients with symptomatic, diabetic distal symmetric polyneuropathy. The details of the referral patterns and the methods for randomization and concealment were not explained. Inclusion criteria included patients between 18 and 74 years with type 1 or 2 diabetes mellitus of at least 1 year's duration, an HbA1c <10%, symptomatic DSP attributable to diabetes, a total symptom score (TSS) >7.5 points, neuropathy impairment score (NIS) subscore for lower limbs of >=2 points, presence of neuropathic pain, and reduced or absent sensation on pinprick test. A 1-week run-in phase was used to ensure that eligible subjects were compliant with the medication, continued to be symptomatic, and did not demonstrate a substantial change from baseline scores. The primary end point was the TSS, a summation of the presence, severity, and duration of the four main neuropathic sensory symptoms (lancinating pain, burning, paresthesia, and asleep numbness). This scale ranges from 0 to 14. TSS was assessed at screening, baseline, and after 1, 2, 3, 4, and 5 weeks of treatment. A treatment difference of 1.83 points of TSS was considered a clinically meaningful change. Neurologic assessments and all scoring were conducted by trained and certified blinded neurologists.

Table 9.2 Efficacy of ALA for treatment of neuropathic symptoms of diabetic DSP. Estimated NNTs, NNHs, and 95% CIs were calculated based on the published data [20]

	Placebo	ALA 600 mg	ALA 1,200 mg	ALA 1,800 mg
≥50% reduction in TSS	26%	62%	50%	56%
		RD=36%	RD=24%	RD=30%
		NNT, (95% CI)	NNT, (95% CI)	NNT, (95% CI)
		2.7 (1.8–5.8)	4.1 (2.3–20.2)	3.2 (2.0–8.6)
Global satisfaction rating; good/very good	29%	62%	56%	71%
		RD=33%	RD=27%	RD=42%
		NNT, (95% CI)	NNT, (95% CI)	NNT, (95% CI)
		3.0 (1.9–7.5)	3.7 (2.1–13.8)	2.4 (1.6–4.3)

From [20]. Reprinted with kind permission from Wolters Kluwer Health
RD Risk difference or ARR (absolute risk reduction), *NNT* Number needed to treat

One hundred and sixty-six patients with symptomatic diabetic neuropathy were assessed. Baseline characteristics of the subjects in the four arms (43 placebo, 45 ALA600, 47 ALA1200, and 56 ALA1800) did not differ significantly, apart from treatment with oral hypoglycemic agents and BMI. Overall, the subjects' mean age was 58 years, 40% male, 83% type 2 diabetes mellitus, mean duration of diabetes 14 years, mean HbA1c 7.7%, and mean duration of neuropathy 4.9 years. An intention-to-treat analysis demonstrated a statistically significant and nondose-dependent response rate (all $p < 0.05$), consisting of a greater than 50% reduction in TSS after 5 weeks that was 62% for ALA600, 50% for ALA1200, and 56% for ALA1800 versus 26% for placebo. The reduction was significant for the lancinating and burning pain subsets of the TSS. Patient self-rated global estimates of efficacy were good or very good in 62% for ALA600, 56% for ALA1200, 71% for ALA1200, and 29% for placebo (Table 9.2).

Of the 181 randomized patients, 15 discontinued during the treatment period (1/43 in placebo arm and 14/138 in the ALA arms) mostly due to adverse events. Adverse effects, including nausea (0, 13, 21, and 48%), vomiting (0, 2, 4, and 26%), and vertigo (0, 4, 4, and 11%) were experienced in placebo, ALA600, ALA1200, and ALA1800, respectively (Table 9.3).

Clinical Bottom Lines

Does tight glycemic control in DM prevent peripheral neuropathic complications in diabetic neuropathy?

1. Optimal glycemic control can prevent the development of peripheral neuropathy in patients with type 1 diabetes. With intensive treatment to optimize glycemic control, there is a 64% (95% CI, 45–76%)–71% (95% CI 34–87%) risk reduction in the development of neuropathy after 5 years.
2. In treatment-naive type 1 diabetic patients with confirmed clinical neuropathy, optimal glycemic control can reduce the symptoms of peripheral neuropathy.

Table 9.3 Tolerability of ALA for treatment of neuropathic symptoms of diabetic DSP [20]

	Placebo	ALA 600 mg	ALA 1,200 mg	ALA 1,800 mg
Treatment-emergent adverse events	21%	27% RD=6% NNH, (95% CI) 16.6 NS	43% RD=22% NNH, (95% CI) 4.5 (2.4–31.0)	54% RD=33% NNH, (95% CI) 3.0 (1.9–7.1)
Nausea	0%	13% RD=13% NNH, (95% CI) 7.7 (4.3–33.9)	21% RD=21% NNH, (95% CI) 4.8 (3.0–11.3)	22% RD=22% NNH, (95% CI) 4.6 (2.9–10.4)
Vomiting	0%	2% RD=2% NNH, (95% CI) 50 NS	4% RD=4% NNH, (95% CI) 25 NS	26% RD=26% NNH, (95% CI) 3.8 (2.6–7.8)
Vertigo	0%	4% RD=4% NNH, (95% CI) 25 NS	4% RD=4% NNH, (95% CI) 25 NS	11% RD=11% NNH, (95% CI) 9.1 (4.9–60.7)
Treatment cessation due to adverse events	2%	0% NS	11% RD=9% NNH, (95% CI) 11 NS	13% RD=11% NNH, (95% CI) 9.1 (4.6–608.5)

From: [20]. Reprinted with kind permission from Wolters Kluwer Health
RD Risk difference, *NNH* Number needed to harm, *NS* Not statistically significant

There is a 14% risk reduction in continuation of clinical symptoms of neuropathy with intensive therapy compared to conventional therapy. However, changes in electrophysiologic testing may not improve despite clinical improvement.

3. The effect of optimal glycemic control on the development of peripheral neuropathy in patients with type 2 diabetes is unknown.

Is ALA effective in treating painful peripheral neuropathy?

1. Oral ALA in doses of 600, 1,200, and 1,800 mg are all effective in reducing neuropathic symptoms of diabetic peripheral neuropathy as assessed by the TSS (>=50% reduction), with NNTs (95% CI) of 2.7 (1.8–5.8), 4.1 (2.3–20.2), and 3.2 (2.0–8.6), respectively [20].
2. Oral ALA in doses of 600, 1,200, and 1,800 mg are all effective in providing good/very good patient self-rated global satisfaction, with NNTs (95% CI) of 3.0 (1.9–7.5), 3.7 (2.1–13.9), and 2.4 (1.4–4.3), respectively.
3. Adverse events, including nausea, vomiting, and vertigo, were identified but occurred most frequently with ALA doses of 1,200 and 1,800 mg. Overall, treatment-emergent adverse events for ALA 600 mg were not significantly different than placebo, but ALA 1,200 and 1,800 mg had NNHs (95% CI) of 4.5 (2.4–31.0) and 3.0 (1.9–7.1), respectively.
4. The evidence supporting the efficacy of oral ALA is based on a single RCT, and several methodological weaknesses have been identified that may partly erode its validity.

Summary

Intensive glycemic control in type 1 diabetes delays or prevents the development of symptomatic peripheral neuropathy. A multicenter, randomized, prospective study by the Diabetes Control and Complications Trial Research Group using primary prevention and secondary intervention cohorts was performed to compare the effect of intensive metabolic therapy with conventional therapy on the development and progression of chronic diabetic complications. While the initial study primarily focused on the complications of retinopathy and nephropathy, the development of peripheral neuropathy was also assessed and the details of the study that specifically related to peripheral neuropathy were detailed in a separate publication. The study was methodologically sound with few limitations. The study population was limited to patients with type 1 diabetes. Patients were randomized to intensive or conventional therapy groups, and patients' adherence to their assigned treatment groups was high. Patients who were assigned to the intensive therapy group received the assigned therapy during more than 98% of the study, and similarly patients assigned to conventional treatment received the assigned therapy during more than 97% of the study. Investigators and patients were not masked to the treatment assignment, although the investigators who performed the neurologic examination, neurophysiologic studies, and reviewed and graded the outcome data were masked.

   At the end point of the study, the primary outcome was the development of confirmed clinical neuropathy, which consisted of evidence of neuropathy from a clinical and electrophysiologic data. This included the presence of subjective neuropathic symptoms; therefore, "confirmed clinical neuropathy" may have identified only more severe stages of neuropathy. However, the investigators did assess patients with "subclinical neuropathy," based only on abnormal neurophysiologic testing and found a 44% (95% CI 34–53) risk reduction with intensive therapy for patients with only nerve conduction study abnormalities and a 53% (95% CI 24–70) risk reduction for patients with only autonomic testing abnormalities.

   Finally, reversibility of established clinical neuropathy by type of intervention was not well-addressed in the trial. A small number ($n=92$) of patients had clinical neuropathy at study entry. While a smaller percentage of these patients who were treated with intensive therapy continued to have clinical neuropathy after 5 years compared to those who received conventional therapy, statistical analysis is limited due to the sample size.

   Oral ALA may improve neuropathic symptoms in diabetic DSP. A single, modestly valid RCT demonstrated that 600 mg was an effective and well-tolerated dose. The number needed to treat to significantly reduce neuropathic pain over a 5-week period was 2.7. Comparison of ALA with other, commonly used medications for neuropathic pain has not been studied. ALA's role in the treatment of painful diabetic neuropathy remains unclear.

   The study had several methodological limitations. First, it was unclear whether or not the subjects were completely treatment-naive or already refractory to multiple medications for neuropathic pain, and concomitant use of other medications for neuropathic pain during the study was not addressed. Second, the authors made no reference to reliability, validation, or usefulness studies of the TSS, upon which they based their outcome [21]. Additionally, details regarding the blinding process were not provided. Third, the subjects' disease phase was not well-described, and the subjects had variable durations of diabetes and peripheral neuropathy. It is possible that the treatment would be more effective in those with early disease and less irreversible damage. Fourth, follow-up was felt not to be sufficiently long. Although 8% failed to complete the treatment course, there were no subjects lost to follow-up. The authors presented the NNT of 600 mg dose ALA, but did not publish the NNTs or NNHs with corresponding 95% CIs for the other doses.

Inflammatory Myopathies

Introduction

Inflammatory myopathies include the three major disorders, polymyositis (PM), dermatomyositis (DM), and inclusion body myositis (IBM). These diseases differ clinically and pathologically [22, 23]. Several diagnostic criteria have been proposed, relying upon various clinical, laboratory, electrophysiological, and histological features [24–27]. Immunotherapy is the mainstay of treatment for these diseases, but they also differ in their response to treatment with IBM being generally refractory. This chapter subtopic focuses on an evidence-based evaluation of specific issues related to the diagnosis and treatment of inflammatory myopathies.

Diagnosis

Introduction

IBM is the most common muscle disease in patients over the age of 50. It typically presents with slowly progressive proximal and distal anterior compartment weakness with quadriceps atrophy [22, 23, 26]. The clinical presentation can be subtle initially, however, and diagnosis is often delayed. Muscle biopsy is diagnostic and characteristically shows autoaggressive inflammation with invasion of nonnecrotic muscle fibers, vacuolated fibers, and congophilic deposits representing inclusions [26, 28, 29]. In some patients, the clinical presentation is compatible with IBM, but muscle biopsy does not display all diagnostic features.

Clinical Case Example

A 52-year-old man presents with approximately 1.5 years of weakness. He initially noticed difficulty going down stairs, and then rising from low-seated positions. He has been losing muscle mass in his thighs. More recently, he has had problems manipulating small objects with his fingers, buttoning his shirts, and opening doors. Physical examination demonstrates bilateral thigh atrophy. There is moderate weakness of knee extension and finger flexion, and mild weakness of elbow flexion and ankle dorsiflexion. CK is elevated at 460 U/L. Electrodiagnostic testing shows findings of a myopathy with fibrillation potentials in weak muscles, and long duration motor unit potentials are seen in the thigh muscles. His physician discusses the clinical suspicion for IBM and recommends a muscle biopsy to confirm the diagnosis. The patient asks what happens if the biopsy does not show what the physician is looking for. He also asks that if the physician's suspicions are confirmed, is there any treatment.

Clinical Question

How useful is a muscle biopsy that does not display characteristic features of IBM in making the diagnosis of IBM?

Search Strategy

Ovid MEDLINE database was searched for the time period from 1950 to May, Week 3, 2009. MeSH terms "inclusion body myositis" (yield 539 articles), "muscle biopsy" (yield 5,069 articles), and "correlation" (yield 395,224 articles) were searched and combined using the Boolean "AND." This yielded a single article by Chahin and Engel [30]. This was considered too restrictive and the search was extended to include the MeSH terms "inclusion body myositis" and "muscle biopsy" combined using the Boolean "AND." After limiting the retrieval to English language and human subjects, the yield was 68 articles. After title and abstract review of this set, the same article by Chahin and Engel and an article by Dahlbom et al. [31] were selected as they specifically addressed the correlation between specific muscle biopsy findings and diagnosis of IBM in cohorts of patients with clinical or pathological features of IBM. PubMed and the Cochrane Library databases were also searched utilizing the same strategy of MeSH terms. No additional relevant articles were found.

Biopsy

The two studies identified address muscle biopsy findings in patients thought to have IBM. Dahlbom et al. retrospectively studied muscle biopsies from 43 patients diagnosed with "definite" IBM according to morphological criteria, including (1) inflammatory cell invasion of nonnecrotic muscle fibers, (2) presence of "rimmed" vacuoles, and (3) intracytoplasmic inclusions identified by electron microscopy or on Congo Red stain, as delineated by Griggs et al. [26]. All 43 patients had at least one biopsy fulfilling all three morphological criteria. Nineteen patients had a single biopsy, nine had two biopsies from different muscles on a single occasion, and three of these patients and 15 others had two or more biopsies at different times. In total,

86 muscle biopsies were analyzed. The study focused only on cumulative biopsy findings in a cohort of patients with biopsy-proven IBM. Nineteen of eighty-six biopsies failed to fulfill criteria 1 and 2; in 14 autoaggressive inflammation was absent, in nine vacuolated fibers were absent, and in four both autoaggressive inflammation and vacuolated fibers were absent. Therefore, at least 22% of muscle biopsies failed to demonstrate confirmatory muscle biopsy findings of IBM (sensitivity 78%). The authors also mention that vacuolated fibers were least likely to be found in biopsies taken from the deltoid muscle, and most likely in those taken from the vastus lateralis and tibialis anterior muscles. Of the 18 patients who underwent two biopsies on different occasions, ten showed different features, but the authors do not specify whether the second biopsy was confirmatory in cases where the first was not.

In a second study, Chahin and Engel retrospectively examined clinical information and muscle biopsy findings in 107 patients diagnosed with PM or IBM on muscle biopsy. Criteria for the diagnosis of IBM included clinical and pathological features, including (1) slowly progressive weakness with specific weakness in the finger flexors and/or quadriceps muscles, (2) EMG findings, (3) vacuolated fibers, (4) autoaggressive inflammation, and (5) congophilic deposits. Utilizing these criteria, the authors identified a group of patients (16/107, 15%) with clinical features of IBM but pathological features of PM, termed PM/IBM. This group was similar to the group of patients fulfilling criteria for IBM in age at disease onset, mean duration of symptoms, distribution of weakness, serum CK level, and lack of response to immunotherapy, but similar to the PM group in gender distribution. Invasion of nonnecrotic fibers was more common in IBM and PM/IBM patients than PM patients. Furthermore, cytochrome c oxidase negative fibers were seen in 63/64 IBM patients and all 16 PM/IBM patients, but only 20/27 PM patients. Thus, the combined absence of nonnecrotic fibers invaded by inflammatory cells and of cytochrome c oxidase negative fibers may provide some evidence against IBM or PM/IBM. Three PM/IBM patients underwent repeat biopsies, none of which showed features diagnostic of IBM. The authors emphasize that muscle biopsy is not flawless in its ability to diagnose IBM, that it is necessary to exclude other diagnoses in the patient suspected clinically to have IBM, and that the ultimate diagnosis must rely not only on morphological criteria but on clinical and electrodiagnostic criteria as well.

Clinical Bottom Lines

1. False-negative muscle biopsies occur in patients with IBM, some possibly related to muscle biopsy site selection (sensitivity 78%).
2. Certain features on muscle biopsy, such as the presence of prominent inflammatory cell invasion of nonnecrotic fibers and cytochrome c oxidase negative fibers, although not specific, provide evidence supporting the diagnosis while their absence raises the possibility of an alternate diagnosis.
3. A muscle biopsy that does not fulfill classic criteria for IBM is insufficient to exclude the diagnosis and should be interpreted in the context of clinical and electrodiagnostic findings.

Summary

Muscle biopsy is clearly accepted as indicated in the diagnosis of IBM. There is the possibility of a nondiagnostic muscle biopsy in the evaluation of any patient with a possible muscle disease. Studies investigating not just the characteristics, but the utility of muscle biopsies and issues surrounding nonconfirmatory muscle biopsies, are difficult to interpret, particularly when investigating the lack of salient features required for a diagnosis. In some disorders, there are no established diagnostic criteria or the criteria are disputed. Muscle biopsies are susceptible to sampling error which may be due to selectivity of muscle involvement, the patchy nature of pathological abnormalities, or variability in the timing of development of abnormalities. Nonetheless, the studies presented confirm that nondiagnostic biopsies occur in patients both with definite IBM (possibly due to muscle biopsy site selection) and in patients who clinically behave as having IBM. Therefore, when counseling a patient with clinical features of IBM but a nonconfirmatory biopsy, the clinician must explain this fact, must look for certain clues in the biopsy that support but do not confirm the diagnosis, and must discuss the potential need for a repeat muscle biopsy.

Treatment

Introduction

Although the exact etiologies of the inflammatory myopathies are unknown, autoimmune bases are presumed. Therefore, treatment rests on immune suppression and immune modulation. The goal is to arrest progression, induce remission, and avoid complications of the disease. Various medications and regimens have been utilized in the different inflammatory myopathies with varying success [23, 32, 33]. In PM and DM, corticosteroids serve as first-line therapy and most patients respond to treatment. Some patients, however, do not respond to corticosteroids, relapse while on corticosteroids, or develop intolerable side effects or complications during treatment. Therefore, alternative noncorticosteroid agents are necessary adjuncts to or replacements of corticosteroid therapy. Some agents are potentially toxic and long-term risks are not always fully established. Some patients also become refractory to even noncorticosteroid agents. In general, PM and DM are responsive to immunotherapy, but IBM is not (despite the findings of autoaggressive inflammation on muscle biopsy) [23, 32, 33]. Intravenous immunoglobulin (IVIG) is a pooled human plasma-derived product with a range of immunomodulating effects [34]. It has been shown to be beneficial in treating a range of autoimmune diseases, and may have a positive effect on the inflammatory myopathies.

Clinical Case Example

A 36-year-old woman presents with 3 months of subacutely progressive proximal muscle weakness. She has had about 4 months of dry cracked cuticles and a photosensitive rash on her scalp, malar region, shoulders, chest, and thighs. Three weeks ago, she started choking on solids and liquids and has lost 7 pounds of weight. Three days ago, she was admitted to the hospital with shortness of breath. CK was 760 U/L. EMG demonstrated fibrillation potentials in weak muscles and small, rapidly recruited motor unit potentials. Muscle biopsy showed findings compatible with dermatomyositis. She was started on prednisone 2.5 months ago, and azathioprine and then methotrexate were added as she worsened. She and her family ask if there is anything more "powerful" she can be given.

Clinical Questions

1. Is IVIG an effective treatment in DM?
2. Is IVIG an effective treatment in IBM?

Search Strategy

Ovid MEDLINE database was searched for the time period from 1950 to May, Week 3, 2009. MeSH terms "dermatomyositis" (yield 5,320 articles) and "IVIG" (yield 7,121 articles) were searched and combined using the Boolean "AND." After limiting the retrieval to English language and human subjects, the yield was 97 articles. Following title and abstract review of this set, a single double-blind, randomized, placebo-controlled trial of IVIG as treatment in DM by Dalakas et al. was selected [35]. PubMed and the Cochrane Library databases were also searched utilizing the same strategy of MeSH terms. No additional relevant articles were found.

Ovid MEDLINE database was searched for the time period from 1950 to May, Week 3, 2009. MeSH terms "inclusion body myositis" (yield 540 articles) and "IVIG" (yield 7,121 articles) were searched and combined using the Boolean "AND." After limiting the retrieval to English language and human subjects, the yield was 25 articles. Following title and abstract review of this set, three double-blind, randomized, placebo-controlled trials of IVIG in the treatment of IBM were identified [36–38]. One of these was excluded because it assessed the treatment effect of IVIG given with high-dose prednisone rather than IVIG alone [38]. Two trials were crossover studies [36, 37]. PubMed and the Cochrane Library databases were also searched utilizing the same strategy of MeSH terms. No additional relevant articles were found.

IVIG in DM

A single double-blind, randomized, placebo-controlled trial by Dalakas et al. has assessed the effectiveness of IVIG in DM [35]. Fifteen patients were block randomized according to disease severity, eight to the treatment arm, and seven to the placebo arm. All were deemed to be treatment resistant, defined as unresponsive or poorly responsive to corticosteroids or "therapeutic doses" of other immune suppressants for at least 4–6 months. IVIG was infused monthly for 3 months at a dose of 2 g/kg divided into two doses given over 2 days. After a washout period of 1 month, four patients crossed over to the placebo arm and four to the treatment arm for another 3 months. Prior immune suppression was left unchanged throughout the study. All patients were followed for up to 3 months after their final infusion. Improvement was considered "major" if neuromuscular symptom scores and MRC scores improved by 5 or more grades each and mild if they improved by 2–4 grades each. Five patients with major improvement also had repeat muscle biopsies performed.

During the randomized phase, patients were relatively well-matched. The treatment group had a statistically significant improvement in muscle strength ($p < 0.018$) and neuromuscular symptoms ($p < 0.035$). Five patients with severe weakness had major improvement. Their mean MRC score increased by 12 grades, mean neuromuscular symptom score by 14 grades, and ADL scores increased to 100. Two patients in the treatment arm had mild improvement with a mean MRC score increase of 2.5 grades and a mean neuromuscular symptom score increase of 4 grades. One patient remained unchanged. The placebo group had no change. Three patients worsened with a mean MRC score decrease of 3 grades and mean neuromuscular score decrease of 5 grades. Two patients had no change, and two had mild improvement with mean MRC and neuromuscular score increases of 2.5.

During the crossover phase, patients crossing to the placebo arm either worsened or remained stable. The patients not crossing over to the placebo arm all lost the beneficial effect of the therapy. The patients crossing over to the treatment arm all had major improvement.

Improvement with treatment was seen 2 weeks after the first infusion, and maximal improvement occurred mostly after the second infusion. Eight treated patients had marked improvement in their rash and their serum CK levels were reduced. Patients receiving placebo saw no improvement in CK levels, and in patients crossing over to the placebo arm serum CK returned to baseline levels after several weeks. IVIG treatment was well-tolerated, and beneficial effects outweighed side effects for those treated.

Repeat muscle biopsies following treatment all showed improvement of histological abnormalities. There was a mean increase in muscle fiber diameter ($p < 0.04$), absence of inflammatory infiltrates other than sparse CD8+ cells in two biopsies, mean capillary number increased and capillary mean diameter decreased ($p < 0.01$), and the muscle fiber to capillary ratio increased and normalized in three patients.

IVIG in IBM

Two double-blind, randomized, placebo-controlled trials have assessed the effectiveness of IVIG in IBM. The first, by Dalakas et al., included 22 patients who were block randomized according to disease severity [36]. Three patients failed to complete the study and 19 patients were analyzed, nine in the treatment arm and ten in the placebo arm. Data on the three patients not analyzed were not published. Study design was comparable to that described in the study presented in the previous section, performed by the same group. All patients crossed over, except one patient initially randomized to the treatment arm. The primary outcome measure was the modified MRC scale (maximum score = 200), and strength was also assessed by the Maximum Voluntary Isometric Contraction (MVIC) method in 11 patients. Ultrasound swallowing was used to assess bulbar function, and swallowing function was examined using a patient questionnaire, oromotor examination, videofluoroscopy, and ultrasound swallowing, although ultrasound swallowing was used for statistical analysis. Patients also assessed their therapy by attempting to specify which therapy they received during which phase, whether they experienced any improvement, to rate overall change, and to define whether any improvement was meaningful. Following the study, a limb-by-limb comparative analysis was undertaken to assess regional muscle function.

During the randomized and crossover phases, no statistically significant changes in MRC or MVIC scores were seen between the two groups. Six individual patients (28%), however, had an MRC score increase of at least 10 points, three following initial randomization to the treatment arm and three following crossover to the treatment arm. In limb-by-limb analysis, there was a statistically significant improvement in some lower extremity muscles ($p < 0.05$), but some muscles continued to worsen. Swallow function as measured as the mean duration of ultrasound swallows in seconds (three dry swallows and three wet swallows) showed a barely significant ($p = 0.05$) improvement when compared to baseline in patients randomized to the treatment arm and when compared to placebo in patients who crossed over to the treatment arm. This data is somewhat conflicting, however, in that for some swallows there was actually improvement after randomization to placebo and worsening when randomized or crossed over to IVIG. Sixteen of nineteen patients correctly defined their treatment phase, and 13 indicated some improvement during IVIG. Six patients reported worsening after crossing over to placebo. Nine patients sought to continue IVIG following the study due to perceived difference in ADLs and quality of life during treatment. Repeat muscle biopsies were performed in patients who responded objectively to IVIG, and there were no qualitative differences seen.

The second paper by Walter et al. also reports a double-blind, randomized, placebo-controlled trial of IVIG in IBM [37]. In this study, 22 patients were block randomized according to disease duration of 6 months of monthly IVIG infusions of 2 g/kg over 2–5 days or placebo, with crossover after the 6 months. One patient in each group refused further treatment after the first study infusion. Nineteen patients had been on prior therapy, and six patients in each group remained on prestudy medication. Included patients had to fulfill clinical and histological criteria for IBM, and muscle biopsy had to be taken within the previous 3 years. Evaluation was by the modified MRC scale (maximum score = 180) at baseline and at 6 and 12 months, comparing changes from baseline between groups and comparing starting and ending points. ADLs were assessed via the Neuromuscular Symptoms and Disability Functional Score (NSS, maximum score = 42). EMG was also done at the same time points, testing three muscles and using abnormal spontaneous activity as a marker for disease activity.

Through the duration of the study, there was a significant mean MRC improvement in strength in both groups ($p = 0.003$), with either stabilization or improvement seen in 90% of patients ($p = 0.001$) but no significant difference between IVIG or placebo treatment periods. There was no difference when analyzing upper and lower limb muscles separately. There was no correlation between response to treatment and serum CK level or extent of inflammation on muscle biopsy. Comparing NSS scores initially to end-of-treatment phase (either at randomization or after crossover), there was a significant improvement in each group ($p < 0.05$). There were also significant differences in NSS scores between treatment and placebo groups at month 6 ($p < 0.05$). There was a trend toward improvement in patient assessment of weakness during treatment only, but without significance. A nonsignificant decline in abnormal spontaneous activity was seen in each group over the 12-month course of the study. In patients with a baseline serum CK >500 U/l at baseline, there was a nonsignificant trend to decreasing levels during treatment only. Following the study, ten patients who elected to remain on therapy and three who did not were available for further follow-up. Both groups lost strength as measured by the MRC scale as compared to the end-of-study evaluation, and this was more marked in the untreated group without reaching significance. The NSS also stabilized in the treated group and worsened in the untreated group without reaching significance.

Clinical Bottom Lines

Is IVIG an effective treatment in DM?
Monthly IVIG at a total dose of 2 g/kg is effective in treatment-resistant DM in improving strength, neuromuscular symptoms, and rash (NNT to prevent a lack of improvement = 2 after randomization, = 1 after crossover, = 2 overall).
Improvement may be seen following the first infusion of IVIG, but patients may require additional infusions to see clear benefit.
IVIG can lead to improvement in muscle biopsy abnormalities.
Is IVIG an effective treatment in IBM?
Monthly IVIG at a total dose of 2 g/kg has not been shown to be significantly effective in improving strength in patients with IBM.
IVIG may have a mild beneficial effect in a minority of individual patients with IBM and may positively affect quality of life, but improvements may be seen

only in certain muscle groups and no factors have been identified to predict the beneficial effect.

IVIG may have a beneficial effect in swallowing function in patients with IBM.

Summary

There is a paucity of blinded, controlled trials investigating specific treatments for the inflammatory myopathies. All of the presented studies have small sample sizes and this limits the ability to generalize conclusions to larger populations of patients. Likewise, the individual and regional improvement seen in some patients cannot be generalized to the larger patient population, but the level of improvement presented can lead to individual functional benefit (although not to a statistically significant degree). In all crossover studies involving IVIG, a lagging treatment effect of IVIG can confound results in the crossover to placebo group which can limit the significance of the findings when compared to the crossover to treatment group. The etiology of the overwhelming patient stability or improvement in the study by Walker et al. as compared to untreated patients historically is unclear – is IVIG implicated, is the study design and the 12 months of physiotherapy provided to be credited, or is there some other undefined difference between this group of patients with IBM and those presented elsewhere? In both studies by Dalakas et al., the definition of "major" improvement is somewhat arbitrary, weakening the argument for significance of effect.

Due to the cost of IVIG and the efforts necessary in its administration, the risk:benefit analysis should be individualized to each patient. It should be considered in patients with DM, particularly those refractory to other treatments. The available data do not support its use in patients with IBM in general. Patients with dysphagia should receive special consideration, however. The single study assessing swallowing function in IBM did find some benefit in some swallowing times (but not in others). There is no mention of symptoms of dysphagia in the patients included in the study, and there is no assessment of improvement or worsening of dysphagia in the patients in the study.

Myasthenia Gravis

Introduction

Myasthenia gravis (MG) is an autoimmune disease that causes muscle weakness and fatigue due to T-cell-dependent, antibody-mediated attack at the neuromuscular junction (NMJ). The majority of patients with MG develop fatiguable, ocular symptoms, such as blurred vision, diplopia, or ptosis. When symptoms remain confined to ocular muscles, a patient is considered to have ocular myasthenia gravis. Patients with generalized MG may develop symptoms, such as fatiguable limb weakness, dysarthria, dysphagia, or dyspnea. These symptoms may develop in conjunction with ocular symptoms, evolve after the development of ocular symptoms, or rarely may occur in the absence of ocular symptoms.

The diagnosis of MG is established through the demonstration of antibodies in the serum to acetylcholine receptors (AChRs) or muscle-specific kinase (MUSK), and through electrodiagnostic testing, including repetitive nerve stimulation (RNS) studies and single-fiber EMG. Treatment is directed toward improving neuromuscular transmission through the use of acetylcholinesterase inhibitors, which increase the availability of acetylcholine at the NMJ and immunomodulating therapy.

Epidemiology

MG is considered to be a relatively rare disease with a complicated epidemiologic profile that has been studied since the 1950s. The epidemiologic profile of MG has changed from the 1950s to the 1990s likely due in part to increased case ascertainment and mortality reduction due to more efficacious, immunomodulatory therapy [39, 40].

Clinical Case Scenario

A 32-year-old female reports a 2-month history of fatiguable diplopia and ptosis. More recently, she has developed fatiguable limb weakness and dysarthria. She reports no other medical problems and has no family history of neurological disease. However, there is a strong family history of autoimmune disease, including thyroid disease in her mother and rheumatoid arthritis in a maternal aunt. Her neurological examination shows fatiguable ptosis and a flaccid dysarthria, with moderately severe facial weakness. Manual muscle strength testing shows moderate weakness of neck flexors and proximal upper limb muscles, with normal deep tendon reflexes and a normal sensory examination. Serologic testing shows normal thyroid function, and elevated AChR antibodies. RNS shows a decrement in accessory and facial compound muscle action potentials.

Clinical Questions

1. What is the incidence of myasthenia gravis?
2. What is the prevalence of myasthenia gravis?

Search Strategy

Ovid MEDLINE database was searched since its inception to June of 2009. MeSH terms "incidence and prevalence" and "myasthenia gravis" were searched and combined using the Boolean "AND." After limiting the retrieval to English and human, 47 items were reviewed. From this set of articles, three articles were reviewed. One systematic review analyzed the incidence and prevalence data from 33 population-based studies [39] while a later study from the same author analyzed the prevalence for an additional 13 studies, but did not report incidence data [41]. A population-based study of incidence and prevalence data in Greece was included in this analysis because it is the single largest population-based study ever reported [40]. For a relatively rare condition, such as MG, larger population-based studies are more likely to provide more accurate epidemiologic data. Unfortunately, this study includes only seropositive cases of MG (does not include seronegative or patients with MUSK antibodies).

It has generally been assumed that MG is a worldwide disease. Epidemiologic studies have been numerous and fairly uniform over time. The majority of these studies are European, however, and certain areas, such as China and Sub-Saharan Africa, have been incompletely studied [41]. Furthermore, none of the population-based studies have been sufficient to identify racial or ethnic differences in MG prevalence [41].

Incidence

An analysis of 33 population-based studies performed worldwide from 1950 to 1995 reported a cumulative, worldwide incidence of 4.6 per million from studies reported in the 1980s [39]. This incidence was slightly higher than that of 2.1 per million reported in studies from the 1950s. This increase in incidence has been attributed to improvement in diagnostic capabilities, resulting in higher case ascertainment. Incidence figures have been fairly uniform worldwide, though higher incidence rates were reported in some areas, such as Virginia and Cyprus. In the single largest study to date of seropositive myasthenia gravis patients identified in Greece, the incidence of MG was 4.80 per million, comparable to other studies [40].

Prevalence

Two studies reviewed worldwide prevalence data from population-based studies reported from 1950 to 1995 [39] and from 1989 to 2002 [41]. Based upon these studies, it is clear that the prevalence of MG has increased over time from a worldwide cumulative prevalence rate of 22.2 per million in the 1950s to 93.9 per million from studies in the 1990s through 2002. This increase in prevalence has outpaced the increase in MG incidence over time and has been attributed to increased survival, in addition to increasing longevity of the general population [41].

The prevalence of seropositive MG in Greece was similar at 70.6 per million (a total of 746 cases) in 1997 [40].

Clinical Bottom Lines

1. The incidence of MG is approximately 4 per million people, and appears fairly uniform worldwide. There are, however, areas with higher incidence rates. Incidence rates have increased over time, likely resulting from improved diagnostic capabilities.
2. The prevalence rate of MG is approximately 93.9 per million people, and has increased steadily over time since the first reported epidemiologic studies on MG in the 1950s.

Summary

There have been a large number of population-based studies of MG that have provided valuable epidemiologic information. A number of limitations in these studies, however, suggest the need for further research. Some areas of the globe have not been studied. Racial or ethnic differences have not been well-studied in population-based studies. Population-based studies of MUSK-positive MG patients have been incompletely studied.

Diagnosis

The diagnosis of MG can be challenging due to a number of factors. Typical MG symptoms, such as fatigue and weakness, can also be seen in a host of other general medical and neurological conditions. A thoughtful history and careful neurological examination are crucial in the initial evaluation of the patient with suspected MG. A history of fluctuating, fatiguable limb weakness and fatiguable ocular or bulbar symptoms would suggest possible MG. The presence of significant pain, sensory loss, or symptoms of bowel or bladder impairment should prompt consideration of an alternate condition. Neurological examination findings of ataxia, sensory loss, or upper motor neuron signs are not expected in MG.

In a patient with suspected MG, antibodies against AChRs provide laboratory confirmation of MG. A minority of patients with otherwise typical clinical and electrodiagnostic findings of MG do not have AChR antibodies in their serum, but may have antibodies to MUSK. A small minority of patients have no demonstrable antibodies to either ACh or MUSK and are considered to have seronegative MG. EMG is performed to rule out other conditions, to prove the existence of an NMJ disorder, and to characterize the nature and severity of the condition. RNS of peripheral motor nerves is the primary EMG method to establish the presence of an NMJ disorder, but may be normal in up to 40% of patients with MG. In such cases, single-fiber EMG is performed in order to establish the presence of an NMJ disorder.

Clinical Questions

1. What is the sensitivity of ACh antibodies in the diagnosis of MG?
2. What is the sensitivity of single-fiber EMG in the diagnosis of MG?

Search Strategy

Ovid MEDLINE database was utilized, with MeSH terms "myasthenia gravis" (yield 12,723 articles), "acetylcholine" (yield 71,636 articles), and "autoantibodies" (yield 55,918 articles). These terms were searched and combined using the Boolean "AND." After limiting the retrieval to English and human, the yield was 1,046 citations. Two articles were chosen, an article by Koon Ho Chan et al. reporting the sensitivity of AChR antibody testing generalized MG [42] and an article by Husain et al. reporting AChR antibody sensitivity in ocular MG [43]. EMBASE, PubMed, and Cochrane Library databases were also searched using the same search strategy, and no additional articles were identified.

Ovid MEDLINE database was utilized, with MeSH terms "myasthenia gravis" (yield 12,723 articles) and electromyography (yield 57,578 articles). These terms were searched and combined using the Boolean "AND." After limiting the retrieval to English and human, the yield was 447 citations. Three articles were selected, including an article by Ho et al., which was a prospective study looking at the sensitivity of single-fiber EMG and other diagnostic tests in MG [44]; an article by Sanders et al., which reported single-fiber EMG sensitivity in a large cohort of patients with MG and in patients with other conditions [45]; and a third article by Padua et al. reporting the sensitivity of single-fiber EMG in patients with ocular MG [46]. EMBASE, PubMed, and Cochrane Library databases were also searched using the same search strategy, and no additional articles were identified.

The Sensitivity of AChR Antibodies in the Diagnosis of MG

A large study evaluated the frequency of seronegativity in 562 adults with acquired, generalized MG [42]. Positive AChR binding or AChR-modulating antibodies were seen in 91.8% of patients (95% confidence interval 93.8–90.4). Specificity was not reported in this study, though the authors report that antibodies to the AChR were not identified in 178 healthy subjects. However, it is well-recognized that patients with other medical and neurological conditions can have antibodies to AChRs.

Examples of such conditions include autoimmune liver disease, graft-versus-host disease, and other autoimmune conditions, such as systemic lupus erythematosus. Therefore, AChR antibodies are helpful in the confirmation of patients with clinically or electrodiagnostically suspected MG, but must be interpreted with caution in patients without clinical or EMG features of MG.

It has been well-established that patients with ocular MG are less likely to have AChR antibodies. One retrospective study was selected to review the frequency of AChR seropositivity in ocular MG [43]. In this study, the sensitivity of AChR antibodies in 102 patients diagnosed with ocular MG was 59%. Specificity was not reported.

The Sensitivity of Single-Fiber EMG in the Diagnosis of MG

The diagnostic sensitivity of single-fiber EMG was reported in a large study of 120 patients with MG, the majority studied prospectively [44]. Single-fiber EMG was abnormal in 92% of patients, though was abnormal in only 80% of patients with ocular MG. Single-fiber EMG was abnormal in 94% of patients with generalized MG, and was abnormal in all 33 patients with moderate or severe MG [44]. No control group was utilized. Another study reported single-fiber EMG findings in 127 patients with MG, 26 normal controls, and in various other conditions, including spinal muscular atrophy (six subjects), peripheral neuropathy (seven subjects), polymyositis (12 subjects), ragged red-fiber disease (four subjects), and asymptomatic thymoma (three subjects) [45]. Single-fiber EMG was normal in all 26 normal controls, but was abnormal in 17/32 of the subjects with other neuromuscular conditions or asymptomatic thymoma.

The sensitivity of SFEMG in a large cohort of 86 cases with suspected ocular MG was reportedly 100% [46]. Patients were classified as having ocular MG if they met at least two of the three criteria, including positive AChR antibody titer, positive response to anticholinesterase, or abnormal response on RNS or single-fiber EMG. Patients who met less than two of these criteria were classified as "undiagnosed," and in this group single-fiber EMG was abnormal in 21% of the 43 patients in this category. Single-fiber EMG was abnormal in all 34 patients diagnosed with ocular MG.

These studies confirm the high sensitivity of single-fiber EMG in the diagnosis of MG, particularly generalized MG. Single-fiber EMG is less sensitive in diagnosing ocular MG and milder forms of generalized MG. Furthermore, single-fiber EMG is frequently abnormal in other neuromuscular conditions, such as peripheral neuropathy, myopathy, and anterior horn cell disease. Given this limited specificity, routine NCS and needle EMG are necessary to rule out other neuromuscular conditions. Another important methodological point is that all of these reported studies looking at large cohorts of MG patients have utilized a standardized single-fiber EMG electrode. Most institutions are no longer using these electrodes currently, and are instead using concentric EMG needles for single-fiber studies. Preliminary data suggests reliability with the concentric needle [47, 48], but further larger studies are necessary to confirm this.

Clinical Bottom Lines

1. AChR antibodies are seen in the serum of nearly 92% of patients with generalized MG and in 59% of patients with ocular MG.
2. Single-fiber EMG is abnormal in 92% of patients with MG, though has limited specificity given that it is frequently abnormal in patients with various other neuromuscular conditions.

Summary

The diagnosis of MG can prove challenging, particularly in patients with mild, generalized ocular MG or seronegative disease. The diagnostic gold standard rests on compatible clinical signs and symptoms, antibody testing, and EMG studies. Furthermore, the limited specificity of the various tests utilized in the diagnosis of MG must be considered, particularly in those patients with atypical signs or symptoms.

Treatment

Treatment of MG involves the use of anticholinesterase inhibitors, such as pyridostigmine, and immune-modulating therapy. Pyridostigmine can offer some relief in some patients with MG, and is often used first-line particularly in those patients with mild or ocular symptoms. Immunomodulating therapy in MG is targeted toward the antibody-mediated, T-cell-dependent attack on the NMJ. Therapies, such as prednisone, azathioprine, mycophenolate mofetil, cyclosporine, intravenous immune globulin, and plasma exchange, have been used primarily in the treatment of generalized MG.

Clinical Questions

1. Is mycophenolate mofetil effective in the treatment of myasthenia gravis?
2. Is thymectomy effective in the treatment of myasthenia gravis?

Search Strategy

Ovid MEDLINE database was utilized, with MeSH terms "myasthenia gravis" (yield 12,723 articles) and "mycophenolate mofetil" (yield 4,349 articles). These terms were searched and combined using the Boolean "AND." After limiting the retrieval to English and human, the yield was 39 citations. Two articles were chosen, including an international, phase III trial assessing the efficacy of mycophenolate mofetil as a steroid-sparing agent in MG [49] and another that evaluated mycophenolate mofetil as initial therapy in MG [50]. EMBASE, PubMed, and Cochrane Library databases were also searched using the same search strategy, and no additional articles were identified.

Ovid MEDLINE database was utilized, with MeSH terms "myasthenia gravis" (yield 12,723 articles) and "thymectomy" (yield 7,713 articles). These terms were searched and combined using the Boolean "AND." After limiting the retrieval to English and human, the yield was 2,334 citations. From these, an evidenced-based review of thymectomy in MG was selected [51]. EMBASE, PubMed, and Cochrane Library databases were also searched using the same search strategy, and no additional articles were identified.

Mycophenolate Mofetil in the Treatment of MG

Prednisone is the initial immunosuppressant medication used in the treatment of most patients with MG. While prednisone is typically effective in the treatment of MG, most patients accrue a significant number of adverse effects with long-term prednisone use. As a consequence, there is great interest in alternative immunosuppressant agents that have the potential to lessen the exposure to prednisone therapy. Mycophenolate mofetil is an inhibitor of inosine monophosphate dehydrogenase, which is a crucial enzyme in the pathway for guanosine nucleotide synthesis. Mycophenolate mofetil inhibits antibody response.

A multicenter, double-blind, placebo-controlled, parallel-group trial compared moderate-dose prednisone alone to combined mycophenolate mofetil and moderate-dose prednisone, in a group of 80 patients with mild–moderate MG [50]. The quantitative MG score at 12 weeks was assessed in both groups, and was found to be similar in both. Furthermore, in an additional 24-week open-label phase, prednisone dose was tapered at a similar rate in both groups.

An international, prospective, randomized, double-blind, placebo-controlled, parallel-group, 36-week trial evaluated efficacy of mycophenolate mofetil as a steroid-sparing agent in the treatment of mild–moderate, generalized, seropositive MG [49]. One hundred and thirty-six patients taking corticosteroids were randomized to mycophenolate mofetil or placebo, with the primary outcome measure being achievement of minimal (disease) manifestations or pharmacologic remission, with reduction in corticosteroid dosage. Secondary outcomes evaluated included disease severity, quality of life scores, and safety. There were no differences in primary and secondary outcomes between the treatment groups with prednisone tapering.

These two rigorous trials suggest that mycophenolate mofetil may not be effective as a steroid-sparing agent in the treatment of MG, findings that have surprised many clinicians and researchers who use this agent regularly in MG. Furthermore, previous, less-rigorous studies have suggested a beneficial effect of mycophenolate mofetil in MG. Short study duration, too small sample size, robust response of patients to prednisone, and entry of milder disease patients have been raised as potential reasons for study conclusions that appear to contradict clinical experience and findings suggesting benefit in previous, smaller, less-rigorous studies.

Thymectomy in MG

There have been numerous retrospective studies over the last 50 years reporting the beneficial effects of thymectomy in MG. To date, no prospective, randomized clinical trial to evaluate the effectiveness of thymectomy in MG has been completed. Studies reported to date have been hampered by a number of methodologic flaws, including the absence of randomized treatment allocation, lack of standardized outcome measures, and the confounding difference in baseline characteristics [51].

An evidenced-based review by Gronseth and Barohn comprehensively analyzed studies evaluating the efficacy of thymectomy in MG between 1966 through 1998 [51]. Twenty-eight Class II studies were analyzed. Patients in these studies were not randomized to thymectomy or nonthymectomy. A number of studies did not report the surgical technique. Length of follow-up was quite variable as was patient lost to follow-up. There were no blinded assessment of outcomes, and nonstandard definitions of remission were used. In all but three of the studies analyzed, patients who underwent thymectomy were more likely to achieve mediation-free remission, become asymptomatic, and improve than patients who did not undergo thymectomy. A number of potentially confounding variables were identified. Patients who underwent thymectomy were younger, more often women, and were more likely to have more severe MG. The studies were not adequately able to control for confounders or baseline subject characteristics. Effects of medical therapy on treatment response, timing of surgery, and effect of differing surgical techniques could not be adequately assessed. The need for a prospective, randomized clinical trial was emphasized.

The general consensus is that thymectomy is likely beneficial in patients with myasthenia gravis. Despite the vast numbers of studies reporting benefit, methodologic flaws and particularly lack of randomization do not permit conclusive evidence of efficacy. At the time of this writing, a prospective, randomized clinical trial is underway to better address this issue.

Summary

Two recent clinical trials evaluating the efficacy of mycophenolate mofetil in conjunction with prednisone failed to demonstrate any improvement in clinical status versus prednisone alone and failed to show any steroid-sparing effect. These findings contradict previous, less-rigorous studies and suggest that mycophenolate mofetil might not be beneficial in the treatment of MG. A large of number of class II studies have reported a beneficial effect of thymectomy in MG, though these studies harbor a number of serious methodologic flaws. It is anticipated that a prospective, randomized clinical trial will provide more definitive answers.

Clinical Bottom Lines

1. Mycophenolate mofetil may offer no additional therapeutic benefit as a steroid-sparing agent in the treatment of MG.
2. Thymectomy is likely effective in the treatment of MG, though a prospective, randomized clinical trial has not proven this definitively.

References

1. Sorenson E, Stalker A, Kurland L, Windebank A. Amyotrophic lateral sclerosis in Olmsted County, Minnesota, 1925–1998. Neurology. 2002;59:280–2.
2. Fang F, Valdimarsdóttir U, Bellocco R, Ronnevi L, Sparén P, Fall K, et al. Amyotrophic lateral sclerosis in Sweden, 1991–2005. Arch Neurol. 2009;66(4):515–9.
3. Zoccolella S, Beghi E, Palagano G, et al. Analysis of survival and prognostic factors in amyotrophic lateral sclerosis: a population based study. J Neurol Neurosurg Psychiatry. 2008;79:33–7.
4. Mandrioli J, Faglioni P, Nichelli P, et al. Amyotrophic lateral sclerosis: prognostic indicators of survival. Amyotrophic Lateral Sclerosis. 2006;7:217–26.
5. Bensimon G, Lacomblez L, Meninger V, et al. A controlled trial of Riluzole in amyotrophic lateral sclerosis. N Engl J Med. 1994;330:585–91.
6. Miller RG, Mitchell JD, Lyon M, Moore DH. Riluzole for amyotrophic lateral sclerosis (ALS)/motor neuron disease (MND). Cochrane Database Syst Rev. 2007:CD001447.
7. Fagius J. Chronic cryptogenic polyneuropathy. The search for a cause. Acta Neurol Scand. 1983;67:173–80.
8. Prineas J. Polyneuropathies of undetermined cause. Acta Neurol Scand. 1970;46:1–72.
9. Smith AG, Singleton JR. The diagnostic yield of a standardized approach to idiopathic sensory-predominant neuropathy. Arch Intern Med. 2004;164:1021–5.
10. Genuth S, Alberti KG, Bennett P, et al. Follow-up report on the diagnosis of diabetes mellitus. Diabet Care. 2003;26:3160–7.
11. Singleton JR, Smith AG, Bromberg MB. Increased prevalence of impaired glucose tolerance in patients with painful sensory neuropathy. Diabet Care. 2001;24:1448–53.
12. Hoffman-Snyder C, Smith BE, Ross MA, Hernandez J, Bosch EP. Value of the oral glucose tolerance test in the evaluation of chronic idiopathic axonal polyneuropathy. Arch Neurol. 2006;63:1075–9.
13. Centers for Disease Control and Prevention (CDC). The prevalence of diabetes and impaired fasting glucose in adults – United States 1999–2000. MMWR Morb Mortal Wkly Rep. 2003; 52:833–7.
14. Novella SP, Inzucchi SE, Goldstein JM. The frequency of undiagnosed diabetes and impaired glucose tolerance in patients with idiopathic sensory neuropathy. Muscle Nerve. 2001;24: 1229–31.
15. Sumner CJ, Sheth S, Griffin JW, Cornblath DR, Polydefkis M. The spectrum of neuropathy in diabetes and impaired glucose tolerance. Neurology. 2003;60:108–11.
16. Low PA. Symptomatic treatment of painful neuropathy. JAMA. 1998;280:1863–4.
17. Ziegler D, Nowak H, Kempler P, Vargha P, Low PA. Treatment of symptomatic diabetic polyneuropathy with antioxidant alpha-lipoic acid: a meta-analysis. Diabet Med. 2004;21:114–21.
18. The Diabetes Control and Complications Trial Research Group. The effect of intensive diabetes therapy on the development and progression of neuropathy. Ann Intern Med. 1995;122:561–8.
19. Ziegler D, Ametov A, Barinov A, Dyck PJ, Gurieva I, Low PA, et al. Oral treatment with alpha-lipoic acid improves symptomatic diabetic polyneuropathy: The SYDNEY 2 Trial. Diabet Care. 2006;29:2365–70.

20. Tang J, Wingerchuk D, Crum B, Rubin DI, Demaerschalk BM. Alpha-lipoic acid may improve symptomatic diabetic polyneuropathy. Neurologist. 2007;13:164–7.
21. Dyck PJ, Karnes JL, O'Brien PC, Litchy WJ, Low PA, Melton 3rd LJ. The Rochester Diabetic Neuropathy Study: reassessment of tests and criteria for diagnosis and staged severity. Neurology. 1992;42:1164–70.
22. Dalakas MC. Polymyositis, dermatomyositis and inclusion body myositis. N Engl J Med. 1991;325:1487–98.
23. Amato AA, Barohn RJ. Idiopathic inflammatory myopathies. Neurol Clin. 1997;15:615–48.
24. Bohan A, Peter JB. Polymyositis and dermatomyositis (first of two parts). N Engl J Med. 1975;292:344–7.
25. Bohan A, Peter JB. Polymyositis and dermatomyositis (first of two parts). N Engl J Med. 1975;292:403–7.
26. Griggs RC, Askanas V, DiMauro S, et al. Inclusion body myositis and myopathies. Ann Neurol. 1995;38:705–13.
27. Hoogendijk JE, Amato AA, Lecky BR, et al. 119th ENMC international workshop: trial design in adult idiopathic inflammatory myopathies, with the exception of inclusion body myositis, 10–12 October 2003, Naarden, The Netherlands. Neuromuscul Disord. 2004;14:337–45.
28. Lotz BP, Engel AG, Nishino H, et al. Inclusion body myositis. Observations in 40 patients. Brain. 1989;112:727–47.
29. Mendell JR, Sahenk Z, Gales T, et al. Amyloid filaments in inclusion body myositis. Novel findings provide insight into nature of filaments. Arch Neurol. 1991;48:1229–34.
30. Chahin N, Engel AG. Correlation of muscle biopsy, clinical course, and outcome in PM and sporadic IBM. Neurology. 2008;70:418–24.
31. Dahlbom K, Lindberg C, Oldfors A. Inclusion body myositis: morphological clues to correct diagnosis. Neuromuscul Disord. 2002;12:853–7.
32. Choy EHS, Hoogendijk JE, Lecky B, et al. Immunosuppressant and immunomodulatory treatment for dermatomyositis and polymyositis. Cochrane Database Syst Rev. 2005;3:CD003643. doi:10.1002/14651858.CD003643.pub2.
33. Griggs RC. The current status of treatment for inclusion-body myositis. Neurology. 2006; 66:S30–2.
34. Brannagan 3rd TH. Current treatments of chronic immune-mediated demyelinating polyneuropathies. Muscle Nerve. 2009;39:563–78.
35. Dalakas MC, Illa I, Dambrosia JM, et al. A controlled trial of high-dose intravenous immune globulin infusions as a treatment for dermatomyositis. N Engl J Med. 1993;329:1993–2000.
36. Dalakas MC, Sonies S, Dambrosia JM, et al. Treatment of inclusion-body myositis with IVIg: a double-blind, placebo-controlled study. Neurology. 1997;48:712–6.
37. Walter MC, Lochmuller H, Toepfer M, et al. High-dose immunoglobulin therapy in sporadic inclusion body myositis: a double-blind, placebo-controlled study. J Neurol. 2000;247:22–8.
38. Dalakas MC, Koffman B, Fujii M, et al. A controlled study of intravenous immunoglobulin combined with prednisone in the treatment of IBM. Neurology. 2001;56:323–7.
39. Phillips LH, Torner JC. Epidemiologic evidence for a changing natural history of myasthenia gravis. Neurology. 1996;47:1233–8.
40. Poulas K, Tsibri E, Kokla A, Papanastasiou D, Tsouloufis T, Marinou M, et al. Epidemiology of seropositive myasthenia gravis in Greece. J Neurol Neurosurg Psych. 2001;71:353–6.
41. Phillips LH. The epidemiology of Myasthenia Gravis. Ann NY Acad Sci. 2003;998:407–12.
42. Chan KH, Lachance DH, Harper CM, Lennon VA. Frequency of seronegativity in adult-acquired generalized myasthenia gravis. Muscle Nerve. 2007;36:651–8.
43. Husain AM, Massey JM, Howard JF, Sanders DB. Acetylcholine receptor antibody measurements in acquired myasthenia gravis. Ann NY Acad Sci. 1998;841:471–4.
44. Oh SJ, Kim DE, Kuruoglu R, Bradley RJ, Dwyer D. Diagnostic sensitivity of the laboratory tests in myasthenia gravis. Muscle Nerve. 1992;15:720–4.
45. Sanders DB, Howard JF, Johns TR. Single-fiber electromyography in myasthenia gravis. Neurology. 1979;29:68–76.

46. Padua L, Stalberg E, LoMonaco M, Evoli A, Batocchi A, Tonali P. SFEMG in ocular myasthenia gravis diagnosis. Clin Neurophysiol. 2000;111:1203–7.
47. Farrugia ME, Weir AI, Cleary M, Cooper S, Metcalfe R, Mallik A. Concentric and single fiber needle electrodes yield comparable jitter results in myasthenia gravis. Muscle Nerve. 2009;39(5):579–85.
48. Benatar M, Hammad M, Doss-Riney H. Concentric-needle single-fiber electromyography for the diagnosis of myasthenia gravis. Muscle Nerve. 2006;34(2):163–8.
49. Sanders DB, Hart IK, Mantegazza R, Shukla SS, Siddiqi ZA, De Baets MHV, et al. An international phase II randomized trial of mycophenolate mofetil in myasthenia gravis. Neurology. 2008;71:400–6.
50. Muscle Study Group. A trial of mycophenolate mofetil with prednisone as initial immunotherapy in myasthenia gravis. Neurology. 2008;71:394–9.
51. Gronseth GS, Barohn RJ. Practice parameter: Thymectomy for autoimmune myasthenia gravis (an evidence-based review). Report of the quality standards subcommittee of the American Academy of Neurology. Neurology. 2000;55:7–15.

Chapter 10
Neuropathic Pain

Brent P. Goodman

Keywords Postherpetic neuralgia • Neuropathic pain • Herpes zoster • Shingles • Central pain • Vaccine • Diabetic neuropathy • Peripheral neuropathy • Diabetes

Neuropathic pain has been defined by the International Association for the Study of Pain as pain that is "initiated or caused by a primary lesion or dysfunction in the nervous system" [1]. It has been estimated that chronic pain affects 2–3% of the general population [2, 3], and has been estimated to cost $40 billion per year in the USA [4]. Neuropathic pain is a heterogenous condition that can result from disorders affecting the central or peripheral nervous system. Postherpetic neuralgia, painful peripheral neuropathy, and central pain conditions are some of the more commonly encountered neuropathic pain disorders and are the focus of this chapter. These conditions have the potential to cause major impairment in quality of life, and can significantly impact social and occupational functioning.

Herpes Zoster and Postherpetic Neuralgia

Herpes zoster (also known as shingles) results from reactivation of the varicella zoster virus. Following primary infection with the varicella virus (chicken pox), the varicella virus remains latent in dorsal root and cranial sensory ganglia. With reactivation, the virus travels along sensory nerves to the skin, resulting in a painful, vesicular rash. The lesions evolve in a dermatomal, unilateral pattern, most frequently involving thoracic segments and the ophthalmic division of the trigeminal nerve.

B.P. Goodman (✉)
Neurology Department, EMG Laboratory, Mayo College of Medicine, Mayo Clinic,
13400 East Shea Blvd., Scottsdale, AZ 85259, USA
e-mail: goodman.brent@mayo.edu

J.G. Burneo et al. (eds.), *Neurology: An Evidence-Based Approach*,
DOI 10.1007/978-0-387-88555-1_10, © Springer Science+Business Media, LLC 2012

Postherpetic neuralgia is a distinctive, often disabling pain syndrome following resolution of the rash. The definition of postherpetic neuralgia has evolved over time, and this term is now applied to individuals with pain persisting for more than 120 days following the resolution of the zoster rash. Pain within 30 days of zoster onset is classified as acute herpetic neuralgia, and pain between 30 and 120 days following rash as subacute herpetic neuralgia [5].

The diagnosis of zoster is clinical based upon the characteristic features of the rash in the distinctive, unilateral, dermatomal distribution. If there is clinical uncertainty about the diagnosis, shell vial viral culture, viral polymerase chain reaction testing, or other tests, such as direct fluorescent antibody staining, immunoperoxidase staining, and Tzanck smear, can be used to establish a diagnosis [6].

Treatment efforts have been focused on prevention of varicella through vaccination, treatment of varicella with antiviral therapy in order to reduce the likelihood of developing postherpetic neuralgia, and treatment of postherpetic neuralgia symptoms with topical and oral pain medications.

Epidemiology

It has been estimated that there are nearly 1 million new cases of zoster annually in the USA [7–9]. A recently reported population-based study from Olmsted County, Minnesota, estimated that the annual medical care cost of treating zoster is $1.1 billion [8]. Furthermore, most of the health care costs are estimated to affect immunocompetent individuals older than 50 years of age.

Clinical Case Example

A 65-year-old man is referred for evaluation of disabling, left-sided thoracic region pain. He reports a history of suffering from a painful rash 6 months previously that was evaluated in an urgent-care clinic and thought to be consistent with shingles. The rash resolved within 3 weeks; however, he reported persistent, severe burning pain in the distribution of the rash. His neurological examination was remarkable for diminished sensation and allodynia in a T10 distribution on the left, but was otherwise unremarkable.

Clinical Questions

1. What is the incidence of zoster?
2. What is the prevalence of postherpetic neuralgia?

Search Strategy

Ovid MEDLINE database was searched since its inception to September of 2009. Medical Subject Heading (MeSH) terms "incidence" and "zoster" were searched and combined using the Boolean "AND." After limiting the retrieval to English and human excluding letters and editorials, a final set of 790 citations were obtained. From this set, one article was selected, a population-based study of an Olmsted County, Minnesota community, and results from a closely followed placebo group enrolled in the Shingles Prevention Study [7, 10]. EMBASE, PubMed, LILACS, and the Cochrane Library databases were also searched implementing the same strategy of MeSH terms and keywords. No additional articles were identified.

Ovid MEDLINE database was searched since its inception to September of 2009. MeSH terms "incidence" and "postherpetic neuralgia" were searched and combined using the Boolean "AND." After limiting the retrieval to English and human excluding letters and editorials, a final set of 151 citations were reviewed, and from these citations one article was selected for review. This study from a primary care medical database in the UK reported the prevalence of postherpetic neuralgia and three other neuropathic pain conditions (Hall GC). EMBASE, PubMed, LILACS, and the Cochrane Library databases were also searched implementing the same strategy of MeSH terms and keywords. No additional articles were identified.

Incidence of Herpes Zoster

A population-based study of residents of Olmsted County, Minnesota, reported an incidence rate of 3.6 per 1,000 patient years [7]. Sixty percent of the patients were women, and the mean age of diagnosis was 59 years. In this report, the incidence of zoster and the rate of complications associated with zoster were much higher in individuals older than 50 years of age. In the Shingles Prevention Study discussed later in this chapter, the incidence of zoster in patients older than 60 years of age was 11.8 cases per 1,000 patient years in the placebo group [10]. There is some question as to whether the incidence of shingles may actually be increasing over time. A decrease in cell-mediated immunity is thought to be the cause of increased incidence of zoster in elderly individuals.

Incidence of Postherpetic Neuralgia

In a recently published study of general practice records from the UK from May 2002 through May of 2005, the incidence of postherpetic neuralgia was 28.2 per 100,000 patient years [2]. As is true with zoster, the frequency of postherpetic neuralgia increases with age. In individuals younger than 60 years of age, the frequency of postherpetic neuralgia is 5%, and increases to 33% in individuals aged 79 and older [7].

Summary

Herpes zoster is relatively common medical condition that is estimated to affect nearly 1 million people annually in the USA with medical care costs estimated at over $1 billion annually. The incidence of zoster has been estimated in one recent population-based study at 3.6 per 1,000 patient years. Zoster is more common in individuals aged 50 and over, and complications related to zoster, including postherpetic neuralgia, are more common in this age group. The incidence of postherpetic neuralgia in the UK was estimated at 28.2 per 100,000 patient years.

Clinical Bottom Lines

1. The incidence of zoster ("shingles") is 3.6 per 1,000 patient years, but is much higher in older patients.
2. The incidence of postherpetic neuralgia is 28.2 per 100,000 patient years. The frequency of postherpetic neuralgia increases with age from 5% in patients younger than 60 years of age to 33% in those aged 79 and older.

Prevention of Postherpetic Neuralgia

Clinical Case Example

A 76-year-old female presents for evaluation of a painful rash. She reports that 4 days ago she developed a stabbing pain involving her left cheek, and the day prior to presentation she noticed numbness and tingling in conjunction with a painful rash. On examination, a vesicular rash was noted in the right V2 distribution of the trigeminal nerve. Facial zoster is diagnosed. The patient asks what can be done to treat her condition and prevent any potential complications.

Clinical Questions

1. Does antiviral therapy prevent the development of postherpetic neuralgia?
2. Does the zoster vaccine prevent the development of postherpetic neuralgia?

Search Strategy

Ovid MEDLINE database was searched since its inception to September of 2009. MeSH terms "antiviral agents/or antiviral" and "postherpetic neuralgia" were searched and combined using the Boolean "AND." After limiting the retrieval to English and human excluding letters and editorials, a final set of 184 citations were obtained. From this set, four articles were chosen for review. EMBASE, PubMed, LILACS, and the Cochrane Library databases were also searched implementing the same strategy of MeSH terms and keywords. No additional articles were identified.

Ovid MEDLINE database was searched since its inception to September of 2009. MeSH terms "vaccines" or "herpes virus vaccines" and "postherpetic neuralgia" were searched and combined using the Boolean "AND." After limiting the retrieval to English and human excluding letters and editorials, a final set of 100 citations were obtained. From this set, the Shingles Prevention Study was selected for review [10]. EMBASE, PubMed, LILACS, and the Cochrane Library databases were also searched implementing the same strategy of MeSH terms and keywords. No additional articles were identified.

Prevention of Postherpetic Neuralgia with Antiviral Therapy

A recent Cochrane analysis reviewed the effectiveness of antiviral therapy in preventing the development of postherpetic neuralgia [5]. A total of 20 clinical trials were reviewed, and 6 trials involving 1,211 individuals were deemed suitable for inclusion. The primary outcome measure was the presence of postherpetic neuralgia 6 months following the zoster rash. Meta-analysis of five trials reporting acyclovir versus placebo and one of famciclovir versus placebo was performed. The studies included patients treated with antiviral therapy within 72 h of rash onset and included only immunocompetent individuals. The incidence of postherpetic neuralgia at 6 months in placebo groups ranged from 11 to 60%, similar to the 12–58% reported in treatment groups. The authors concluded that acyclovir therapy did not reduce the incidence of postherpetic neuralgia.

Pain scores were reported in only two of the studies beyond 3 months, and in these studies pain was significantly reduced in the acyclovir-treated group. While all six of the clinical trials were randomized, controlled parallel studies, only one was considered high quality by the authors, and the five authors were considered "fair" because of possible bias in several key areas. The authors suggested that further studies of famciclovir or other antiviral therapies would be appropriate, suggesting that better reporting of pain, quality of life measures, and studies of immunocompromised individuals should be included in future studies.

This Cochrane analysis conflicts with other studies reporting a benefit of antiviral therapies in preventing postherpetic neuralgia [11, 12]. A reason for these discrepancies is not entirely clear. In another earlier, systematic review, it was concluded that antiviral therapy reduced the duration but not the incidence of postherpetic neuralgia (four acyclovir trials and one famciclovir trial) [13]. Specifically, it was concluded that there was evidence of a reduction in postherpetic neuralgia incidence at 1–3 months. However, with the Cochrane analysis, postherpetic neuralgia was defined as pain persisting beyond 120 days following zoster reactivation, a definition not adopted in this earlier review.

Prevention of Postherpetic Neuralgia with Zoster Vaccination

The Shingles Prevention Study utilized a live, attenuated zoster vaccine administered to individuals aged 60 and older in order to determine whether the incidence and severity of zoster and postherpetic neuralgia could be reduced in those receiving vaccine compared to placebo [10]. A total of 38,546 individuals were enrolled in this double-blind, placebo-controlled, multiinstitutional clinical trial, and followed for a mean duration of 3.1 years. During the follow-up period, there were a total of 957 confirmed cases of zoster, of which 315 occurred in the vaccine group and 642 in the placebo group. This was a statistically significant reduction in the development of zoster in those receiving placebo ($P < 0.001$), with a number needed to treat (NNT) of 59 (CI 50–72).

A total of 107 cases of postherpetic neuralgia (defined as pain persisting for 90 days or more following rash) were identified, including 27 in the vaccination group and 80 in the placebo group. This was a statistically significant reduction in the development of postherpetic neuralgia ($P < 0.001$), with a reported reduction of incidence from 1.38 cases per 1,000 person-years in the placebo group to 0.46 person-years in the vaccine group. The NNT to prevent postherpetic neuralgia development is 364 (CI 259–577). The duration of pain and severity of illness scores were also significantly reduced in the vaccine group. Injection site side effects were more commonly seen in those receiving vaccine compared to placebo, but otherwise the rate of systemic side effects was similar in both groups.

Summary

At present, available evidence suggests that pain following zoster is reduced with antiviral therapy, but latest meta-analysis of clinical trial data does not confirm a reduction in the development of postherpetic neuralgia with antiviral therapy. At least some of the discrepancies in the literature regarding postherpetic neuralgia prevention might result from differences in disease classification. There appears to be a growing consensus that the designation of postherpetic neuralgia should be applied to individuals with pain persisting for at least 120 days following the resolution of rash. There is sufficient evidence to confirm that the zoster vaccine results in a significant reduction in the likelihood of developing zoster and secondarily, a significant reduction in postherpetic neuralgia.

Clinical Bottom Lines

1. There is no compelling evidence to suggest that acyclovir or famciclovir significantly reduces the likelihood of developing postherpetic neuralgia. There is some evidence to suggest that acute and subacute herpetic neuralgia pain may be reduced with antiviral therapy.

2. Administration of zoster vaccine significantly reduces the risk of developing zoster and postherpetic neuralgia, though NNT is quite high, particularly in postherpetic neuralgia prevention with an NNT of 364.

Treatment of Postherpetic Neuralgia

Clinical Questions

1. Does topical lidocaine reduce postherpetic neuralgia pain?
2. Does anticonvulsant therapy reduce postherpetic neuralgia pain?

Search Strategy

Ovid MEDLINE database was searched since its inception to September of 2009. MeSH terms "lidocaine" and "postherpetic neuralgia" were searched and combined using the Boolean "AND." After limiting the retrieval to English and human excluding letters and editorials, a final set of 93 citations were obtained. EMBASE, PubMed, LILACS, and the Cochrane Library databases were also searched implementing the same strategy of MeSH terms and keywords. No additional articles were identified. The selected article is a recent Cochrane review that supplements an original 2007 review of the same topic [14].

Ovid MEDLINE database was searched since its inception to September of 2009. MeSH terms "anticonvulsants/or pregabalin" and "postherpetic neuralgia" were searched and combined using the Boolean "AND." After limiting the retrieval to English and human excluding letters and editorials, a final set of 93 citations were obtained. EMBASE, PubMed, LILACS, and the Cochrane Library databases were also searched implementing the same strategy of MeSH terms and keywords. No additional articles were identified. The selected article is a recent Cochrane review of anticonvulsant therapy in postherpetic neuralgia [15].

Topical Lidocaine and Postherpetic Neuralgia

Three clinical trials involving 182 lidocaine-treated individuals and 132 subjects in placebo group were included [14]. Meta-analysis of the primary outcome measure, mean pain relief, was possible in only two of the studies and suggested that topical lidocaine was superior to placebo with a P-value of 0.003. Mean reduction in the visual analog scale (VAS) was reported in two of the three studies, showing a statistically significant reduction in one trial ($P=0.03$) and no significant benefit in the other study. Limitations of these studies included the following: small numbers of individuals studied, one of the trials remains unpublished (and not formally peer-reviewed), and all of the reviewed studies were authored by the same first author.

The authors concluded that there is still insufficient evidence to recommend topical lidocaine as first-line therapy in the treatment of postherpetic neuralgia.

Anticonvulsant Therapy for Postherpetic Neuralgia

A trial of gabapentin at dosages up to 3,600 mg was compared to placebo in 229 patients with postherpetic neuralgia [15]. Using a global improvement scale, 43% of patients improved on gabapentin compared to 12% with placebo. The NNT was 3.8 (CI 2.4–8.7). In an earlier study, combination carbamazepine in conjunction with clomipramine was superior to transcutaneous electronic nerve stimulation in postherpetic neuralgia pain reduction. The authors reported that for postherpetic neuralgia and other pain conditions (trigeminal neuropathy and diabetic neuropathy), the NNT for carbamazepine was 2.5 (CI 2.0–3.4) [15].

Summary

Postherpetic neuralgia remains a challenging entity to treat. Meta-analysis of three clinical trials utilizing topical lidocaine in the treatment of postherpetic neuralgia suggested that there is likely some benefit of topical lidocaine in the treatment of this condition, but that there was insufficient evidence to recommend this agent as first-line therapy. Gabapentin and carbamazepine have demonstrated efficacy in significantly reducing postherpetic neuralgia.

Clinical Bottom Lines

1. Topical lidocaine is probably effective in the treatment of postherpetic neuralgia, but there is no sufficient evidence to recommend it as first-line therapy in the treatment of postherpetic neuralgia.
2. Anticonvulsant therapy, including gabapentin and carbamazepine, results in significant pain reduction in patients with postherpetic neuralgia with NNT of 3.8 and 2.5, respectively.

Central Neuropathic Pain

Epidemiology

Central pain is a heterogenous condition that results from trauma or neurological disorders that affect the brain or spinal cord. A myriad of conditions can result in chronic neuropathic pain, including spinal cord injury, traumatic brain injury, multiple sclerosis, stroke, tumors, and epilepsy. Chronic pain can be a major source of disability and has the potential to limit the quality of life in patients with these disorders. An understanding of the mechanisms involved in central pain generation is limited. Furthermore, the identification of central pain and distinction of central neuropathic from nonneuropathic pain can be difficult. These current realities complicate efforts to study and appropriately diagnose and treat patients with central pain.

Central neuropathic pain can be established with certainty in individuals with diagnostic testing identifying a lesion that could produce pain, pain that occurs in a neuroanatomically reasonable pain distribution, and sensory signs that are congruent with somatotropic representation of the body within the central nervous system [16]. The treatment of central neuropathic pain is often challenging and frequently limited by incomplete (or complete lack of) pharmacotherapeutic benefit, drug or treatment side effects, or drug–drug interactions.

Clinical Case Example

A 65-year-old man with a history of stroke 3 months prior to evaluation presents with a history of severe, lancinating right arm pain that began sometime following his stroke. He reports a history of right arm and leg weakness and right-sided hemisensory loss that began abruptly, and he had an MRI scan that confirmed the presence of an acute ischemic stroke. His weakness largely resolved within a few weeks, but he was left with persistent, residual pain and sensory loss primarily involving the right arm. The neurological examination confirms mild upper motor neuron-type weakness affecting the right arm, brisk deep tendon reflexes with an extensor plantar response on the right, and subjective diminution in sensation over the right arm and leg.

Clinical Questions

1. What is the incidence of poststroke pain?
2. What is the prevalence of poststroke pain?

Search Strategy

Ovid MEDLINE database was searched since its inception to September of 2009. MeSH terms "stroke" and "pain" and "incidence" were searched and combined using the Boolean "And". After limiting the retrieval to English and human excluding letters and editorials, a final set of 178 citations were obtained. EMBASE, PubMed, LILACS, and the Cochrane Library databases were also searched implementing the same strategy of MeSH terms and keywords. No additional articles were identified. Of these articles, a prospective study of central poststroke pain by Andersen and colleagues was selected [17].

Ovid MEDLINE database was searched since its inception to September of 2009. MeSH terms "stroke" and "pain" and "prevalence" were searched and combined using the Boolean "AND." After limiting the retrieval to English and human excluding letters and editorials, a final set of 132 citations were obtained. Of these, a population-based study from Sweden and a cross-sectional study over a 3-month period from Singapore were selected for review [18, 19]. EMBASE, PubMed, LILACS, and the Cochrane Library databases were also searched implementing the same strategy of MeSH terms and keywords. No additional articles were identified.

Incidence of Poststroke Pain

There is to our knowledge only one prospective study reporting the incidence of central poststroke pain. This study followed 267 consecutive stroke patients younger than 81 years of age [17]. Two hundred and seven patients survived at least 6 months, and were able to communicate adequately to participate in the study. Evaluations were performed at 1 week, 1 month, 6 months, and 12 months following stroke. The incidence of central poststroke pain in this group of patients was 8%. All but one of these patients had dysesthesia or allodynia on the affected side on sensory testing. CT scans were more likely to show larger ($P < 0.005$) and more acute lesions ($P < 0.005$) in patients with central poststroke pain than those without. Thalamic lesions were noted in 25% of the patients. There was no positive correlation between central poststroke pain and depression.

Prevalence of Poststroke Pain

A recent, population-based study reported the prevalence of central poststroke pain in a Swedish municipality [18]. Three hundred and eighty-eight patients with stroke were registered, and of these 253 patients survived and were examined at 1 year following their stroke. Eleven percent of patients reported pain that was deemed consistent with central, poststroke pain. Contrary to the study reported above, a positive correlation was noted between depression and central poststroke pain, but there was no correlation with stroke type, age, gender, or prestroke risk factors. A positive correlation between stroke severity and central poststroke pain was reported, consistent with the incidence study reported above.

A cross-sectional study of stroke patients attending an outpatient, Singapore, tertiary rehabilitation unit over a 3-month period reported the prevalence of central poststroke pain and impact on quality of life [19]. Of 475 stroke patients seen over the 3-month time period, only 107 patients met inclusion criteria. The primary reasons for exclusion included cognitive or language deficits limiting the clinical evaluation or poststroke follow-up of less than 6 months. Nearly half of the studied patients reported chronic pain, and 12% of patients studied suffered from central poststroke pain. When compared with patients reporting chronic musculoskeletal pain, patients with central poststroke pain were noted to be more likely to suffer from sensory loss involving the affected limb.

Summary

Pain is a common and likely underdiagnosed manifestation of central nervous system disease. Diagnostic distinction of neuropathic from nonneuropathic pain can be challenging and has not only important treatment implications, but also impacts our thoughts about pathophysiologic and epidemiologic aspects of pain occurring in disorders of the central nervous system. Pain has long been recognized as a potential complication of cerebral stroke, and a definitive diagnosis of central, neuropathic pain in this group can be established with greater certainty given that sensory loss often occurs in conjunction with other neurological deficits and that stroke can be visualized on radiographic studies. In a prospective study of a cohort of stroke patients, the incidence of poststroke pain was 8%. A cross-sectional study involving a large number of patients in a Singapore rehabilitation unit reported that nearly half of the patients studied had chronic pain, and of this group 12% of patients were diagnosed with neuropathic, poststroke pain.

Clinical Bottom Lines

1. The incidence of poststroke pain in a prospectively studied group of stroke patients was 8%.
2. The prevalence of neuropathic, poststroke pain was 12%, though nearly half of the patients studied reported chronic pain (remainder deemed nonneuropathic).

Treatment of Central Neuropathic Pain

Clinical Questions

1. Is pregabalin effective in reducing central neuropathic pain?
2. Are tricyclic antidepressants effective in reducing central neuropathic pain?

Search Strategy

Ovid MEDLINE database was searched since its inception to September of 2009. MeSH terms "stroke" and "pain" and "pregabalin" and "anticonvulsant" were searched and combined using the Boolean "AND." After limiting the retrieval to English and human excluding letters and editorials, a final set of 28 citations were obtained. From this set, a Cochrane study was selected for review here. EMBASE, PubMed, LILACS, and the Cochrane Library databases were also searched implementing the same strategy of MeSH terms and keywords. No additional articles were identified.

Ovid MEDLINE database was searched since its inception to September of 2009. MeSH terms "tricyclic," "antidepressive agents, tricyclic" and "neuropathic pain" were searched and combined using the Boolean "AND." After limiting the retrieval to English and human excluding letters and editorials, a final set of 264 citations were obtained. From this set, two articles were selected, including a Cochrane database review. EMBASE, PubMed, LILACS, and the Cochrane Library databases were also searched implementing the same strategy of MeSH terms and keywords. No additional articles were identified.

Pregabalin in Central Neuropathic Pain

A Cochrane review reported data from two studies of pregabalin in the treatment of central neuropathic pain [20]. These studies suggested that 25% of patients treated with pregabalin experienced a 50% reduction in central neuropathic pain symptoms compared to 7% in the placebo group. The NNT for 50% pain reduction was estimated at 5.6 (CI 3.5–14). Pain reduction of at least 30% was reported in 42% of patients compared with 13% of patients in the placebo group, with an NNT of 3.5 (CI 2.3–7.0).

Tricyclic Antidepressants in Central Neuropathic Pain

Reported in a Cochrane review of tricyclic antidepressants in central pain, the authors conclude that there is some indication of effectiveness, but few trials and small numbers of participants prevent "firm recommendations" [21]. In a study of 30 patients with central poststroke pain, 67% of patients treated with amitriptyline experienced partial or complete pain relief compared to only 7% of those in the placebo group. It is unclear why the response rate in the placebo group was so minimal when compared with placebo group response rates in other studies. In another study, clomipramine and nortriptyline were more effective than placebo in the treatment of pain due to various central causes.

Summary

Pregabalin and tricyclic antidepressant medications can be effective in the treatment of central neuropathic pain. In studies of pregabalin, 25% of patients achieved a 50% reduction in central neuropathic pain with an NNT of 5.6. Smaller numbers of trials and enrolled patients precluded definitive recommendations about effectiveness of tricyclic medications, but in 1 study of 30 patients with neuropathic, poststroke pain, 67% of patients achieved partial or complete pain relief compared to only 7% in the placebo-treated group.

Clinical Bottom Lines

1. Pregabalin is effective in the reduction of central neuropathic pain with NNT of 5.6 to achieve a 50% reduction in pain symptoms.
2. Tricyclic medications also appear to be effective in the treatment of central neuropathic pain, though studies are limited.

Painful Peripheral Neuropathy

Neuropathic pain is a potential, disabling manifestation of patients with peripheral neuropathy. Symptoms can consist of painful tingling, aching, burning, or lancinating pain in the extremities. Involvement of somatic sensory $A\delta$(delta) and C peripheral nerve fibers is necessary for the development of neuropathic pain, and neuropathic pain can occur in nearly all types of peripheral nerve diseases, including sensorimotor peripheral neuropathy, polyradiculoneuropathy, sensory neuronopathy, and small-fiber peripheral neuropathy (SFPN). Furthermore, most disorders that cause or are associated with these various types of neuropathy can result in neuropathic pain.

The diagnostic evaluation that is utilized to provide objective, confirmatory evidence of a peripheral neuropathy in patients with neuropathic pain consists of electrodiagnostic testing (EMG), autonomic testing, and skin biopsy. Electrodiagnostic testing is typically unremarkable in patients with SFPN, and autonomic testing or skin biopsy is typically necessary to establish a diagnosis in these patients.

Painful SFPN is one of the more frequently encountered neuropathic pain conditions in clinical practice. Diagnostic confirmation of SFPN is dependent upon the demonstration of physiologic impairment of small-fiber nerves on autonomic testing or loss of small nerve fibers on skin biopsy. Oral and topical pharmacologic medications are the primary treatment options in patients with neuropathic pain in SFPN and other peripheral nerve disorders.

Diabetes mellitus (DM) is one of the more commonly recognized causes of painful peripheral neuropathy, including SFPN. It is now increasingly recognized that SFPN is also associated with impaired glucose tolerance and other features of the metabolic syndrome, particularly hypertriglyceridemia.

Clinical Case Example

A 46-year-old man is referred for evaluation of a 2-year history of burning pain in her distal extremities. The patient first noted loss of sensation in her toes 2 years prior, and over the last year has noted progression of numbness to the ankles bilaterally. She reports constant burning pain in her feet, with superimposed lancinating pains in the feet. More recently, she has noticed numbness in her fingertips bilaterally.

Neurological examination reveals normal manual muscle testing and deep tendon reflexes in the upper and lower extremities with normal proprioception, vibration, and light touch on sensory testing. Reduction in temperature and pinprick sensation to the level of the mid-shins bilaterally is noted. Gait, station, and coordination are normal.

Epidemiology

Incidence and prevalence rates for peripheral neuropathy of all causes are not known. Given that some individuals with peripheral neuropathy are asymptomatic and given the considerable difficulties in objectively demonstrating certain types of peripheral neuropathy (such as SFPN), precise incidence and prevalence data will likely remain elusive. Diabetes mellitus is the most common cause of painful peripheral neuropathy in most populations, and polyneuropathy and neuropathic pain in DM are more amenable to epidemiologic study. However, many epidemiologic studies have not differentiated painful and nonpainful diabetic neuropathy.

The overall prevalence estimate of DM in 2005 in the USA was 7%, but in individuals older than 60 years of age the estimated prevalence was 20.9% [22]. In 2005, the estimated overall incidence for DM was 1.5 million. Prevalence estimates of peripheral neuropathy in patients with DM have ranged between 26 and 47% [23]. The prevalence of neuropathic pain in diabetic neuropathy has not been a primary focus of most epidemiologic studies.

Clinical Question

1. What is the incidence of painful diabetic neuropathy?
2. What is the prevalence of painful peripheral neuropathy in individuals with DM?

Search Strategy

Ovid MEDLINE database was searched since its inception to September of 2009. MeSH terms "incidence" and "neuralgia" or keyword "neuropathic pain" were searched and combined using the Boolean "AND." After limiting the retrieval to English and human excluding letters and editorials, a final set of 342 citations were obtained. From this set, two articles were selected. EMBASE, PubMed, LILACS, and the Cochrane Library databases were also searched implementing the same strategy of MeSH terms and keywords. No additional articles were identified.

Ovid MEDLINE database was searched since its inception to September of 2009. MeSH terms "prevalence" and "neuralgia" or keyword "neuropathic pain" were combined using the Boolean "AND." After limiting the retrieval to English and human excluding letters and editorials, a final set of 88 citations were obtained. An additional search using MeSH terms "diabetic neuropathies" and "neuralgia" or "neuropathic pain" was reviewed. After limiting the retrieval to English and human excluding letters and editorials, a final set of 401 articles were reviewed. From this set, population-based studies from South Wales and Finland were reviewed [24, 25].

EMBASE, PubMed, LILACS, and the Cochrane Library databases were also searched implementing the same strategy of MeSH terms and keywords. No additional articles were identified.

Incidence of Diabetic Neuropathic Pain

A Dutch study reported the incidence rates of various neuropathic pain conditions, including diabetic, painful peripheral neuropathy, by analyzing a national primary care database between 1996 and 2003 [26]. Cases of diabetic neuropathy were not independently verified by the review committee, but rather diagnoses were accepted if they recurred in the record and if "typical" neuropathic pain symptoms were present. Furthermore, diabetic neuropathic pain was only considered if the diagnosis was made following a formal diagnosis of DM. The incidence rate of diabetic neuropathy in the Dutch population was 72.3 per 100,000 person-years. Also of note, there was an increase in the incidence of diabetic neuropathy over the study period.

A similar study reported from the UK also reported painful diabetic neuropathy incidence rates from general practice in the UK between 1992 and 2001 [2]. Primary care records from the Health Information Network database were reviewed. The incidence rate in this population was 27 per 100,000 years.

Prevalence of Neuropathic Pain in Diabetic Neuropathy

A population-based study from South Wales in the UK reported a neuropathic pain prevalence rate of 26.4% in individuals with type II DM [24]. Average duration of DM in this study was 8 years. All patients with type II DM were identified in a database and sent a screening questionnaire, inquiring about the presence of neuropathic pain. Individuals who responded were invited for a clinical examination. The response rate was high, with all but 27 of 353 potentially eligible individuals responded. There are some questions about the generalizability of this data given that the population studied was almost exclusively Caucasian and that the study area is geographically "circumscribed." In an earlier population-based study from Finland, 144 patients with newly diagnosed DM type II were evaluated at baseline, and nearly two-thirds of the cohort was examined again at 10 years following the diagnosis of DM [25]. At baseline, 6% of this cohort had neuropathic pain, and at 10 years 20% of patients reported neuropathic pain.

Summary

Population-based epidemiologic studies of diabetic neuropathy are quite limited, particularly in regard to incidence and prevalence rates for painful diabetic neuropathy. The prevalence of neuropathic pain clearly increases with increasing DM disease duration. The prevalence is as high as 26% in a cohort of diabetic patients with average disease duration of 8 years. General incidence rates of diabetic neuropathic pain in the population may be as high as 72.3 per 100,000 years. Very little is known about racial or ethnic differences in the prevalence of neuropathic pain in DM. There is some suggestion that the incidence of diabetic neuropathic pain is increasing, likely related to increasing rates of DM in the studied populations.

Clinical Bottom Lines

1. The incidence of painful diabetic neuropathy ranges from 27 to 72 per 100,000 person-years.
2. The prevalence of painful peripheral neuropathy in DM increases with increasing DM disease duration, but may occur in as many as 26% of diabetic patients.

Treatment

The treatment of painful peripheral neuropathy is often challenging. There are no medications that are universally effective in reducing neuropathic pain, and medications may result in incomplete pain resolution, particularly in cases of moderate to severe neuropathic pain. Furthermore, neuropathic pain medications may have dose limiting side effects, have the potential to interact with other medications, and can be costly for patients.

Clinical Questions

1. Are tricyclic medications effective in the treatment of painful peripheral neuropathy?
2. Is pregabalin effective in the treatment of painful peripheral neuropathy?
3. Is gabapentin effective in the treatment of painful peripheral neuropathy?

Search Strategy

Ovid MEDLINE database was searched since its inception to September of 2009. MeSH terms "antidepressive agents, tricyclic," and "diabetic neuropathy" were combined using the Boolean "AND." After limiting the retrieval to English and human excluding letters and editorials, a final set of 103 citations were obtained. An additional search using MeSH terms "antidepressive agents, tricyclic" and "neuralgia" was performed, and 176 citations were obtained. A Cochrane review was selected for analysis [21]. EMBASE, PubMed, LILACS, and the Cochrane Library databases were also searched implementing the same strategy of MeSH terms and keywords. No additional articles were identified.

Ovid MEDLINE database was searched since its inception to September of 2009. MeSH terms "anticonvulsants/or pregabalin" and "neuralgia" were combined using the Boolean "AND." After limiting the retrieval to English and human excluding letters and editorials, a final set of 372 citations were obtained. An additional search using MeSH terms "anticonvulsants/or pregabalin" and "diabetic neuropathies" was performed, and 148 citations were obtained. A Cochrane review was selected for analysis [20]. EMBASE, PubMed, LILACS, and the Cochrane Library databases were also searched implementing the same strategy of MeSH terms and keywords. No additional articles were identified.

Ovid MEDLINE database was searched since its inception to September of 2009. MeSH terms "anticonvulsants/or gabapentin" and "diabetic neuropathy" were combined using the Boolean "AND." After limiting the retrieval to English and human excluding letters and editorials, a final set of 179 citations were obtained. An additional search using MeSH terms "anticonvulsants/or gabapentin" and "neuralgia" was performed, and 495 citations were obtained. Two articles were selected for analysis, including a Cochrane review of anticonvulsant therapy in neuropathic pain and recent clinical trial of combination gabapentin and tricyclic medications in the treatment of neuropathic pain [27, 28]. EMBASE, PubMed, LILACS, and the Cochrane Library databases were also searched implementing the same strategy of MeSH terms and keywords. No additional articles were identified.

Tricyclic Medications Are Effective in the Treatment of Painful Diabetic Neuropathy

A recent Cochrane review reported the results of meta-analysis of five placebo-controlled trials evaluating the effectiveness of tricyclic medications in the treatment of diabetic neuropathy [21]. Tricyclic medications relieved neuropathic pain in all five studies, with an NNT of 1.3 (CI 1.2–1.5). Amitriptyline was evaluated in three of these studies, imipramine was evaluated in two of the studies, and desipramine was analyzed in the fifth study. Of 101 patients studied in these five clinical trials, only four patients reportedly withdrew from the studies due to adverse side effects. However, this review also examined other neuropathic pain conditions and studied other antidepressant medications, including selective serotonin reuptake inhibitors and serotonin and noradrenaline reuptake inhibitors for these various conditions, reporting a study drop-out rate of 13% from active treatment groups. The number needed to harm (NNH) for the cumulative tricyclic medication studies was 6 (CI 4.2–10.7) for minor side effects.

Pregabalin Is Effective in the Treatment of Painful Diabetic Neuropathy

Pregabalin was the focus of a recent Cochrane review of acute and chronic pain treatment in adults [20]. Meta-analysis of seven placebo-controlled clinical trials of pregabalin in painful diabetic neuropathy was reported. A total of 2,086 individuals participated in these trials. At a dose of 600 mg daily, 45% of patients achieved a

50% reduction in neuropathic pain compared to 25–30% in the placebo group. The calculated NNT was between 5 and 6 (CI 4–10). The most commonly reported side effects for this medication included somnolence and dizziness, which were reported in 15 and 46% of patients, respectively, on a 600-mg daily dose. NNH (CI) was calculated at 8.8 (CI 7–12) and 2.8 (CI 2.5–3.2).

Gabapentin Is Effective in the Treatment of Painful Diabetic Neuropathy

Gabapentin was studied in a placebo-controlled clinical trial of 165 patients with painful diabetic neuropathy using up to 3,600 mg daily [27]. Fifty-nine percent of patients receiving gabapentin reported improvement on the global impression of change compared to 33% in the placebo group, and 26% of patients in the gabapentin group reported complete pain relief versus 15% in the placebo group. The NNT for this study was 3.8 (CI 2.4–8.7).

A double-blind, crossover trial involving 56 individuals evaluated the efficacy of either gabapentin, nortriptyline, or a combination of these medications in patients with painful diabetic neuropathy or postherpetic neuralgia [28]. Patients were randomized to receive consecutive sequences of these medications during three 6-week treatment periods, with the primary outcome being mean daily pain reduction at the maximum tolerated dose. Forty patients with diabetic peripheral neuropathy and 16 patients with postherpetic neuralgia were studied. In patients with diabetic peripheral neuropathy, pain reduction was greater with combination therapy using gabapentin and nortriptyline when compared to treatment with either drug alone. Moderate pain relief was achieved in 65% of those on gabapentin, 76% in the nortriptyline group, and 84% in those treated with combination therapy.

Summary

Tricyclic antidepressant medications, pregabalin, and gabapentin result in significant neuropathic pain relief in patients with peripheral neuropathy. A recently reported clinical trial directly compared nortriptyline to gabapentin in patients with diabetic neuropathy and postherpetic neuralgia, and nortriptyline was slightly superior. Furthermore, nortriptyline and gabapentin in combination resulted in significant pain relief when compared with these medications individually. Given different putative pharmacotherapeutic mechanisms, it is possible that these medications have a synergistic effect in reducing neuropathic pain.

Clinical Bottom Lines

1. Tricyclic antidepressant medications are effective in reducing neuropathic pain associated with diabetes mellitus with an NNT of 1.3.

2. Pregabalin results in significant reduction in neuropathic pain in patients with diabetic polyneuropathy with NNT between 5 and 6.
3. Gabapentin is effective in reducing neuropathic pain in patients with diabetic polyneuropathy with NNT of 3.8.
4. Combination gabapentin and nortriptyline is effective in neuropathic pain reduction in patients with diabetic polyneuropathy.

References

1. Merskey H, Bogduk N. Classification of chronic pain: descriptions of chronic pain syndromes and definitions of pain terms. 2nd ed. Seattle, WA: IASP; 1994. p. 212.
2. Hall GC, Carroll D, McQuay HJ. Primary care incidence and treatment of four neuropathic pain conditions: a descriptive study, 2002–2005. BMC Fam Pract. 2008;9:26.
3. Bouhassira D, Lanteri-Minet M, Attal N, Laurent B, Touboul C. Prevalence of chronic pain with neuropathic characteristics in the general population. Pain. 2008;136:380–7.
4. Turk DC. Clinical effectiveness and cost-effectiveness of treatments for patients with chronic pain. Clin J Pain. 2002;18:355–65.
5. Li Q, Yang J, Zhou M, Zhang Q, He L. Antiviral treatment for preventing postherpetic neuralgia. Cochrane Database Syst Rev. 2009;4.
6. Sampathkumar P, Drage LA, Martin DP. Herpes Zoster (Shingles) and postherpetic Neuralgia. Mayo Clin Proc. 2009;84(3):274–80.
7. Yawn BP, Saddier P, Wollan P, St Sauver JL, Kurland MJ, Sy LS. A population-based study of the incidence and complication rates of herpes zoster before zoster introduction. Mayo Clin Proc. 2007;82(11):1341–9.
8. Yawn BP, Itzler RF, Wollan PC, Pellisier JM, Sy LS, Saddier P. Health care utilization and cost burden of herpes zoster in a community population. Mayo Clin Proc. 1009;84(9):787–94.
9. Insinga RP, Itzler RF, Pellissier JP, Saddier P, Nikas AA. The incidence of herpes zoster in a United States administrative database. J Gen Intern Med. 2005;20(8):748–53.
10. Oxman MN et al. A vaccine to prevent herpes zoster and postherpetic neuralgia in older adults. N Engl J Med. 2005;352(22):2271–84.
11. Crooks RJ, Jones DA, Fiddian AP. Zoster-associated chronic pain: an overview of clinical trials with acyclovir. Scand J Infect Dis. 1991;80:62–8.
12. Wood MJ, Kay R, Dworkin RH. Oral acyclovir therapy accelerates pain resolution in patients with herpes zoster: a meta-analysis of placebo-controlled trials. Clin Infect Dis. 1996;22(2): 341–7.
13. Alper BS, Lewis PR. Does treatment of acute herpes zoster prevent or shorten postherpetic neuralgia? J Fam Pract. 2000;49(3):255–64.
14. Khaliq W, Alam S, Puri NK. Topical lidocaine for the treatment of postherpetic neuralgia. Cochrane Database Syst Rev. 2009;3.
15. Wiffen PJ, Collins S, McQuay HJ, Carroll D, Jadad A, Moore RA. Anticonvulsant drugs for acute and chronic pain (Review). Cochrane Database Syst Rev. 2009;3.
16. Treeded RD, Jensen TS, Campbell JN, et al. Neuropathic pain: redefinition and a grading system for clinical and research purposes. Neurology. 2008;70:1630–5.
17. Andreson G, Vestergaard K, Ingeman-Nielson M, Staehelin Jensen T. Incidence of post-stroke pain. Pain. 1995;61:187–93.
18. Appelros P. Prevalence and predictors of pain and fatigue after stroke: a population-based study. Int J Rehab Res. 2006;29:329–33.
19. Kong KH, Woon VC, Yang SY. Prevalence of chronic pain and its impact on health-related quality of life in stroke survivors. Arch Phys Med Rehab. 2004;85:35–40.
20. Moore RA, Straube S, Wiffen PJ, Derry S, McQuay HJ. Pregabalin for acute and chronic pain in adults (Review). Cochrane Database Syst Rev. 2009;3.

21. Saarto T, Wiffen PJ. Antidepressants for neuropathic pain (Review). Cochrane Database Syst Rev. 2007;4.
22. Centers for Disease Control and Prevention. Diabetes: Disabling, deadly, and on the rise. GA, USA:CDC; 2005.
23. Barrett AM, Lucero MA, Le T, Robinson RL, Dworkin RH, Chappell MD. Epidemiologic, public health burden, and treatment of diabetic peripheral neuropathic pain: a review. Pain Med. 2007;8(S2):S50–62.
24. Davies M, Williams R, Brophy S, Taylor A. The prevalence, severity, and impact of painful diabetic peripheral neuropathy in type 2 diabetes. Diabet Care. 2006;29(7):1518–22.
25. Partanen J, Niskanen L, Lehtinen J, Mervaala E, Siitonen O, Uusitupa M. Natural history of peripheral neuropathy in patients with non-insulin dependent diabetes mellitus. NEJM. 1995;333:89–94.
26. Dieleman JP, Kerklaan J, Huygen FJPM, Bouma PAD, Sturkenboom MCJM. Incidence rates and treatment of neuropathic pain conditions in the general population. Pain. 2008;137: 681–8.
27. Backonja M, Betdoun A, Edwards KR, Schwarz SI, Fonseca V, et al. Gabapentin for the symptomatic treatment of painful neuropathy in patients with diabetes mellitus. JAMA. 1998;280(21): 1831–6.
28. Gilron I, Bailey JM, Dongsheng T, Holden RR, Jackson AC, Houlden RL. Nortriptyline and gabapentin, alone and in combination for neuropathic pain: a double-blind, randomized controlled crossover trial. Lancet. 2009;374:1252–61.

Chapter 11
Acute Therapies and Disease-Modifying Therapies for Multiple Sclerosis

Khurram Bashir and Dean M. Wingerchuk

Keywords Multiple sclerosis • Optic neuritis • Disease modifying therapy • Clinically isolated syndrome • Epidemiology • Diagnosis • Treatment • Prognosis • Evidence-based medicine

Introduction

We summarize the evidence for several diagnostic and therapeutic questions about multiple sclerosis (MS), the most common nontraumatic disabling neurological disease in young adults [1]. A putative autoimmune disease but with as yet unknown antigen(s), MS presents in 85% of patients with an "attack" ("exacerbation"; "flare") of neurological symptoms and signs that evolve over days to weeks, plateau, and then often spontaneously improve partially or completely. Recurrent attacks or detection of new magnetic resonance imaging (MRI) lesions compatible with MS upon follow-up defines relapsing–remitting MS (RRMS) [2–4]. The remaining 15% of patients are present with a progressive, unremitting neurological syndrome, typically a myelopathy, and are deemed to have primary progressive multiple sclerosis (PPMS). Approximately two-thirds of RRMS patients will eventually develop secondary progressive multiple sclerosis (SPMS), usually after a latency of 1–2 decades, although there is substantial variability in this latency. Lasting neurological impairment may occur as a result of repeated attacks (relapses) but most significant disability, such as the need for cane, walker, or wheelchair, is accrued during the progressive phase of MS. The underlying immunopathology of MS is heterogeneous, and it is possible that diagnostic imaging techniques and other biomarkers may eventually allow more precise, biologically based diagnosis and the management of disease subtypes currently all labeled as "MS."

D.M. Wingerchuk (✉)
Neurology Department, Mayo Clinic, 13400 East Shea Boulevard, Scottsdale, AZ 85259, USA
e-mail: wingerchuk.dean@mayo.edu

J.G. Burneo et al. (eds.), *Neurology: An Evidence-Based Approach*,
DOI 10.1007/978-0-387-88555-1_11, © Springer Science+Business Media, LLC 2012

We consider the supportive evidence for specific interventions for the management of acute attacks and use of disease-modifying therapies (there are six Food and Drug Administration-approved drugs) to prevent attacks and slow disability progression. In all search strategies, we utilized the Ovid MEDLINE and Cochrane systematic review databases, searched from 1990 to 2010, and employed filters for systematic reviews, meta-analyses, and randomized controlled trials (RCTs) where possible.

Treatment of Acute Attacks of Optic Neuritis and Multiple Sclerosis

Introduction

Optic neuritis is a common inflammatory demyelinating syndrome that has been extensively investigated in isolation and in the context of established MS. Focal areas of inflammation and demyelination in the CNS cause the acute symptoms and signs of optic neuritis or other MS attacks. Therefore, rapid-onset anti-inflammatory strategies have typically been used in both settings with a view to halting the inflammatory cascade, ameliorating attack symptoms, and speeding recovery.

Acute Attacks

Clinical Case Example 1

An otherwise healthy 25-year-old man presents with right visual loss and is diagnosed with optic neuritis.

Clinical Questions

1. In patients with optic neuritis, does treatment with corticosteroids improve (a) rate of clinical recovery or (b) final visual outcome compared with placebo?
2. In patients with optic neuritis, does treatment with corticosteroids reduce the risk of recurrent optic neuritis or other relapse (future MS development)?

Search Strategy

We used the medical subject heading (MeSH) terms "optic neuritis," and "adrenal cortex hormones" and the keyword "corticosteroids" to search for relevant primary literature and systematic reviews.

Evidence

We found a systematic review that addressed the questions [5]. It included 566 patients from three RCTs, the primary one of which was the optic neuritis treatment trial (ONTT) [6]. The placebo-controlled ONTT randomized 457 acute optic neuritis patients to either intravenous methylprednisolone (IVMP) 1,000 mg for 3 days plus an oral prednisone taper ($n = 151$) or oral prednisone 1 mg/kg/day for 14 days plus a tapering dose ($n = 156$). Outcome assessments included proportion of patients with complete visual recovery at 8 days, 30 days, and longer (6–36 months) as well as number with recurrent optic neuritis or clinically definite MS at 2 and 5 years. Other RCTs studied adrenocorticotropic hormone (ACTH) versus placebo and were targeted to visual outcome. For purposes of meta-analysis, 100 mg of IVMP was considered equivalent to 80 mg oral prednisone or 16 units of ACTH. Heterogeneity between RCTs was noted in the meta-analysis.

High-dose IVMP (>500 mg/day) plus a prednisone taper or ACTH therapy resulted in faster visual recovery at 1 month but not at 6 months; oral prednisone alone had no benefit. High-dose IVMP also reduced risk of relapse at 2 years but not 5 years in data derived from the ONTT. Major side effects included depression, acute pancreatitis, and rash (approximately 1–7% incidence).

Clinical Bottom Lines

1. Compared with placebo, the treatment of acute optic neuritis with high dose (>500 mg/day IVMP for 3 days plus an oral prednisone taper) or ACTH for 30 days is associated with improved visual acuity at 1 month (NNT = 11) but not 6 months after onset.
2. Compared with placebo, the treatment of acute optic neuritis with high-dose IVMP (as above), but not low-dose IVMP, reduced the risk of recurrent optic neuritis or other clinical relapse at 2 years (NNT = 14) but not 5 years after the onset.

Summary

High-dose corticosteroids speed recovery from acute optic neuritis but do not enhance long-term visual outcome. They also appear to temporarily reduce the risk of recurrent symptomatic demyelinating disease for up to 2 years. Therefore, such treatment is reasonable for most patients with optic neuritis, especially those who do not have medical contraindications to corticosteroids.

Clinical Case Example 2

A 31-year-old woman with established RRMS presents with a new myelitis attack consisting of moderate lower extremity weakness, a sensory level, and bladder incontinence.

Clinical Questions

1. Compared with placebo, does treatment with corticosteroids improve clinical outcome from multiple sclerosis relapses?
2. Compared with placebo, does treatment with intravenous immune globulin (IVIG) improve clinical outcome from multiple sclerosis relapses?
3. Compared with sham exchange, does treatment with plasma exchange improve clinical outcome from multiple sclerosis relapses?

Search Strategy

We used the MeSH terms "multiple sclerosis," "adrenal cortex hormones," "immunoglobulins, intravenous," "plasmapheresis," and "plasma exchange" and the keywords "corticosteroids," "attack," "relapse," "flare," and "exacerbation" to search for relevant primary literature and systematic reviews. We found systematic reviews and Cochrane reviews that addressed the questions about corticosteroids and IVIG and an RCT that compared plasmapheresis against sham exchange for patients with severe, corticosteroid-refractory attacks of CNS demyelinating disease.

Evidence

Two systematic reviews considered the effect of corticosteroids [5, 7]. A Cochrane review included data from 377 participants in six placebo-controlled RCTs [7]. Interventions ranged from IVMP, oral methylprednisolone, and ACTH, all of which reduced the risk of attack worsening or failure to improve at 5 weeks after therapy (NNT=4). There was a somewhat greater effect for high-dose (1 g/day) IVMP but the difference compared with other therapies was not statistically significant. Only one trial, which utilized oral MP, evaluated long-term benefit on neurological impairment. It found a significant benefit at 8 weeks but equivocal benefit at 1 year. There were no important differences between intravenous and oral dosing otherwise and short (3 days) versus longer (up to 15 days) treatment courses also did not differ. In the meta-analysis, there were fewer psychiatric and gastrointestinal adverse events in the IVMP-treated groups compared with oral MP groups.

Two studies of adjunctive IVIG with IVMP for acute MS relapses showed no benefit over placebo [8, 9]. A small RCT ($n=22$) with a crossover design studied the potential benefit of plasmapheresis against sham exchange as rescue therapy for corticosteroid-refractory attacks of CNS demyelination [10]. The study included 12 patients with typical MS and a severe, steroid-refractory attack. Four patients experienced important clinical improvement during active plasmapheresis compared with one during sham exchange. This was not significant. The overall results of the RCT, which included patients with recurrent myelitis, acute disseminated encephalomyelitis, neuromyelitis optica, and other CNS inflammatory demyelinating conditions, did show significant benefit for plasmapheresis response (42%) versus sham exchange (6%).

Clinical Bottom Lines

1. Compared with placebo, administration of high-dose methylprednisolone for 3–15 consecutive days, either by intravenous or oral route, increases the likelihood of better neurological outcome at 5 weeks (NNT = 4) but does not convincingly improve long-term neurological recovery.
2. Administration of adjunctive IVIG does not speed recovery or improve neurological outcome after MS relapse in patients being treated with corticosteroids.
3. In patients with severe, corticosteroid-refractory attacks of CNS demyelinating disease, rescue therapy with plasma exchange may increase the proportion of patients who respond (42%) compared with sham exchange (6%; NNT = 3), but more research is needed specifically for MS.

Summary

Although mild attacks (e.g., focal numbness) may be managed without active intervention, moderate or severe attacks warrant consideration of treatment with corticosteroids to speed recovery. There is no established role for IVIG in the treatment of acute MS attacks. Patients with severe attacks (e.g., paraplegia, blindness) and who do not improve significantly with corticosteroid therapy could be offered plasma exchange; a typical course consists of seven exchanged performed at an every-other-day frequency. None of these therapies have been approved specifically for the treatment of MS attacks. Future research opportunities may include combination therapies and tailoring treatment options to underlying immunological mechanisms, if radiological and other biomarkers of specific disease patterns are validated.

Disease-Modifying Therapies for Multiple Sclerosis

There are six approved therapies for MS as of early 2010. These include three interferon beta (IFNβ) drugs (intramuscular IFNβ-1a, subcutaneous IFNβ-a, and subcutaneous IFNβ-1b), glatiramer acetate, mitoxantrone, and natalizumab. The indications for each drug vary and depend on the classification of the disease course as a clinically isolated syndrome (CIS) (first-ever demyelinating event), relapsing–remitting disease, or a progressive form of MS.

Clinically Isolated Syndromes

Introduction

Increased access to neurologists and MRI has resulted in a substantial proportion of patients presenting for diagnosis during or after their first-ever clinical event. However, confirmation of an MS diagnosis requires dissemination in space (either a second clinical attack or development of new MRI lesions) and time. Until those criteria are met, the sentinel neurological event is deemed to be a "clinically isolated syndrome" if it is determined that the patient is at significant future risk for confirmed MS. Risk stratification is accomplished mainly with brain MRI data; the presence of >1 lesion typical of demyelination portends a future risk of clinical relapse of nearly 90% at 14 years, whereas if the scan is normal, the risk of MS is only about 20% [1]. The revised McDonald criteria allow confirmation of dissemination in space and time after detection of new MRI abnormalities or a new clinical attack ("relapse") during follow-up, therefore defining a "relapsing–remitting" MS course [4].

Conceptually, treating CIS patients with a disease-modifying therapy that reduces the risk of future inflammatory demyelinating lesions could delay official conversion the MS diagnosis and, more importantly, preserve neurological function.

Clinical Case

An otherwise healthy 28-year-old woman develops right optic neuritis. Brain MRI reveals six white matter lesions, all periventricular, and two lesions enhance following intravenous gadolinium administration. She is diagnosed with CIS (optic neuritis with high risk for future development of MS) and is advised to consider initiating disease-modifying therapy.

Clinical Question

1. Compared with placebo, does treatment with INF-β or glatiramer acetate (GA) reduce the rate of conversion to definite multiple sclerosis?

Search Strategy

We used MeSH terms "multiple sclerosis," "clinically isolated syndrome," "interferon," and "glatiramer acetate," to find RCTs that addressed the clinical questions.

Evidence

We detected RCTs for each of intramuscular INFβ-1a, low-dose subcutaneous IFNβ-1a, subcutaneous IFNβ-1b, and glatiramer acetate in which CIS patients were randomized to either the interferon therapy or placebo. In each study, the primary outcome was conversion to MS, either "clinically definite" MS (defined as occurrence of a second clinical attack) or fulfillment of the "McDonald criteria" for MS, which allows for either new MRI lesions or a clinical event to achieve the dissemination criteria.

Intramuscular IFNβ-1a

Two large, RCTs showed efficacy of intramuscular IFNβ-1a for prevention or delay of the second clinical attack that defines "clinically definite" MS [11, 12]. The CHAMPS study was a randomized, double-blind, placebo-controlled RCT of 383 patients with CIS [11]. Participants had ≥2 brain MRI lesions and received 30 µg of intramuscular IFNβ-1a or placebo for 3 years after initial therapy with 3 days of IV methylprednisolone and 15 days of oral prednisone. The IFN group MS conversion rate (second clinical attack) was lower (35%) than that of the placebo arm (50%). Clinical disability was not assessed. MRI measures were significantly better in the interferon group (median T2-weighted lesion volume at 18 months, mean number of new or enlarging lesions, mean number of gadolinium-enhancing lesions). The ETOMS CIS study ($n=309$) compared subcutaneous IFNβ-1a at a lower dose (22 µg weekly) than typically used in RRMS with placebo [12]. There was no standard corticosteroid treatment protocol at the onset. Interferon treatment reduced the clinically definite MS conversion rate to 34% versus 45% for placebo.

One large RCT addressed the efficacy of subcutaneous IFNβ-1b for prevention or delay "clinically definite" MS or for the establishment of MS diagnosis by McDonald criteria. The BENEFIT study compared IFNβ-1b 250 µg s.c. every other day ($n=292$) with placebo ($n=176$) in CIS patients [13]. The coprimary efficacy outcomes were time to clinically definite MS by modified Poser criteria and time to MS according to McDonald criteria. INFβ-1b prolonged time to CDMS (618 days compared to 255 days with placebo; relative risk reduction of 48%) and time to McDonald MS. IFNβ-1b treatment reduced the cumulative probability of CDMS to 28% from 45% at 2 years in the placebo group and the cumulative probability of McDonald MS to 69% from 85%. Expected MRI benefits were also seen and treatment was well tolerated.

A large RCT studied the efficacy of glatiramer acetate in 481 CIS patients with unifocal clinical manifestation and two or more T2-weighted brain lesions measuring 6 mm or more [14]. They were randomly assigned to receive either subcutaneous glatiramer acetate 20 mg per day or placebo for up to 36 months, unless they converted to CDMS. The primary endpoint was time to conversion to CDMS. Glatiramer acetate significantly reduced the risk of developing CDMS by 45% compared with placebo. The time for 25% of patients to convert to CDMS was prolonged by 115%, from 336 days for placebo to 722 days for glatiramer acetate. The proportion of patients having a second attack was similarly reduced from 42.9% in the placebo group to 24.7% in the glatiramer acetate group (Table 11.1).

Table 11.1 Disease modifying therapies for clinically isolated syndromes

Outcome	Trial	NNT vs. Placebo
Conversion to CDMS	CHAMPS (s.c. IFNβ-1a)	6.7 over 3 years
	ETOMS (s.c. IFNβ-1a low dose)	9.1 over 2 years
	BENEFIT (s.c. IFNβ-1b)	5.9 over 2 years
	PreCISe (s.c. glatiramer acetate)	5.5 over 3 years
Conversion to "McDonald MS"	BENEFIT (s.c. IFNβ-1b)	6.3 over 2 years

Clinical Bottom Lines

1. Compared with placebo, conversion to CDMS after CIS presentation may be delayed by the treatment with intramuscular IFNβ-1a (NNT 6.7 over 3 years), subcutaneous IFNβ-1b (NNT = 5.9 over 2 years), or glatiramer acetate (NNT = 5.5 over 3 years).

Summary

Intramuscular IFNβ-1a, subcutaneous IFNβ-1b, and glatiramer acetate are indicated for the delay of a second attack that establishes an MS diagnosis. It remains unknown whether such early treatment strategies impact the long-term course of the disease and resulting neurological impairment. The decision to start one of these disease-modifying therapies should involve discussion of the available short-term efficacy data, uncertain long-term benefits and adverse effects of the drugs, as well as incorporate the patient's preferences.

Treatment of SPMS and PPMS

MS is an immune-mediated, demyelinating disease of the central nervous system (CNS) that shows a range of clinical features and clinical disease courses. Based on the presence or absence of relapses and remissions and/or progression of neurologic deficits, MS patients may be categorized into different clinical types [2]. PPMS presents with "disease progression from the onset with occasional plateaus and temporary minor improvements" but without relapses or remissions during its course [2]. SPMS patients begin with a pattern of RRMS that later undergoes a transition to a progressive course with or without superimposed relapses [2]. PPMS patients are reported to differ from those with RRMS and SPMS in their clinical, genetic, laboratory, imaging, and pathological characteristics, as well as in their response to therapeutic agents [15–17]. The incidence of PPMS subtype is reported to be around 10% (between 8 and 37%) of all MS patients [18–21]. PPMS is relatively more common in patients who present at a later age (i.e., after the age of 40 years), and in men [15]. The most common presentation in PP disease is a chronic progressive myelopathy [15]. A prerequisite for establishing a diagnosis of definite MS in these patients is to demonstrate a clinical disease course of greater than 1 year, the dissemination of lesions by cranial MRI and/or evoked potentials (EP), and inflammatory changes in cerebrospinal fluid (CSF) [22, 23]. Strict adherence to these criteria may lead to the diagnosis of PPMS being missed because of the reported observation of normal cranial MRI [24] and absent oligoclonal bands (OCB) in PPMS patients. Spinal cord MRI may demonstrate abnormalities in cases where the cranial MRI is normal [24]. Pathologically, PPMS has less perivascular cuffing and parenchymal cellular infiltration compared to SPMS [25]. PPMS has a prognosis for severe disability and no therapeutic intervention has been proven to arrest or slow its relentlessly progressive course.

Treatment of SPMS

IFNβ Therapies

IFNβ agents used for treating MS patients are recombinant proteins produced in *E. coli* or Chinese hamster ovarian cells. These agents are approved for use in relapsing forms of MS and in the CISs. Their utility is SPMS is controversial and currently open to debate.

Interferon Beta-1b

In a large, multicenter, randomized trial in Europe, IFNβ-1b was compared to placebo in 718 SPMS patients with EDSS of 3.0–6.5 and evidence of clinically active disease. Initially designed as a 3-year study, this trial was stopped at 2 years at the recommendation of the independent monitoring board because of "overwhelming efficacy" determined at the time of the preplanned interim analysis. The primary endpoint for SPMS trial, which was the time to confirmed disability progression, measured as an increase in EDSS score confirmed at 3 months and was significantly delayed. This delay in progression was apparent at nine and became statistically significant at 12 months after 2 years of treatment. With IFNβ-1b treatment, both the proportion of patients becoming wheelchair bound and the time to becoming wheelchair bound were significantly decreased. The salutary effect of IFNβ-1b on relapses and MRI parameters noted in the phase III RRMS trial [26, 27] was again noted in this European IFNβ-1b SPMS study. IFNβ-1b treatment also showed a statistically significant effect on the patient reported health-related quality of life measures [28]. A second phase III trial of IFN β-1b in SPMS in North America failed to demonstrate a significant therapeutic effect of this agent on slowing disease progression. In this trial, 939 SPMS patients were randomly assigned to two different doses of IFNβ-1b or to placebo administered as a subcutaneous injection every other day. The primary endpoint was identical to the one in the European IFNβ-1b SPMS trial. This lack of effect persisted even when patients were stratified by variables that included baseline degree of disability and relapse rate. However, the reduction in annualized and mean relapse rates, number of moderate to severe relapses, relapse duration, hospitalizations, number of treatment courses with glucocorticoids all favored treatment with IFNβ-1b. On cranial MRI, T2 lesion volume, new or enlarging T2 lesions, and new or enlarging gadolinium-enhancing lesions were significantly less in the treated group. The difference in outcome of the European and North American trials is believed to be due to the different patient characteristics despite similar entry criteria [29]. The patients in the European study were younger, had shorter duration of MS, had a more recent transition to the progressive course, were more likely to have relapses superimposed on their progressive course, and had a greater number of gadolinium-enhancing lesions on their cranial MRI at study entry. Thus, in the SPMS patients enrolled in the European trial, "inflammatory activity," as measured by clinical relapses and gadolinium-enhancing lesions on MRI, was still a major component of their pathophysiological disease process.

Subcutaneous IFNβ-1a

In SPECTRIMS study, 618 SPMS patients were randomly treated with either subcutaneous IFNβ-1a or placebo three times a week for a period of 3 years [30]. The primary outcome of the study was time-to-confirmed sustained progression, and this was not significantly different between the treated and placebo groups at the end of the study period. However, treatment with subcutaneous IFNβ-1a demonstrated a significant benefit on the relapse rate, other relapse related secondary outcome measures, median number of active lesions per patient per scan, and the accumulation of T2 lesion load [30, 31]. Post-hoc analysis suggested a greater benefit in patients with greater than one clinical relapse in the 2 years prior to study entry and in women.

Intramuscular IFNβ-1a

The efficacy of intramuscular IFNβ-1a in SPMS patients was studied in a randomized, double-blind, placebo-controlled study of 436 patients (IMPACT Trial) [32]. As the opposed to the other therapeutic SPMS trials, the investigators for this study chose multiple sclerosis functional composite (MSFC), a relatively new and less well-established disability measure, as the primary outcome. Compared to placebo weekly intramuscular injections of IFNβ-1a were shown to reduce the median MSFC z-score by 40.4%; this difference in outcomes between the two groups was statistically significant. However, an evaluation of the individual components of the

MSFC demonstrated that the only significant effect was on the measure of upper extremity function (nine-hole peg test). The other components of MSFC, including those measuring cognition and lower extremity function did not show a statistically significant therapeutic effect. Also, the treatment with intramuscular IFNβ-1a did not appear to alter the rate of disability progression as measured by EDSS. There were statistically significant effects noted on the mean number of relapses, new or enlarging T2 hyperintense lesions, number of gadolinium-enhancing lesions and quality of life measures. Because of the fact that a beneficial effect of intramuscular IFNβ-1a could not be demonstrated on EDSS, this drug has not been approved for use in SPMS by the FDA in the USA.

Summary of IFNβ Trials in SPMS

Of the four, large, randomized, double-blind, placebo-controlled trials of IFNβ in SPMS, only the European IFNβ-1b trial demonstrated a beneficial therapeutic effect. The other three trials failed to show an effect on the accumulation of sustained disability measured by EDSS following IFNβ treatment. These contradictory results appear to be, at least in part, due to differences in patient populations enrolled in these studies. An analysis of the European and North American IFNβ-1b SPMS studies showed that younger patients, patients with shorter duration of secondary progressive disease, patients with recent relapse activity, and patients with greater than average EDSS progression over the 2 years prior to study entry were more likely to benefit from IFNβ treatment [29].

Common side effects of IFNβ therapy are lymphopenia, elevated serum transaminases, injection site reactions (with subcutaneous preparations), depression, and flu-like symptoms. The incidence of flu-like symptoms is highest at the start of therapy and tends to decrease over time; these flu-like symptoms may be lessened by premedication with acetaminophen or nonsteroidal anti-inflammatory drugs (NSAIDs). Depression may appear and in some of the initial trials doubled over that seen with placebo in the years 3 through year 5 (10% vs. 5%). Postmarketing studies have not shown depression to be a significant issue with IFNβ-1b, and in the European and North American SPMS trials, depression did not occur more commonly in the treated than the placebo groups.

Glatiramer Acetate

GA is a synthetic polymer of four amino acids found in the myelin basic protein. Glatiramer acetate has not been studied in patients with SPMS in a large, randomized, double-blind, placebo-controlled trial.

Natalizumab

Natalizumab is a humanized monoclonal antibody against $\alpha4$-integrin. Natalizumab has not been studied in patients with SPMS in a randomized, double-blind, placebo-controlled fashion. Because of the potential risk of PML and strict monitoring requirements as well as the difficulty in differentiating PML symptoms from those of progressive MS, natalizumab use in SPMS is not advisable.

Mitoxantrone

Mitoxantrone is an anthracenedione derivative, which was developed as an antineo-plastic agent and has been used to treat a variety of malignant conditions [33]. It interacts with topoisomerase-2 and intercalates the DNA resulting in cytotoxic and immunosuppressive effects [34, 35]. An early randomized, double-blind trial compared the effect of mitoxantrone to that of IVMP over a 32-month period in patients with relapsing SPMS [36]. The treatment with mitoxantrone administered intravenously at a dose of 12 mg/m^2 body surface area resulted in significant improvement in EDSS. The proportion of patients with an EDSS greater than 5.0 decreased to 42% from a baseline of 71% after the treatment for 1 year. The total number of gadolinium-enhancing lesions was also significantly lower in the mitoxantrone group. This led to a phase III investigator-blinded, randomized, placebo-controlled study of mitoxantrone in worsening RRMS and SPMS patients (the "MIMS Trial") [37]. A total of 194 patients were randomly assigned to mitoxantrone 12 mg/m^2, mitoxantrone 5 mg/m^2, or placebo administered intravenously every 3 months for 2 years. The primary endpoint was a multivariate composite of five clinical measures, including change in EDSS, ambulation index (AI), and standardized neurological status (SNS) from baseline, median time to first relapse, and number of relapses treated with steroids. The mean EDSS scores decreased by 0.3 steps compared to a 0.23 step increase in EDSS in the placebo group. The median time to first treated relapse, and the mean number of steroid-treated relapses also favored the treatment group. This treatment effect was maintained 12 months after the last treatment. In addition, the proportion of patients with confirmed neurological progression, annualized relapse rate, proportion of relapse-free patients, and number of hospitalizations were all lower in the mitoxantrone group. An assessment of the quality of life measures demonstrated a significantly less worsening in the treated group versus the placebo group. In a subset of patients who underwent MRI assessments, the number of gadolinium-enhancing and new T2 lesions was decreased with treatment. In this study, the majority of the patients with SPMS experienced relapses superimposed on their disease course while 25.5% of the patients had slow worsening of disability without relapses. The study was not powered to detect differential effects of treatment on the two subgroups.

Based on these results, mitoxantrone has been approved for use in worsening RRMS (RRMS patients with frequent relapses followed by incomplete recovery) and SPMS. The treatment is administered intravenously at a dose of 12 mg/m^2 body surface area every 3 months over 30–45 min. The treatment duration is limited by a maximum lifetime dose of 140 mg/m^2 because of the potential risk of cardiac toxicity. Overall, the risks associated with mitoxantrone are generally considered acceptable in the clinical settings where this therapy is employed. The potential serious adverse effects of therapy include infections, congestive heart failure, asymptomatic drop in left ventricular ejection fraction, acute leukemia, tissue damage in case of accidental paravasation, and infertility. Careful monitoring of laboratory and cardiac assessments is recommended before, during and after the treatment with mitoxantrone [33, 38].

Intravenous Immunoglobulin

Based on some promising results from several small trials, a large multicenter, randomized, placebo-controlled study of IVIG was carried out in 318 patients with SPMS [39]. In this trial, IVIG 1 g/kg/month was compared to placebo over a 27-month period. The primary outcome was the time to confirmed progression measured by EDSS. The IVIG treatment did not demonstrate a beneficial effect on the time to confirmed EDSS progression, the annual relapse rate, the change in T2-lesion load, or any of the other clinical outcome measures.

Clinical Bottom Lines

1. In the treatment of SPMS, IFNβ therapy is more likely to reduce relapses and prevent disability in patients who are younger, have a shorter duration of disease, and demonstrate clinical or radiographic relapses.
2. In the treatment of SPMS, IFNβ is unlikely to benefit patients who are older with no superimposed relapses.
3. Mixoxantrone is more likely to improve disability and reduce relapses in patients with SPMS with a more rapid disease progression and signs of relapses.
4. IVIg did not demonstrate any benefit in patients with SPMS.

Summary of Randomized Clinical Trials in SPMS

Current evidence suggests that SPMS patients who are relatively younger, have a shorter duration of disease, have recently transitioned to secondary progressive course, and demonstrate superimposed clinical relapses or gadolinium-enhancing lesions on MRI are likely to benefit from IFNβ therapy. Patients who are older and have a slowly and "purely" progressive course with no superimposed inflammatory activity appear to derive little or no benefit from IFNβ treatment. SPMS patients with more rapid progression of disease and those with on-going inflammatory disease (clinical relapses or gadolinium-enhancing lesions) seem to derive the most benefit from mitoxantrone. Other agents have either not been studied or have failed to modify the disease course in SPMS patients. A summary of the randomized clinical trials done in SPMS cohorts is given in Table 11.2.

Table 11.2 Summary of pivotal RCT in SPMS

Drug/Study	Effect on primary endpoint	Effect of secondary endpoint	Comments
IFNβ-1b (European SPMS Trial)	*Positive* effect on disability progression as measured by EDSS	*Positive* effect on relapses and MRI measures	This study led to approval of IFNβ-1b for SPMS in Europe and Canada
IFNβ-1b (North American SPMS Trial)	*Negative* effect on disability progression as measured by EDSS	*Positive* effect on relapses and MRI measures	Results of this study contradicted the European study results because of differences in patient population
Subcutaneous IFNβ-1a (SPECTRIMS Trial)	*Negative* effect on disability progression as measured by EDSS	*Positive* effect on relapses and MRI measures	Patient population similar to that enrolled in the North American SPMS study
Intramuscular IFNβ-1a (IMPACT Trial)	*Positive* effect on disability progression as measured by MSFC	*Negative* effect on disability progression as measured by EDSS *Positive* effect on relapses and MRI measures	The beneficial effect on MSFC mostly a result of the effect on upper extremity function; no significant effect on cognition or lower extremity function
Mitoxantrone (MIMS Trial)	*Positive* effect on disability progression as measured by composite score of five different measures	*Positive* effect on relapses and MRI measures	Currently approved for SPMS, worsening RRMS, and progressive relapsing MS (PRMS)
Intravenous immunoglobulin	*Negative* effect on disability progression as measured by EDSS	*Negative* effect on relapses and MRI measures	No beneficial effect noted on any clinical outcome measure

Treatment of PPMS

Currently, there is no proven therapy for the treatment of PPMS. A number of large, multicenter therapeutic clinical trials have demonstrated disappointing results in this MS subtype.

Interferon Beta

Two small pilot trials of intramuscular IFN β-1a compared to placebo in 50 PPMS patients [40] and of IFNβ-1b in combined PPMS plus transitional MS patient population [41] failed to show a beneficial effect on the disease course. No large, placebo-controlled, randomized trial of IFNβ agents has been conducted in patients with PPMS.

Glatiramer Acetate

Glatiramer acetate was studied in 943 patients with PPMS over 3 years in a double-blind, placebo-controlled trial [42]. The primary end point in this trial was time to one point EDSS change sustained for 3 months in patients with EDSS of 3.0–5.0 at the time of study-entry, and 0.5-point EDSS change sustained for 3 months in patients with EDSS of 5.5–6.5 at study entry. The trial was stopped early at the recommendation of an independent data safety monitoring board because of a lack of beneficial treatment effect on the primary outcome measure. MRI analysis demonstrated a statistically significant reduction on gadolinium-enhancing lesions at 1 year and on T2 lesion volume at year 3 compared to placebo. A post-hoc subgroup analysis showed a possible beneficial effect among male PPMS patients. A slower than expected rate of disability progression in the placebo group resulted in erroneous power calculations and effects size, ultimately contributing to the negative result in this trial.

Natalizumab

Natalizumab has not been studied in PPMS and is not recommended for use in this MS subtype.

Mitoxantrone

To date, no large randomized, double-blind, placebo-controlled, multicenter study has evaluated the role of mitoxantrone therapy in PPMS. Kita et al. reported no clinical benefit of mitoxantrone therapy in PPMS patients in a phase II clinical trial [43]. Another open-label, observational study reported the effect of treatment in nine PPMS patient out of a total of 94 progressive patients treated with 20 mg of mitoxantrone (not weight based) in combination with 1 g of methylprednisolone given once a month. Over the course of 6-month follow-up, seven of the nine patients continued to worsen while two remained stable on this regimen [44]. Another open-label study evaluated the effect of two different dosing protocols in 64 PPMS. The investigators reported a modest beneficial effect of mitoxantrone on disease progression in patients with baseline EDSS score of less than six using the more aggressive dosing regimen [45].

Rituximab

Rituximab is a chimeric anti-CD20 monoclonal antibody that selectively depletes B cells [46]. Rituximab was evaluated in 439 PPMS patients over a 96-week period in a double-blind, placebo-controlled, randomized clinical trial [47]. The primary endpoint was time to confirmed disease progression measured as worsening of EDSS sustained for 3 months. Despite a trend favoring treatment with rituximab, a statistically significant effect on disease progression could not be demonstrated. As with the GA trial, a beneficial effect was noted on T2 lesion volume compared to placebo; however, the treatment with rituximab did not reduce progression of brain atrophy. Post-hoc subgroup analysis of this trial demonstrated a suggestion of beneficial effect in patients younger than 51 years of age and those with gadolinium-enhancing lesions on their baseline MRI scans. In contrast to the GA trial, there was no preferential effect of rituximab in PPMS patient of either gender. Rituximab treatment was more frequently associated with serious infections and infusion-related reactions compared to placebo.

Clinical Bottom Lines

1. No therapeutic agent has been found to slow disability or reduce relapses in PPMS.

Summary of Randomized Clinical Trials in PPMS

Despite a greater risk of progression in PPMS patients, none of the therapeutic agents studied in this MS subtype have shown a beneficial effect in slowing or stopping further accumulation of disability. A summary of clinical trials done to date in PPMS cohorts is given in Table 11.3. Despite negative results, these trials suggest that GA may have a potential beneficial effect in men with PPMS, and rituximab

Table 11.3 Summary of pivotal RCT in PPMS

Drug/Study	Effect on primary endpoint	Effect of secondary endpoint	Comment
Glatiramer Acetate (PROMiSE Trial)	*Negative* effect on disability progression as measured by EDSS	*Positive* effect on MRI measures	Post-hoc analysis suggested a beneficial effect on disease progression in men
Rituximab (OLYMPUS Trial)	*Negative* effect on disability progression as measured by EDSS	*Positive* effect on T2 lesion volume on MRI *Negative* effect on brain volume on MRI	Post-hoc analysis suggested a beneficial effect in patients <51 years of age and those with gadolinium-enhancing lesions

may have a favorable influence on the disease course in younger patients and those with gadolinium-enhancing lesions. However, as these suggestions are based on post-hoc analyses, further studies are needed to be confident about the validity of these observations.

References

1. Compston A, Coles A. Multiple sclerosis. Lancet. 2008;372:1502–17.
2. Lublin FD, Reingold SC. Defining the clinical course of multiple sclerosis: results of an international survey. Neurology. 1996;46:907–11.
3. Poser CM, Paty DW, Scheinberg L, McDonald WI, Davis FA, Ebers GC, et al. New diagnostic criteria for multiple sclerosis: guidelines for research protocols. Ann Neurol. 1983;13:227–31.
4. Polman CH, Reingold SC, Edan G, Filippi M, Hartung HP, Kappos L, et al. Diagnostic criteria for multiple sclerosis: 2005 revisions to the "McDonald Criteria". Ann Neurol. 2005;58:840–6.
5. Brusaferri F, Candelise L. Steroids for multiple sclerosis and optic neuritis: a meta-analysis of randomized controlled clinical trials. J Neurol. 2000;247:435–42.
6. Beck RW, Cleary PA, Anderson Jr MM, et al. A randomized, controlled trial of corticosteroids in the treatment of acute optic neuritis. N Engl J Med. 1992;326:581–8.
7. Filippini G, Brusaferri F, Sibley WA, Citterio A, Ciucci G, Midgard R, Candelise L. Corticosteroids or ACTH for acute exacerbations in multiple sclerosis. Cochrane Database Syst Rev. 2000;4:CD001331.
8. Sorensen PS, Haas J, Sellebjerg F, Olsson T, Ravnborg M. TARIMS Study Group. IV immunoglobulins as add-on treatment to methylprednisolone for acute relapses in MS. Neurology. 2004;63:2028–33.
9. Visser LH, Beekman R, Tijssen CC, Uitdehaag BM, Lee ML, Movig KL, et al. A randomized, double-blind, placebo-controlled pilot study of i.v. immune globulins in combination with i.v. methylprednisolone in the treatment of relapses in patients with MS. Mult Scler. 2004;10:89–91.
10. Weinshenker BG, O'Brien PC, Petterson TM, et al. A randomized trial of plasma exchange in acute CNS inflammatory demyelinating disease. Ann Neurol. 1999;46:878–86.

11. Jacobs LD, Beck RW, Simon JH, et al. Intramuscular interferon beta-1a therapy initiated during a first demyelinating event in multiple sclerosis. N Engl J Med. 2000;343:898–904.
12. Comi G, Filippi M, Barkhof F, et al. Effect of early interferon treatment on conversion to definite multiple sclerosis: a randomised study. Lancet. 2001;357:1576–82.
13. Kappos L, Polman C, Freedman MS, et al. Treatment with interferon beta-1b delays conversion to clinically definite and McDonald MS in patients with clinically isolated syndromes. Neurology. 2006;67:1242–9.
14. Comi G, Martinelli V, Rodegher M, et al. Effect of glatiramer acetate on conversion to clinically definite multiple sclerosis in patients with clinically isolated syndrome (PreCISe study): a randomised, double-blind, placebo-controlled trial. Lancet. 2009;374:1503–11.
15. Thompson AJ, Polman CH, Miller DH, et al. Primary progressive multiple sclerosis. Brain. 1997;120:1085–96.
16. Weiner HL, Mackin GA, Orav EJ, et al. Intermittent cyclophosphamide pulse therapy in progressive multiple sclerosis: Final report of the Northeast Cooperative Multiple Sclerosis Treatment Group. Neurology. 1993;43:910–8.
17. Goodkin DE, Rudick RA, Medendorp SV, et al. Low-dose (7.5 mg) oral methotrexate reduces the rate of progression in chronic progressive multiple sclerosis. Ann Neurol. 1995;37:30–40.
18. Confavreux C, Aimard G, Devic M. Course and prognosis of multiple sclerosis assessed by the computerized data processing of 349 patients. Brain. 1980;103(2):281–300.
19. Minderhoud JM, van der Hoeven JH, Prange AJA. Course and prognosis of chronic progressive multiple sclerosis. Acta Neurol Scand. 1988;78:10–5.
20. Runmarker B, Andersen O. Prognostic factors in a multiple sclerosis incidence cohort with twenty-five years of follow-up. Brain. 1993;116:117–34.
21. Weinshenker BG, Bass B, Rice GPA, et al. The natural history of multiple sclerosis: a geographically based study. I. Clinical course and disability. Brain. 1989;112:133–46.
22. Poser CM, Paty DW, Scheinberg L, et al. New diagnostic criteria for multiple sclerosis: guidelines for research protocols. Ann Neurol. 1983;13:227–31.
23. Polman CH, Reingold SC, Edan G, et al. Diagnostic criteria for multiple sclerosis: 2005 revisions to the "McDonald Criteria". Ann Neurol. 2005;58(6):840–6.
24. Thorpe JW, Kidd D, Moseley IF, et al. Spinal MRI in patients with suspected multiple sclerosis and negative brain MRI. Brain. 1996;119(Part 3):709–14.
25. Revesz T, Kidd D, Thompson AJ, Barnard RO, McDonald WI. A comparison of the pathology of primary and secondary progressive multiple sclerosis. Brain. 1994;117(4):759–65.
26. Group TIMSS. Interferon beta-1b is effective in relapsing-remitting multiple sclerosis. I. Clinical results of a multicenter, randomized, double-blind, placebo-controlled trial. Neurology. 1993;43:655–61.
27. Group IMSGatUoBCMMA. Interferon beta-1b in the treatment of multiple sclerosis: Final outcome of the randomized controlled trial. Neurology. 1995;45:1277–85.
28. Freeman JA, Thompson AJ, Fitzpatrick R, et al. Interferon-beta1b in the treatment of secondary progressive MS: impact on quality of life. Neurology. 2001;57(10):1870–5.
29. Kappos L, Weinshenker B, Pozzilli C, et al. Interferon beta-1b in secondary progressive MS: a combined analysis of the two trials. Neurology. 2004;63(10):1779–87.
30. Randomized controlled trial of interferon- beta-1a in secondary progressive MS: Clinical results. Neurology. 2001;56(11):1496–504.
31. Li DK, Zhao GJ, Paty DW. Randomized controlled trial of interferon-beta-1a in secondary progressive MS: MRI results. Neurology. 2001;56(11):1505–13.
32. Cohen JA, Cutter GR, Fischer JS, et al. Benefit of interferon beta-1a on MSFC progression in secondary progressive MS. Neurology. 2002;59(5):679–87.
33. Neuhaus O, Kieseier BC, Hartung HP. Therapeutic role of mitoxantrone in multiple sclerosis. Pharmacol Ther. 2006;109(1–2):198–209.
34. Huff AC, Kreuzer KN. Evidence for a common mechanism of action for antitumor and antibacterial agents that inhibit type II DNA topoisomerases. J Biol Chem. 1990;265(33): 20496–505.

35. Fesen MR, Kohn KW, Leteurtre F, Pommier Y. Inhibitors of human immunodeficiency virus integrase. Proc Natl Acad Sci USA. 1993;90(6):2399–403.
36. van de Wyngaert FA, Beguin C, D'Hooghe MB, et al. A double-blind clinical trial of mitoxantrone versus methylprednisolone in relapsing, secondary progressive multiple sclerosis. Acta Neurol Belg. 2001;101(4):210–6.
37. Hartung HP, Gonsette R, Konig N, et al. Mitoxantrone in progressive multiple sclerosis: a placebo-controlled, double-blind, randomised, multicentre trial. Lancet. 2002;360(9350):2018–25.
38. Neuhaus O, Kieseier BC, Hartung HP. Mitoxantrone in multiple sclerosis. Adv Neurol. 2006;98:293–302.
39. Hommes OR, Sorensen PS, Fazekas F, et al. Intravenous immunoglobulin in secondary progressive multiple sclerosis: randomised placebo-controlled trial. Lancet. 2004;364(9440):1149–56.
40. Leary SM, Miller DH, Stevenson VL, Brex PA, Chard DT, Thompson AJ. Interferon beta-1a in primary progressive MS: an exploratory, randomized, controlled trial. Neurology. 2003;60(1):44–51.
41. Montalban X. Overview of European pilot study of interferon beta-Ib in primary progressive multiple sclerosis. Mult Scler. 2004;10(Suppl 1):S62; discussion 62–64.
42. Wolinsky JS, Narayana PA, O'Connor P, et al. Glatiramer acetate in primary progressive multiple sclerosis: results of a multinational, multicenter, double-blind, placebo-controlled trial. Ann Neurol. 2007;61(1):14–24.
43. Kita M, Cohen JA, Fox RJ. A phase II trial of mitoxantrone in patients with primary progressive multiple sclerosis. Paper presented at 56th Annual Meeting of the American Academy of Neurology2004, San Francisco, CA.
44. Debouverie M, Vandenberghe N, Morrissey SP, et al. Predictive parameters of mitoxantrone effectiveness in the treatment of multiple sclerosis. Mult Scler. 2004;10(4):407–12.
45. Coustans M, Le Page E, Leray E, Fanorena E, Cormier B, Edan G. Clinical impact of mitoxantrone in 64 primary progressive multiple sclerosis patients. Paper presented at 55th Annual Meeting of the American Academy of Neurology 2003, Honolulu, HI, USA.
46. Reff ME, Carner K, Chambers KS, et al. Depletion of B cells in vivo by a chimeric mouse human monoclonal antibody to CD20. Blood. 1994;83(2):435–45.
47. Hawker K, O'Connor P, Freedman MS, et al. Rituximab in patients with primary progressive multiple sclerosis: results of a randomized double-blind placebo-controlled multicenter trial. Ann Neurol. 2009;66(4):460–71.

Chapter 12
Infections of the Nervous System

Nicholas L. King and Jorge G. Burneo

Keywords Bacterial meningitis • Herpes encephalitis • Neurocysticercosis • Fungal meningitis • Treatment • Diagnosis

Bacterial Meningitis

Introduction

Bacterial meningitis occurs when pathogenic bacteria enter the subarachnoid space of a susceptible individual. The mechanism by which bacteria gain entry into the subarachnoid space is poorly understood as the process occurs in both immunocompromised and immunocompetent individuals. The bacteria cause the release of chemotactic factors in the host, leading to a massive influx of leukocytes into the CSF [1]. In the case of bacterial meningitis, the predominant cells are polymorphonuclear leukocytes, which release multiple cytotoxic agents leading to a purulent inflammation in the subarachnoid space. Neurological damage and death may ensue due to multiple mechanisms, some of which are treatable and others that are inevitable despite the best treatment.

N.L. King (✉)
Clinical Neurology, Indiana University School of Medicine,
10335 Bronze Dr., Noblesville, IN 46060, USA
e-mail: nilking@iupui.edu

J.G. Burneo et al. (eds.), *Neurology: An Evidence-Based Approach*,
DOI 10.1007/978-0-387-88555-1_12, © Springer Science+Business Media, LLC 2012

Epidemiology

Introduction

Although dozens of species of bacteria can cause meningitis in humans, the majority of cases are caused by two to five different species. Age, immune status, and history of intracranial instrumentation all affect the risk of getting bacterial meningitis, as well as the most likely causative agent.

Clinical Case Example

A 42-year-old man who was previously in a good state of health presented to his primary care physician for 3 days of increasing headache, stiff neck, and irritability. He has felt feverish for the last 2–3 days as well. Some of his coworkers have been sick and he thinks he caught their cold. In the office, his temperature was 102.3°F, and he was slightly tachycardic. His examination revealed nuchal rigidity with meningismus, but was otherwise unremarkable. The primary care physician sent him to the local emergency department for antibiotics and a lumbar puncture (LP). He received appropriate therapy and had a lumbar puncture performed, which revealed a neutrophilic pleocytosis, elevated protein, and low glucose. The neurology service was consulted for further management. The patient was told he had bacterial meningitis. The emergency room physician wanted to know what the most likely pathogen was so they could consider prophylactic treatment of close contacts if necessary. The patient wanted to know how he got bacterial meningitis.

Clinical Questions

1. What is the incidence of bacterial meningitis?
2. What are the most common causative organisms?
3. What are the risk factors that predispose a person to bacterial meningitis?

Search Strategy

Ovid MEDLINE database was searched since its inception to March 2009. Medical Subject Heading (MeSH) term "bacterial meningitis" was searched using the "focus" limiter and limiting to only the "epidemiology" subheading (*Meningitis, Bacterial/ep [Epidemiology]). After limiting the retrieval to English and human, a set of 226 citations were obtained. Many of these studies were performed in Africa, Europe, and Asia. This set of citations was combined with MeSH term "exp United States/" using the Boolean "AND." This revealed a set of 15 citations. From this set,

Table 12.1 Age-specific incidence of bacterial meningitis (cases per 100,000 persons in each age group)

Age group	H. influenzae	S. pneumoniae	N. meningitidis	Group B Streptococcus	L. monocytogenes
<1 month	0	15.7	0	125.0	39.2
1–23 months	0.7	6.6	4.5	2.8	0
2–29 years	0.1	0.5	1.1	0.1	0.04
30–59 years	0.2	1.0	0.3	0.05	0.1
≥60 years	0.07	1.9	0.1	0.1	0.6

Source: Modified from Schuchat et al. [2]

four articles were reviewed; one was a surveillance of bacterial meningitis in adults and children in 22 counties representing a population of about 10 million people [2], one was a 10-year retrospective analysis of adults with bacterial meningitis [3], and two were retrospective reviews in children [4, 5]. PubMed and the Cochrane Library databases were also searched implementing the same strategy and no additional relevant articles were detected.

Epidemiology: Incidence

Prior to 1990, *Haemophilus influenzae* type b was a major cause of bacterial meningitis in the USA [2]. Each of the studies reviewed examined data after the routine use of the *H. influenzae* type b vaccine. In the surveillance study, the authors compared their data to a similar surveillance performed before the use of the vaccine in 1986. This study found the overall incidence of bacterial meningitis to be 2.4 cases per 100,000 persons. The most common organisms were (per 100,000 persons), *Streptococcus pneumoniae*, 1.1; *Neisseria meningitidis*, 0.6; group B streptococcus, 0.3; *Listeria monocytogenes*, 0.2; and *H. influenzae*, 0.2 [2]. The incidence of a particular pathogen varied greatly among age groups. Table 12.1 shows the extrapolated data for the number of cases of meningitis for each pathogen per 100,000 persons in each age group. When compared to the 1986 data, there was an 87 and 40% decrease in meningitis cases among the 1–23-month age group and 2–18-year age group, respectively [2].

The article that performed the retrospective analysis in adults did not give absolute incidence data, but did reveal a higher percentage of gram-negative rods causing meningitis (16% of cases) in the older population compared to the surveillance study. They also found that an immunocompromised state, recent neurosurgical procedure, and diabetes mellitus were the most common predisposing factors to bacterial meningitis (Table 12.2) [3]. The two retrospective analyses in children also do not present absolute incidence data, but do report similar percentages of causative organisms as in the other articles.

Table 12.2 Conditions predisposing patients to bacterial meningitis

Predisposing factor	Frequency	Percent of cases
Immunocompromised	12	31.6
Neurosurgical procedure	9	23.6
Sinusitis	9	23.6
Diabetes mellitus	5	13.2
None	2	5.3

Modified from Pizon et al. [3]

Clinical Bottom Lines

1. The overall incidence of bacterial meningitis in the USA is roughly 2.4 cases per 100,000 persons.
2. The causative organism varies by age group. Group B streptococcus is the most common cause of bacterial meningitis in infants, and *S. pneumoniae* and *N. meningitidis* are the two most common causes in all other age groups.
3. An immunocompromised state, diabetes mellitus, and recent neurosurgical procedure are the most common predisposing factors to the development of bacterial meningitis.

Summary

There are many studies that report the percentage of bacterial meningitis caused by a specific species of bacteria, but there are few population studies that can estimate the incidence. The study by Schuchat et al. revealed an incidence similar to those estimated previously in older texts. The recent studies that report percentages of causative organisms are all very similar which differ greatly from articles published before the use of the *H. influenzae* vaccine. Future data may show a similar decrease in the incidence of *S. pneumoniae* meningitis after the routine use of the pneumococcal vaccine.

Diagnosis

Introduction

Once a diagnosis of meningitis is suspected, confirming a diagnosis of bacterial meningitis requires a lumbar puncture. Initial studies on the spinal fluid can be highly suggestive of bacterial meningitis and identification of the specific pathogen can be made by various methods.

Clinical Case Example

The same 42-year-old man above is ready to have the lumbar puncture. The emergency room physician consulted neurology to ask if they needed to do a computed tomography (CT) scan of the patient's head prior to doing a lumbar puncture and to ask what tests to perform on the spinal fluid.

Clinical Questions

1. Is a CT scan of the head required before performing a lumbar puncture in patients with suspected bacterial meningitis?
2. What initial studies should be performed on spinal fluid and how do the results aid in diagnosis?

Search Strategy

Ovid MEDLINE database was searched since its inception to March 2009. MeSH terms "spinal puncture" and "Tomography, X-Ray Computed" were searched using the "focus" limiter. These were combined using the Boolean "AND," which revealed a final set of 57 citations. Three of the most recent articles were reviewed; one was a prospective study [6] and two were reviews [7, 8]. PubMed and the Cochrane Library databases were also searched implementing the same strategy and no additional relevant articles were detected.

The Evidence

CT

Hasbun et al. performed a prospective analysis of patients with suspected meningitis who would be candidates for a lumbar puncture. The emergency room physician was allowed to make the decision of whether or not to perform a head CT after the patients were enrolled in the study. Of the 301 patients enrolled in the study, 66 patients did not have a head CT and did not have complications from the lumbar puncture. Of the 235 patients that did have a head CT, 11 had mass effect. In 7 of the 11 patients that had mass effect, the physicians felt that the mass effect was not sufficient to preclude lumbar puncture. None of the seven had brain herniation 1 week after the lumbar puncture. Of the four that did not receive a lumbar puncture, two died of brain herniation despite not having a lumbar puncture. None of the remaining patients with abnormalities on head CT had brain herniation 1 week after lumbar puncture [6].

Additionally, there was a subset of patients that were more likely to have an abnormal head CT: patients at least 60 years of age or immunocompromised, patients with a history of central nervous system (CNS) disease, and patients who had a seizure within 1 week before presentation. Of the remaining patients, only 3 of 96 had an abnormal head CT; all had a lumbar puncture and none had brain herniation [6]. Two retrospective studies provided similar criteria for choosing when to perform a head CT before LP, but they add papilledema as an additional criterion [7, 8].

Lab Studies

The typical cerebrospinal fluid (CSF) profile for a bacterial meningitis is a polymorphonuclear pleocytosis, an elevated CSF protein, low CSF glucose, and an elevated serum procalcitonin. Of these, the procalcitonin level is the most sensitive and specific for differentiating bacterial from nonbacterial meningitis [9]. Pretreatment with antibiotics for less than 12 h prior to lumbar puncture is not associated with a change in the CSF profile. However, pretreatment for more than 12 h prior to lumbar puncture results in higher CSF glucose and lower CSF protein despite a persistently elevated white blood cell count [10].

Detection of the causative microorganism is achieved in 70–90% of CSF samples by Gram stain or blood culture [11]. One study evaluated the use of polymerase chain reaction (PCR) for rapid detection of the causative bacterial pathogen in suspected meningitis [12]. The researchers used 141 CSF samples from patients with suspected bacterial meningitis. In 28 samples, the Gram stain or culture identified the causative bacterial pathogen and in 113 samples, the organism was not identified by microscopy or culture. The PCR test identified the pathogen in all 28 positive samples and in 5 of the negative samples. Of those five, three met the researchers' other criteria for bacterial meningitis and were identified as true positives while the other two were identified as false positives [12]. These data provided 100% sensitivity and 98% specificity for identifying bacterial meningitis by PCR.

Clinical Bottom Lines

1. In patients with suspected bacterial meningitis, head CT should be performed if the patient is at least 60 years of age or immunocompromised, has a history of CNS disease, has papilledema, or had a seizure within 1 week before presentation.
2. Spinal fluid polymorphonuclear pleocytosis, elevated CSF protein, low CSF glucose, and elevated serum procalcitonin help differentiate bacterial meningitis from other forms of meningitis.
3. Spinal fluid PCR is highly sensitive and specific for detection of the bacterial pathogen in suspected bacterial meningitis.

Summary

A lumbar puncture should be performed on all patients with suspected meningitis. A head CT should be performed in selected patients to assess the risk of herniation. The initial routine spinal fluid studies may suggest bacterial meningitis, but a definitive diagnosis requires culture or pathogen-specific PCR testing.

Treatment

Introduction

Treatment of bacterial meningitis is different from treatment of infections in other organ systems. The blood–brain barrier acts as a filter that entirely prevents some antibiotics from reaching the meninges and decreases the penetration of other antibiotics. Therefore, the choice of antibiotics depends not only on the infecting organism, but also on the amount of antibiotic that would reach the site of infection. Additionally, inflammation of the meninges can interfere with the treatment of bacterial meningitis and medications that reduce the amount of inflammation may improve outcomes.

Clinical Case Example

The same 42-year-old man above is in the emergency department ready to have the lumbar puncture. The emergency room physician asked the neurologist when they should initiate therapy and which drugs to choose.

Clinical Questions

1. When should antimicrobial therapy be initiated in suspected bacterial meningitis?
2. Which drugs should be initiated for suspected bacterial meningitis?

Search Strategy

Ovid MEDLINE database was searched since its inception to August 2009. MeSH term "bacterial meningitis" was exploded and subsequently limited to therapy (exp Meningitis, Bacterial/th). After limiting the retrieval to English and human, a set of 357 citations were obtained. Because the treatment of bacterial meningitis evolves rapidly, this set was limited to the years 2004–2009 and a final set of 106 citations were obtained. The most recent reference, an overview of Cochrane reviews, was reviewed. A practice guideline from 2004 was also reviewed.

The Evidence

Antibiotics

Tunkel et al. outline the recommended empirical antibiotics for patients with suspected bacterial meningitis. All patients without head trauma or a history of neurosurgical procedures should receive vancomycin and a third-generation cephalosporin. Patients over the age of 50 years should also receive ampicillin to cover for *L. monocytogenes*. Patients that have had a recent neurosurgical procedure, penetrating head trauma, or a CSF shunt should receive vancomycin plus either ceftazidime, cefepime, or meropenem [13]. These recommendations are classified as A-III, meaning there is good evidence from opinions of respected authorities, clinical experience, descriptive studies, or reports of expert committees. A Cochrane review examined studies comparing ceftriaxone alone to chloramphenicol and found no significant difference in outcomes. However, the review did not find any randomized controlled trials evaluating the addition of vancomycin to ceftriaxone. The authors of the review concluded that the use of vancomycin plus ceftriaxone was supported by the available evidence as well as experiential evidence that vancomycin improves outcomes in patients infected with penicillin-resistant organisms [14].

Steroids

Tunkel et al. reviewed five trials examining the use of dexamethasone in bacterial meningitis. Four of the studies were not determinative. A prospective, randomized, double-blinded trial compared dexamethasone to placebo in adults. That trial showed a significant reduction in the development of cardiorespiratory failure, seizures, and impairment of consciousness as well as a reduction in mortality in patients with pneumococcal meningitis treated with dexamethasone [15]. Tunkel et al. recommend treating patients with suspected pneumococcal meningitis with dexamethasone 0.15 mg/kg every 6 h for 2–4 days. The first dose should be given 10–20 min before or at least with the first dose of antibiotics [13]. The Cochrane review examined 20 studies of corticosteroid use in acute bacterial meningitis. The reviewers found a significant improvement in outcomes among patients in high-income countries who were treated with dexamethasone, regardless of the causative organism. Their recommendation was to treat all bacterial meningitis patients with dexamethasone before or with the first dose of antibiotics [14].

Clinical Bottom Lines

1. Patients with suspected acute bacterial meningitis should be treated empirically with vancomycin and a third-generation cephalosporin. Patients over the age of 50 years should also receive ampicillin. Patients that have had a recent neurosurgical procedure, penetrating head trauma, or a CSF shunt should receive vancomycin plus either ceftazidime, cefepime, or meropenem.
2. All patients with suspected bacterial meningitis should receive *dexamethasone 0.15 mg/kg every 6 h*. The first dose should be given before or with the first dose of antibiotics.

Summary

Empirical therapy with vancomycin and a third-generation cephalosporin should be initiated in all patients with suspected bacterial meningitis. If the patient is over the age of 50 years, ampicillin should be added. Patients that have had a recent neurosurgical procedure, penetrating head trauma, or a CSF shunt and have a suspected bacterial meningitis should receive vancomycin plus either ceftazidime, cefepime, or meropenem. In addition to antibiotics, all patients with suspected bacterial meningitis should receive dexamethasone before or with the first dose of antibiotics. Even though the available data show a benefit only in patients with pneumococcal meningitis, because of the relative safety of dexamethasone, all patients with bacterial meningitis should receive it until pneumococcal meningitis is ruled out as a causative organism.

Prognosis

Introduction

Left untreated, certain forms of bacterial meningitis including pneumococcal and meningococcal meningitis are highly fatal. Even when treated appropriately, mortality and morbidity are significant and are higher in certain populations. Certain criteria at presentation may predict the outcome.

Clinical Case Example

The same 42-year-old man above is treated appropriately in the emergency department and is diagnosed with bacterial meningitis. The patient has heard that people can die from meningitis. He wants to know if he is going to survive.

Clinical Questions

1. What is the overall mortality of bacterial meningitis?
2. What is the morbidity in survivors of bacterial meningitis?

Search Strategy

Ovid MEDLINE database was searched since its inception to November 2009. MeSH terms "prognosis" and "bacterial meningitis" were exploded, searched, and combined using the Boolean "AND." After limiting the retrieval to English and human between the years 2004 and 2009, a final set of 154 citations were obtained. Three studies were reviewed; one prospective, longitudinal study of adult patients admitted with community-acquired acute bacterial meningitis [16] and two retrospective reviews [17, 18].

The Evidence

Mortality ranged from 20 to 31% and all neurological sequelae, including epilepsy, deafness, hemiparesis, and encephalopathy, ranged from 16 to 23% in the studies reviewed [16–18]. Patients aged 65 years or more had a mortality of 31% compared to 13% in patients under the age of 65 years ($p = 0.00$) [17]. In the prospective study, in patients with acute bacterial meningitis, seven factors were found to be independent predictors of unfavorable outcomes: internal comorbidity (defined as arteriosclerosis or coronary artery disease, diabetes mellitus, malignancy, alcoholic liver disease, chronic renal disease, and immunodeficiency), >48 h to the onset of treatment, coma, hypotension, high CSF protein, low CSF:serum glucose ratio, and an etiology other than meningococcus [16].

Clinical Bottom Lines

1. Mortality among adults with acute bacterial meningitis ranges from 20 to 31% with the highest mortality among patients older than 65 years.
2. Permanent neurological sequelae range from 16 to 23%.
3. Predictors of an unfavorable outcome include internal comorbidity, >48 h to the onset of treatment, coma, hypotension, high CSF protein, low CSF:serum glucose ratio, and an etiology other than meningococcus.

Summary

Mortality from bacterial meningitis ranges from 20 to 31%. Patients over the age of 65 years are more likely to die from bacterial meningitis than younger patients. Among survivors, a significant percentage have permanent neurological sequelae. Several factors can predict an unfavorable outcome in patients with bacterial meningitis.

HSV Encephalitis

Introduction

Viral encephalitis is a relatively rare CNS infection. However, mortality and morbidity in patients with viral encephalitis are relatively high. Herpes simplex virus encephalitis (HSE) is the most commonly identified viral encephalitis. Patients typically present with headache, fever, and alterations in consciousness with or without focal neurological deficits and seizures. Treatment is effective in reducing morbidity and mortality if initiated promptly.

Epidemiology

Introduction

Both HSV-1 and HSV-2 are prevalent and infect 40–80% of individuals worldwide. However, only a minority of infected individuals have clinical evidence of HSV infection at any given time.

HSV-1 is the etiologic agent of 85–95% of cases of HSE, and HSV-2 is the etiologic agent of the remainder [19].

Clinical Case Example

A 45-year-old man presents to the emergency department via ambulance because his family found him having convulsions. The family reported that he had "the flu" for the last 2 days. When asked what they mean by "the flu," they said he had a headache and fever and was complaining of aching all over. They said that for the last few hours, he was acting silly. They said he seemed confused and disoriented. Then, he became agitated and started convulsing. In the emergency department, his temperature was 103.1°F and was awake, but disoriented. He spoke incoherently and did not recognize his family. Otherwise, the physical exam was unremarkable and most of the neurological exam was normal, with the exception of the sensorium.

Clinical Question

1. What is the incidence of herpes encephalitis?

Search Strategy

Ovid MEDLINE database was searched since its inception to March 2009. MeSH terms "incidence or prevalence" and "herpes encephalitis" were searched and combined using the Boolean "AND." A final set of 28 citations were obtained. Two studies were reviewed [20, 21].

The Evidence

A study in Finland examined all adults in the Helsinki area with acute encephalitis between 1967 and 1991. The authors identified 322 patients with acute encephalitis for an overall incidence of 1.4 cases per 100,000 adults per year. Fifty-three patients had confirmed, probable, or suggested HSE. This represents 33% of all cases of encephalitis in which an etiology was identified and 16% of all the cases of encephalitis. This translates to an incidence of at least 2.3 cases of herpes simplex encephalitis per 1,000,000 adults per year [21]. If herpes simplex encephalitis truly represents 33% of all cases of encephalitis, then the incidence would be 4.7 cases per 1,000,000 adults per year. A Swedish retrospective study of all cases of herpes simplex encephalitis revealed an incidence of 2.2 cases per 1,000,000 adults [22]. These estimates are consistent with other reported incidences of herpes encephalitis [19].

Clinical Bottom Line

1. Herpes simplex encephalitis occurs in 2–5 cases per million adults per year.

Summary

Herpes simplex encephalitis is diagnosed in 2–3 out of every 1 million adults per year in developed countries. The actual incidence is almost certainly higher and probably closer to 5 cases per million adults per year. The low rate of confirmed diagnosis of patients with encephalitis limits the ability to accurately estimate the overall incidence of herpes simplex encephalitis.

Diagnosis

Introduction

Patients with HSE present similarly to patients with other forms of viral encephalitis and certain forms of noninfectious encephalitis. The most common presentation is a triad of headache, fever, and altered consciousness. Some patients also have focal neurological deficits or seizures. Because this presentation is common among various forms of encephalitis, making a diagnosis of HSE requires specific tests that can differentiate the various forms of encephalitis.

Clinical Questions

1. Which diagnostic studies aid in the diagnosis of herpes encephalitis?
2. What initial studies should be performed on spinal fluid and how do the results aid in diagnosis?

Search Strategy

Ovid MEDLINE database was searched since its inception to March 2009. MeSH term "herpes encephalitis" was exploded and subsequently limited to diagnosis (exp Encephalitis, Herpes Simplex/di). After limiting the retrieval to English and human and review articles, a final set of 21 citations were obtained. A review article from the *Journal of Neurology* was reviewed [23].

The Evidence

A review of viral encephalitis highlights the importance of PCR in confirming a diagnosis of HSE. As outlined in the review article, patients with HSE typically present with a fever, headache, and altered consciousness with or without seizures and focal neurological deficits. However, as indicated in the article, that presentation is common among many forms of infectious and noninfectious causes of encephalitis. Brain MRI and EEG can be helpful in distinguishing HSE from other forms of encephalitis, but again these studies are only suggestive, not diagnostic. Characteristic findings on an MRI would be hyperintensities in the temporal lobes and the inferior frontal lobes. An EEG may show periodic lateralized epileptiform discharges (PLEDs), but neither the presence nor the absence of PLEDs is helpful in making a diagnosis of HSE [23]. PCR for herpes simplex virus (HSV) in the CSF is 95% specific and, when performed between 48 h and 10 days after the onset of symptoms, is 95% sensitive. The sensitivity drops rapidly before and after that window [23]. The data from this review are similar to data presented in other reviews of the literature [19].

Clinical Bottom Line

1. HSV PCR is the gold standard for diagnosis of HSE. The HSV PCR is 95% specific, and it is 95% sensitive when performed between 48 h and 10 days after the onset of symptoms.

Summary

Clinical presentation with fever, headache, and altered consciousness suggests a possible encephalitic process. MRI and EEG studies may suggest HSE, but a definitive diagnosis can only be made with PCR for HSV on CSF. The HSV PCR is 95% specific, and it is 95% sensitive when performed between 48 h and 10 days after the onset of symptoms.

Treatment

Introduction

HSV encephalitis is a very aggressive form of encephalitis and it is the most common form of encephalitis. When treated quickly and appropriately, mortality and morbidity can be reduced significantly. However, delays in presentation to the hospital and delays in recognizing the diagnosis often lead to a delay in initiation of therapy. Delaying the treatment leads to worse outcomes even if treated with a full course of appropriate antimicrobial agents.

Clinical Case Example

In our 45-year-old man with encephalitis, emergency room physician consults neurology for help with management.

Clinical Questions

1. Which antiviral medication should be used empirically with suspected encephalitis?
2. What is the best therapy for patients with confirmed HSE?
3. Should steroids be used in patients with HSE?

Search Strategy

Ovid MEDLINE database was searched since its inception to March 2009. MeSH term "herpes encephalitis" was exploded and subsequently limited to therapy (exp Encephalitis, Herpes Simplex/th). A final set of 14 citations were obtained, including a review [23].

The Evidence

Based on the review of the literature, an appropriate treatment for HSE was acyclovir 10 mg/kg every 8 h for at least 14 days. Some authors recommended extending treatment to 21 days in patients who are immunocompromised [23]. The recommendation to treat for 21 days is based on a study showing that 20% of patients had a positive PCR result after 14 days of treatment and another study showing that 8% of patients who received 10–14 days of treatment required a second course for a suspected relapse [19, 24, 25]. It is also recommended to treat patients with mannitol or steroids if there is evidence of edema on CT or MRI [23]. However, these are recommendations based on experience without evidence supporting it. Other reviewers have identified small studies that showed reduced morbidity in patients treated with intravenous steroids at the onset of symptoms [26, 27]. However, these studies were insufficient to make a clear recommendation.

Clinical Bottom Lines

1. Acyclovir is the mainstay of treatment in HSE and is dosed 10 mg/kg every 8 h. The duration of therapy should be at least 14 days, but a 21-day course should be considered.
2. There is insufficient evidence to support the use of steroids in HSE.

Summary

Patients with suspected encephalitis should receive acyclovir empirically unless specifically contraindicated. If a diagnosis of HSE is confirmed or highly suggested, patients should receive at least 14 days of acyclovir. Steroids may be beneficial in patients that have evidence of edema on neuroimaging, but studies do not support the use of steroids in all patients with HSE.

Prognosis

Introduction

HSV encephalitis is nearly universally fatal if left untreated. Even with appropriate therapy, morbidity and mortality are high. Certain factors may predict the outcome in patients with HSE.

Clinical Case Example

Our 45-year-old man was diagnosed with herpes encephalitis and treated appropriately. The family wants to know if he will survive and, if so, will he get back to normal?

Clinical Questions

1. What is the mortality of herpes encephalitis?
2. What is the morbidity in survivors of herpes encephalitis?

Search Strategy

Ovid MEDLINE database was searched since its inception to March 2009. MeSH terms "prognosis" and "herpes encephalitis" were searched and combined using the Boolean "AND." A final set of 28 citations were obtained. One retrospective analysis was reviewed [28].

The Evidence

In a large, retrospective, multicenter study, 93 patients were identified as having HSE between 1991 and 1998. Fifteen percent of the patients died as a result of the HSE. Twenty percent had a severe disability, 28% had a moderate disability, 23% had a mild disability, and 14% fully recovered [28]. The authors found no difference in outcomes based on age, MacCabe score, presence of focal neurological deficits or seizures, need for mechanical ventilation, serum sodium concentration, and CSF values. They found two factors that did predict outcomes. Patients with a Simplified Acute Physiology Score greater than 27 at admission and who had a delay of more than 2 days between hospital admission and initiation of acyclovir therapy were statistically significantly more likely to have a severe disability or death at 6 month follow-up [28].

Clinical Bottom Lines

1. Mortality from HSE at a large medical center is about 15% [28].
2. The majority of patients who survive HSE have permanent sequelae with only about 15% of patients making a full recovery.

Summary

Mortality among patients with HSE is about 15% even when treated appropriately with acyclovir. Among survivors, the majority have at least some permanent disability. Presentation to the hospital in the early stages of the infection and early initiation of acyclovir therapy help to reduce the mortality and morbidity in patients with HSE.

Neurocysticercosis

Introduction

Neurocysticercosis (NCC) is the most common parasitic infection of the CNS and the most common cause of epilepsy worldwide, especially in countries where sanitary infrastructure is deficient. In Latin American countries, the frequency of NCC is very high [29–31], and it is becoming increasingly common in developed countries because of immigration from endemic regions [32, 33]. It is acquired by the ingestion of food contaminated of *Taenia solium* (pork tapeworm) eggs usually from food contaminated by people with taeniasis.

Clinical Presentation

The most common clinical manifestation is a seizure, but patients may also present with headache and/or signs of increased intracranial pressure. The clinical presentation is affected by the number and location of cysts in the brain parenchyma and/or in the basilar or perimesencephalic cisterns. The course of the disease may remain subacute or chronic for many years, and then present with focal signs of cerebrovascular events secondary to an acute inflammatory response to parasites. Cysticerci can also invade the spinal cord, eyes, and subcutaneous and muscular tissues of the body. Muscular pseudohypertrophy is seen more frequently in patients from Asia who have cysticercosis; it accounts for 0.6% of cases in China. Muscular pseudohypertrophy is extremely rare in America [34].

Clinical Case Example

A 27-year-old man presents for evaluation of a new onset seizure that began with clonic activity in the left upper extremity which was followed by secondary generalization. Cranial CT demonstrated a nonenhancing cystic lesion without edema. A diagnosis of NCC was made and the patient was treated with prednisone, albendazole, and oxcarbazepine.

Clinical Questions

1. Is the efficacy of anticysticidal therapy dependent on the stage of the lesion on neuroimaging?
2. Does faster resolution of cysts with anticysticidal therapy improve outcome?

3. Should corticosteroid therapy be part of the initial regimen?
4. Is the risk of seizure recurrence associated with the length of time to cyst resolution?

Classification of NCC

Cysticercal cysts evolve through four stages. In the vesicular stage, the cyst contains living larva and has the appearance on CT scan of a nonenhancing cystic lesion without edema. As the larva degenerates, a colloidal stage evolves. The CT scan demonstrates a ring-enhancing lesion with edema. Cysts in the vesicular and those in the colloidal stages contain live active cysts that have the appearance of a nodule (invaginated scolex). As the larva continues to degenerate, the size of the cyst becomes smaller and the membrane of the cyst thickens. This is the "granulo-nodular" stage which has the CT appearance of a cyst with ring enhancement. The final stage is the stage of calcification, where a calcified lesion is seen on CT scan [35].

Diagnosis

The diagnosis of NCC is based on the neuroimaging abnormalities described in the above section. The most definitive neuroimaging evidence of NCC is a cystic lesion showing the scolex on neuroimaging or the direct visualization of subretinal parasites on funduscopic examination.

CT is the most commonly used neuroimaging test for the disease and maintains relatively good diagnostic sensitivity when used in disease-endemic areas. Small lesions, especially those situated close to bone or within ventricles, may be missed on CT scans. A magnetic resonance imaging (MRI) scan is, therefore, often added for increased diagnostic sensitivity and accuracy. MRI is also the modality of choice when evaluating patients with intraventricular cysticercosis and when assessing brainstem cysts and small cysts located over the convexity of the cerebral hemispheres. The main shortcoming of MRI is its failure to detect small calcifications.

Lesions regarded as highly suggestive of neurocysticercosis on neuroimaging are the appearance of a cyst without demonstrating the scolex or an enhancing or calcified lesion. The diagnosis is also supported by resolution of the intracranial cystic lesion or lesions with either anticysticidal therapy with albendazole or praziquantel or spontaneous resolution of the lesion. A serum immunoelectrotransfer blot (EITB) can be sent for the detection of anticysticercal antibodies, and an enzyme-linked immunosorbent assay (ELISA) can be performed on CSF [36].

Epidemiologic factors that may lead to a diagnosis of NCC include evidence of household contact with *T. solium*, immigration from an area where the disease is endemic, and a history of repeated travel to disease-endemic regions. Detection of the parasite in a biopsy of a brain or spinal cord lesion is one of the proposed absolute criteria for the diagnosis of NCC [36]. However, the combination of epidemiologic, clinical, and laboratory information may lead to an accurate diagnosis and avoid an invasive diagnostic procedure.

Treatment

Patients most typically become symptomatic when the cyst has evolved to a calcified lesion. They may, however, also become symptomatic in the stage with a ring-enhancing lesion. There is controversy about whether or not to treat a single CT-enhancing lesion as there may be spontaneous resolution of the brain lesion. The most important therapeutic question is whether or not anticysticidal therapy affects the risk of seizure recurrence. In addition, there is concern that cysticidal therapy may result in a marked inflammatory response to the larval antigens resulting in cerebral edema and seizure activity. There is agreement that if a patient presents with a seizure with this type of lesion they should be treated with anticonvulsant therapy. There are few large (greater than 50 patients) double-blind, randomized, controlled clinical trials that address this question.

In one of the few randomized, double-blind, controlled trials comparing albendazole therapy to placebo in 120 adults [37], there was a significant reduction in the number of seizures at 3 month follow-up in patients treated with a 10-day course of albendazole, dexamethasone, and anticonvulsants compared to patients treated with anticonvulsants and placebo. This study has had a major impact on the treatment of NCC. A subsequent meta-analysis of randomized trials published between 1979 and 2005 included 464 patients with cystic lesions and 478 patients with enhancing lesions [34]. The authors of this paper concluded that anticysticidal therapy reduced the risk for seizure recurrence in patients with cystic lesions (44% of patients given specific cysticidal therapy vs. 19% of patients not given treatment, $p = 0.025$) and reduced the rate of generalized seizures in patients with cystic lesions [34].

The recommended doses of anticysticidal therapy are well-accepted, although there is still debate about the duration of treatment: albendazole at a daily dose of 15 mg/kg of body weight for 10–14 days or praziquantel at a daily dose of 50 mg/kg of body weight for either 1 day or 2 weeks. Albendazole is the preferred initial anticysticidal agent based on nonrandomized, controlled trials.

During therapy with anticysticidal agents, there is a risk of a strong inflammatory reaction with the development of cerebral edema. Prednisone might be started either before or with the first dose of anticysticidal therapy and continued throughout the course of treatment.

The efficacy of albendazole plus dexamethasone on reducing the risk of seizure recurrence was demonstrated in a randomized, controlled, open trial of 123 children, the majority of whom had a single lesion on CT [38].

Bottom Lines

1. NCC is the most common parasitic disease of the CNS and is linked to the ingestion of *T. solium* eggs.
2. Common neurological symptoms include epilepsy, headache, and focal neurological signs.
3. Patients with suspected NCC should be given anticysticidal drugs concomitantly with symptomatic medication (e.g., antiepileptics medication in case of recurrent seizures).
4. The use of steroids is not supported by clinical trials.

Fungal Meningitis

Introduction

Fungal meningitis is a rare infection in immunocompetent patients, but it remains a significant cause of morbidity and mortality in immunocompromised patients. Cryptococcal meningitis is the most common form of fungal meningitis, but there are dozens of fungi that can cause meningitis. Certain geographic areas have a higher incidence of certain forms of fungal meningitis based on the relatively higher concentrations of the organism in those areas.

Epidemiology

Introduction

Estimating the incidence of all causes of fungal meningitis is difficult due to the multitude of potential causative organisms, some of which are difficult or impossible to diagnosis. Cryptococcal meningitis is the most common form of fungal meningitis.

Clinical Case Example

A 50-year-old woman with chronic diabetes, on dialysis for chronic renal insufficiency, presented to her primary care physician for 5 weeks of dull, aching headache, malaise, and "just not feeling right." She had a few episodes of fever over the last week, but were not sustained. She also had some muscle aches, especially in her neck. Her general physical examination and neurological examination were normal, except for some neck stiffness. Because of the neck stiffness and intermittent fevers, the primary care physician was worried about meningitis and sent the patient to the local emergency department. There, neurology was consulted for further evaluation.

Clinical Questions

1. What is the incidence of fungal meningitis?
2. What factors predispose patients to fungal meningitis?

Search Strategy

Ovid MEDLINE database was searched since its inception to March 2009. MeSH terms "incidence or prevalence" and "fungal meningitis" were searched and combined using the Boolean "AND." A final set of 26 citations were obtained. None of the articles was a study or review of fungal meningitis in the general population. Most of the articles were studies of specific fungal etiologies. Two articles about general fungal meningitis in special populations were reviewed – one was a review of meningitis in the elderly and one was a retrospective study of causes of meningitis in cancer patients.

The Evidence

Fungal meningitis is a rare form of meningitis, but it is more common in certain populations. A review of meningitis in the elderly estimated the incidence at 2–9 cases per 100,000 persons per year. The same review reported that meningitis due to *Cryptococcus neoformans* comprised 4% of all cases of meningitis in patients aged 60 years and older, which would be 0.8 to 3.6 cases per 1,000,000 [39]. The article did not report the incidence of other forms of fungal meningitis. In an article analyzing causes of meningitis in a small group of patients with a variety of cancers, 7 of the 79 cases of meningitis (9%) were due to fungi. Six of those seven were due to *C. neoformans* [40]. These articles highlight the difficulty of studying fungal meningitis – that fungal meningitis in the general population is so rare, it is difficult to do epidemiological studies.

Clinical Bottom Lines

1. Cryptococcal meningitis comprises 4–8% of all forms of meningitis in the elderly or patients with cancers.
2. Cryptococcal meningitis is the most common cause of fungal meningitis.

Summary

Fungal meningitis is very rare in the general population, but is more common in patients that are immunocompromised, elderly, or with cancer. *C. neoformans* is the most common form of fungal meningitis.

Diagnosis

Introduction

Patients with fungal meningitis often present with an indolent course of headache and stiff neck with or without fevers. The most important factor in diagnosing fungal meningitis is suspecting it. A lumbar puncture helps the clinician to narrow the differential diagnosis, but confirming fungal meningitis requires specific organism-specific testing.

Clinical Questions

1. In a patient with evidence of meningitis, what factors suggest a fungal etiology?
2. How can the diagnosis of fungal meningitis be confirmed?

Search Strategy

Ovid MEDLINE database was searched since its inception to March 2009. MeSH term "fungal meningitis" was exploded and subsequently limited to diagnosis (exp Meningitis, Fungal/di). After limiting the retrieval to English and human articles between 2004 and 2009 and excluding letters and editorials, a final set of 121 citations were obtained. Three studies were reviewed – one was a review of cryptococcal meningitis [41], one was a retrospective analysis of coccidioidal meningitis [42], and one was a review of imaging features in CNS infections in patients with AIDS [43].

The Evidence

Laboratory Studies

The combination of a lymphocytic predominance on CSF cell counts and normal to mildly low glucose suggests a nonbacterial and possibly fungal etiology [11]. However, this profile is not specific to fungal meningitis and further studies are required to confirm the diagnosis. An India ink stain can be helpful in identifying cryptococcal meningitis, but it has a low sensitivity. Various serum and CSF antibody and antigen tests can be used to diagnose specific fungal infections, but again the sensitivity and specificity of these tests are variable [11, 41].

Magnetic Resonance Imaging

A study of imaging findings in coccidioidal meningitis reported that 26 of 48 patients (54%) had abnormalities, but the majority of those were nonspecific changes, including meningeal enhancement and/or hydrocephalus. Only three patients had abscesses [42]. The other studies reported similar nonspecific MRI findings in other forms of fungal meningitis [41, 43].

Clinical Bottom Lines

1. CSF cell count, protein, and glucose may suggest fungal meningitis, but further studies are required to confirm the diagnosis.
2. Serum and CSF antigens and antibodies to specific organisms can confirm a diagnosis if positive, but do not rule out fungal meningitis if negative.
3. MRI can aid in the diagnosis of fungal meningitis, but most patients with fungal meningitis have nonspecific MRI findings.

Summary

Fungal meningitis can be difficult to diagnose. The initial CSF profile may suggest a nonbacterial and nonviral etiology of infection. Neuroimaging can be helpful in making a diagnosis, but confirmation of the diagnosis requires specific antibody or antigen testing on the CSF.

Treatment

Introduction

Fungi as a class of organisms generally respond well to a few broad-spectrum antifungal medications. However, obtaining concentrations in the spinal fluid adequate for treating fungal meningitis is often barred by the toxic side effects of the medications. Treatment of fungal meningitis must balance the morbidity from the organism against the toxicity of the medications.

Clinical Questions

1. What is the most appropriate empirical treatment for suspected fungal meningitis?
2. Once the diagnosis is made, how are specific fungal meningitides treated?

Search Strategy

Ovid MEDLINE database was searched since its inception to March 2009. MeSH term "fungal meningitis" was explored, subsequently limited to therapy (exp Meningitis, Bacterial/th), searched, and combined using the Boolean "AND." After limiting the retrieval to English and human and excluding letters and editorials, a final set of 58 citations were obtained. Because fungal meningitis can be caused by a wide variety of pathogens, each specific form of fungal meningitis should be researched individually. An article covering cryptococcal meningitis was reviewed as a representative article [41].

The Evidence

Randomized, controlled trials for the treatment of fungal meningitis are lacking. In a review of cryptococcal meningitis, the authors recommend treating patients with cryptococcal meningitis with amphotericin B 0.7–1 mg/kg/day and flucytosine 100 mg/kg/day for 2 weeks, followed by fluconazole 400 mg/day for the next 8 weeks, followed by fluconazole 200 mg/day for maintenance therapy [41]. Textbook chapters reviewing the available literature have supported that treatment [11, 44]. The same text recommends either fluconazole or amphotericin B with or without flucytosine for the treatment of all fungal infections [44]. These recommendations come from anecdotal evidence or expert opinions.

Clinical Bottom Lines

1. Fungal meningitis is treated with amphotericin B or fluconazole with or without flucytosine depending on the etiology of the infection.
2. Since cryptococcal meningitis is the most common form of fungal meningitis, treatment with amphotericin B plus fluconazole is an appropriate combination for empirically treating suspected fungal meningitis.

Summary

Fungal infections respond well to amphotericin or fluconazole. However, due to the potential toxicity of the medications, close monitoring is required to ensure adequate treatment while minimizing the side effects of the medication.

Prognosis

Introduction

There are many factors that affect the prognosis in patients with fungal meningitis. Because the majority of patients that get fungal meningitis are immunocompromised, the patient's underlying comorbidities dramatically affect the patient's outcome. Within a given population of immunocompromised patients, certain other factors also influence the outcome after fungal meningitis.

Clinical Questions

1. What is the mortality of fungal meningitis?
2. What are the chances she will get fungal meningitis again?

Search Strategy

Ovid MEDLINE database was searched since its inception to March 2009. MeSH terms "prognosis" and "fungal meningitis" were searched and combined using the Boolean "AND." A final set of nine citations were obtained. There is very little evidence-based research on the prognosis of fungal meningitis. Three articles were reviewed – one article examining neuroimaging as a prognostic indicator for coccidioidal meningitis [45], a review of cryptococcal meningitis [41], and a prospective study of recurrent meningitis in the Netherlands [46].

The Evidence

Mortality

In the article examining neuroimaging in coccidioidal meningitis, those patients with hydrocephalus had a higher mortality rate than patients without hydrocephalus (39% vs. 9%). Patients with no radiographic abnormalities had a mortality rate of 8% [45]. In a review of cryptococcal meningitis, higher mortality was associated with abnormal mental status, high organism burden, and raised CSF opening pressure [41].

Recurrence Risk

In a prospective study of recurrent meningitis in the Netherlands, 153 patients had cryptococcal meningitis in the study. Of those, 12 patients or 8% had a recurrence of cryptococcal meningitis. HIV infection was the greatest risk factor for recurrence [46].

Clinical Bottom Lines

1. Mortality in fungal meningitis varies depending on the clinical presentation. Hydrocephalus in the setting of coccidioidal meningitis and abnormal mental status, high organism burden, and raised CSF opening pressure in the setting of cryptococcal meningitis are risk factors for a higher mortality.
2. Recurrence of cryptococcal meningitis is low, but HIV is a risk factor for recurrence.

Summary

Most patients with fungal meningitis are immunocompromised. The degree of immunocompromise and the reason for it affect the outcome. Certain factors, such as hydrocephalus, altered mental status, and an elevated CSF pressure, increase the risk of an unfavorable outcome.

References

1. Pfister H-W, Roos KL. Bacterial Meningitis. In: Roos KL, editor. Principles of neurologic infectious diseases. New York: McGraw -Hill; 2005. p. 13–28.
2. Schuchat A, Robinson K, Wenger JD, et al. Bacterial meningitis in the United States in 1995. N Engl J Med. 1997;337:970–6.
3. Pizon AF, Bonner MR, Wang HE, Kaplan RM. Ten years of clinical experience with adult meningitis at an urban academic medical center. J Emerg Med. 2006;30:367–70.
4. Dawson KG, Emerson JC, Burns JL. Fifteen years of experience with bacterial meningitis. Pediatr Infect Dis J. 1999;18:816–22.
5. Nigrovic LE, Kuppermann N, Malley R. Children with bacterial meningitis presenting to the Emergency Department during the Pneumococcal conjugate vaccine era. Acad Emerg Med. 2008;15:522–8.
6. Hasbun R, Abrahams J, Jekel J, Quagliarello VJ. Computed tomography of the head before lumbar puncture in adults with suspected meningitis [see comment]. N Engl J Med. 2001; 345:1727–33.
7. Greig PR, Goroszeniuk D. Role of computed tomography before lumbar puncture: a survey of clinical practice. Postgrad Med J. 2006;82:162–5.
8. van Crevel H, Hijdra A, de Gans J. Lumbar puncture and the risk of herniation: when should we first perform CT? J Neurol. 2002;249:129–37.
9. Ray P, Badarou-Acossi G, Viallon A, et al. Accuracy of the cerebrospinal fluid results to differentiate bacterial from non bacterial meningitis, in case of negative gram-stained smear. Am J Emerg Med. 2007;25:179–84.
10. Nigrovic LE, Malley R, Macias CG, et al. Effect of antibiotic pretreatment on cerebrospinal fluid profiles of children with bacterial meningitis. Pediatrics. 2008;122:726–30.
11. Roos KL, editor. Principles of neurologic infectious diseases. New York: McGraw-Hill; 2005.
12. Poppert S, Essig A, Stoehr B, et al. Rapid diagnosis of bacterial meningitis by real-time PCR and fluorescence in situ hybridization. J Clin Microbiol. 2005;43:3390–7.
13. Tunkel Allan R, Hartman Barry J, Kaplan Sheldon L, et al. Practice Guidelines for the Management of Bacterial Meningitis. Clin Infect Dis. 2004;39:1267–84.

14. Prasad K, Karlupia N, Kumar A. Treatment of bacterial meningitis: an overview of Cochrane systematic reviews. Respir Med. 2009;103:945–50.
15. de Gans J, van de Beek D. European dexamethasone in adulthood bacterial meningitis study I. Dexamethasone in adults with bacterial meningitis. N Engl J Med. 2002;347:1549–56.
16. Dzupova O, Rozsypal H, Prochazka B, Benes J. Acute bacterial meningitis in adults: predictors of outcome. Scand J Infect Dis. 2009;41:348–54.
17. Cabellos C, Verdaguer R, Olmo M, et al. Community-acquired bacterial meningitis in elderly patients: experience over 30 years. Medicine (Baltimore). 2009;88:115–9.
18. Ishihara M, Kamei S, Taira N, et al. Hospital-based study of the prognostic factors in adult patients with acute community-acquired bacterial meningitis in Tokyo, Japan. Intern Med. 2009;48:295–300.
19. King NL, Roos KL. Herpesvirus Encephalitis. In: Halperin JJ, editor. Encephalitis: diagnosis and treatment. New York: Informa Healthcare; 2008.
20. Whitley RJ, Gnann JW. The incidence and severity of herpes simplex encephalitis in Sweden, 1990–2001. Clin Infect Dis. 2007;45:881–2.
21. Rantalaiho T, Farkkila M, Vaheri A, Koskiniemi M. Acute encephalitis from 1967 to 1991. J Neurol Sci. 2001;184:169–77.
22. Hjalmarsson A, Blomqvist P, Skoldenberg B. Herpes simplex encephalitis in Sweden, 1990–2001: incidence, morbidity, and mortality. Clin Infect Dis. 2007;45:875–80.
23. Kennedy PGE. Viral encephalitis. J Neurol. 2005;252:268–72.
24. Lakeman FD, Whitley RJ. Diagnosis of herpes simplex encephalitis: application of polymerase chain reaction to cerebrospinal fluid from brain-biopsied patients and correlation with disease. National Institute of Allergy and Infectious Diseases Collaborative Antiviral Study Group. J Infect Dis. 1995;171:857–63.
25. McGrath N, Anderson NE, Croxson MC, Powell KF. Herpes simplex encephalitis treated with acyclovir: diagnosis and long term outcome. J Neurol Neurosurg Psychiatry. 1997;63:321–6.
26. Meyding-Lamade UK, Oberlinner C, Rau PR, et al. Experimental herpes simplex virus encephalitis: a combination therapy of acyclovir and glucocorticoids reduces long-term magnetic resonance imaging abnormalities. J Neurovirol. 2003;9:118–25.
27. Nakano A, Yamasaki R, Miyazaki S, Horiuchi N, Kunishige M, Mitsui T. Beneficial effect of steroid pulse therapy on acute viral encephalitis. Eur Neurol. 2003;50:225–9.
28. Raschilas F, Wolff M, Delatour F, et al. Outcome of and prognostic factors for herpes simplex encephalitis in adult patients: results of a multicenter study. Clin Infect Dis. 2002;35:254–60.
29. Gaffo AL, Guillen-Pinto D, Campos-Olazabal P, Burneo JG. Cysticercosis as the main cause of partial seizures in children in Peru. Rev Neurol. 2004;39:924–6.
30. Garcia HH, Gilman R, Martinez M, et al. Cysticercosis as the major cause of epilepsy in Peru. The Cysticercosis Working Group in Peru (CWG). Lancet. 1993;341:197–200.
31. Roman G, Sotelo J, Del Brutto O, et al. A proposal to declare neurocysticercosis an international reportable disease. Bull World Health Organ. 2000;78:399–406.
32. Wallin MT, Kurtzke JF. Neurocysticercosis in the United States. Neurology. 2004;63:1559–64.
33. Burneo JG, Plener I. Neurocysticercosis and Epilepsy Research Network. Neurocysticercosis in a patient in Canada. CMAJ. 2009;180:639–42.
34. Del Brutto OH, Roos KL, Coffey CS, Garcia HH. Meta-analysis: cysticidal drugs for neurocysticercosis: albendazole and praziquantel. Ann Intern Med. 2006;145:43–51.
35. Murthy JMK, Reddy YVS. Prognosis of epilepsy associated with single CT enhancing lesion: a long term follow up study. J Neurol Sci. 1998;159:151–5.
36. Del Brutto OH, Rajsekhar B, White AC, et al. Proposed diagnostic criteria for neurocysticercosis. Neurology. 2001;57:177–88.
37. Garcia HH, Pretell EJ, Gilman RH, et al. A trial of antiparasitic treatment to reduce the rate of seizures due to cerebral cysticercosis. N Engl J Med. 2004;350:249–58.
38. Kalra V, Dua T, Kumar V. Efficacy of albendazole and short-course dexamethasone treatment in children with 1 or 2 ring-enhancing lesions of neurocysticercosis: a randomized controlled trial. J Pediatr. 2003;143:111–4.

39. Miller LG, Choi C. Meningitis in older patients: how to diagnose and treat a deadly infection. Geriatrics. 1997;52:43–4.
40. Safdieh JE, Mead PA, Sepkowitz KA, Kiehn TE, Abrey LE. Bacterial and fungal meningitis in patients with cancer. Neurology. 2008;70:943–7.
41. Bicanic T, Harrison TS. Cryptococcal meningitis. Br Med Bull. 2004;72:99–118.
42. Drake KW, Adam RD. Coccidioidal meningitis and brain abscesses: analysis of 71 cases at a referral center. Neurology. 2009;73:1780–6.
43. Offiah CE, Turnbull IW. The imaging appearances of intracranial CNS infections in adult HIV and AIDS patients. Clin Radiol. 2006;61:393–401.
44. King NL, Roos KL. Therapy of central nervous system infections. In: Johnston MV, Gross RA, editors. Principles of drug therapy in neurology. Oxford: Oxford University Press; 2008.
45. Arsura EL, Johnson R, Penrose J, et al. Neuroimaging as a guide to predict outcomes for patients with coccidioidal meningitis. Clin Infect Dis. 2005;40:624–7.
46. van Driel JJ, Bekker V, Spanjaard L, van der Ende A, Kuijpers TW. Epidemiologic and microbiologic characteristics of recurrent bacterial and fungal meningitis in the Netherlands, 1988–2005. Clin Infect Dis. 2008;47:e42–51.

Chapter 13
Neurocritical Care

Rajat Dhar and Michael N. Diringer

Keywords Cerebral hemorrhage • Hypertension • Subarachnoid hemorrhage • Intracranial vasospasm • Intracranial aneurysm • Brain ischemia • Recombinant factor VIIa • Craniotomy

Intracerebral Hemorrhage

Introduction

Intracerebral hemorrhage (ICH), bleeding into the brain parenchyma, can be a devastating cerebrovascular event. It accounts for 10% of all strokes, with a case fatality rate as high as 40%.

Epidemiology

Clinical Case

A 45-year-old African–American man with a history of uncontrolled hypertension presents to the emergency department (ED) 1 h after sudden onset of left hemiparesis. Computed tomography (CT) of the head (Fig. 13.1a) reveals a right basal ganglia hemorrhage measuring 3×4 cm (volume 18 ml). Admission blood pressure (BP) is 200/105 mm Hg.

R. Dhar (✉)
Neurology Department (Division of Neurocritical Care),
Washington University School of Medicine, 660 S Euclid Avenue, Box 8111,
St. Louis, MO 63110, USA
e-mail: dharr@neuro.wustl.edu

J.G. Burneo et al. (eds.), *Neurology: An Evidence-Based Approach*,
DOI 10.1007/978-0-387-88555-1_13, © Springer Science+Business Media, LLC 2012

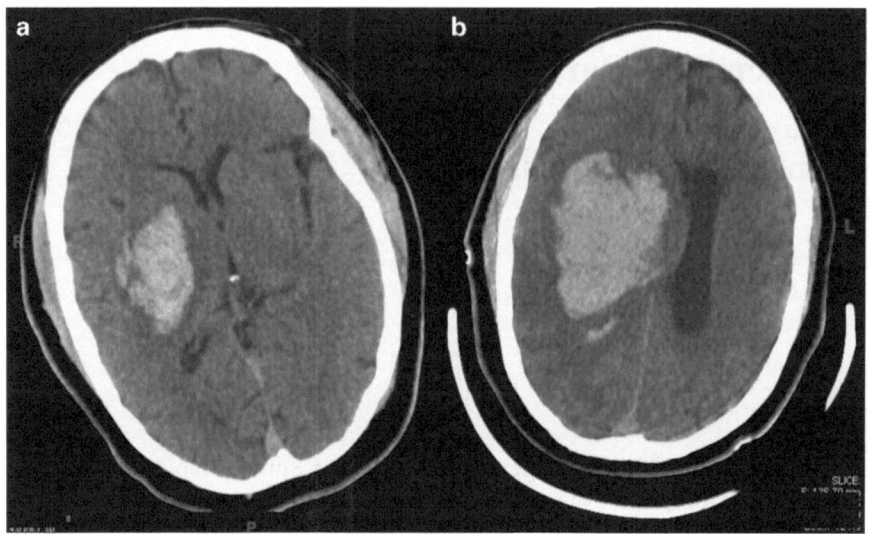

Fig. 13.1 (**a**) Admission CT of the head showing intracerebral hemorrhage in the right basal ganglia. (**b**) Repeat CT 2 h later with significant hematoma expansion, increased mass effect, and new intraventricular hemorrhage

Background

The incidence rate of ICH is 7–11 cases per 100,000 in a white population, but 2.3-fold higher rate in black persons under the age of 75 years [1]. Hypertension is the largest risk factor for ICH with an odds ratio (OR) of 3.7 (95% CI 2.5–5.4) in a systematic review of case-control studies [2]. Rates of ICH have been decreasing over the past decades likely related to better control of blood pressure [3, 4]. This has been partially offset by an increase in ICH related to rising utilization of anti-thrombotic therapies, such as warfarin, especially in the elderly [5].

Clinical Question

1. What is the current attributable risk for *hypertension* in deep (nonlobar) ICH?

Search Strategy

PubMed was searched from 1994 to October 21, 2010. MeSH terms "Cerebral Hemorrhage" and "Hypertension" were combined along with keyword "Attributable Risk." Only one of the three citations retrieved was a contemporary case-control study in ICH [6].

Results

This case-control study examined the population from the Greater Cincinnati region between 1997 and 2000, including 188 cases of ICH. While history of hypertension was not a risk factor for lobar ICH, it was present in 74 of 121 deep ICH cases, yielding an adjusted OR of 4.2 (95% CI 2.3–7.8). It had the highest attributable risk (AR) of all measured variables at 54% (95% CI 40–65%). This study was subsequently expanded to 540 cases, allowing race-specific risks to be compared [7]. While the multivariate OR for nonlobar ICH in whites was 4.1 (95% CI 2.4–7.0) with an AR of 19%, it was 17.7 (5.9–53.1) with AR of 60% (42–76%) in the black population.

Clinical Bottom Line

1. Hypertension remains the most important risk factor for deep ICH in the black population with an attributable risk between 40 and 65%.

Summary

Case-control studies such as this one may be confounded by recall bias and variations in the diagnosis of hypertension among cases and controls (some of whom may have undiagnosed hypertension). However, the effect of hypertension as a powerful risk factor for nonlobar ICH especially in the black population appears robust, arguing that better awareness and control are still needed.

Diagnosis

Clinical Case

He is moved to the neurological intensive care unit 2 h after arrival to the ED. During transfer, he becomes increasingly lethargic, no longer opening his eyes and not moving his right arm spontaneously. Repeat head CT (Fig. 13.1b) reveals significant enlargement of his ICH (volume 30 ml) with increased mass effect.

Background

The traditional belief that ICH was an apoplectic but static event has been challenged by observations over the past 15 years noting evidence of ongoing bleeding associated with neurological deterioration.

Table 13.1 Incidence of hematoma expansion in acute intracerebral hemorrhage

Study	Type	Number	Time to first CT (mean)	Increase in ICH % (ml)	Growth by >33%
Cincinnati [8]	Prospective cohort study	103	<3 h (89 min)	44.5% (6.3 ml)	26% at 1 h 38% by 24 h
F7ICH-1371 [9]	RCT (placebo arm)	96	<3 h (111 min)	29% (8.7 ml)	32%
FAST trial [10]	RCT (placebo arm)	268	<3 h (109 min)	26% (7.5 ml)	N/A
Beijing [11]	Cohort study	126	<4 h	N/A	25.4%

Clinical Questions

1. What is the incidence of *hematoma expansion* (HE) after spontaneous ICH?
2. Is HE predicted by higher admission blood pressure?
3. How does HE impact on outcome after ICH?

Search Strategy

PubMed was searched from inception to October 21, 2010. The MeSH term "Cerebral Hemorrhage" was combined with keywords (hematoma or hemorrhage) AND (expansion OR enlargement OR growth). Retrieval was limited to adult, human studies, yielding 434 citations. There were two prospective cohort studies and two prospective trials (examining treatment with recombinant factor VIIa [rFVIIa], from which we analyzed data on placebo patients). A number of retrospective studies were also reviewed for comparison. The keyword "blood pressure" was added to refine the search to the impact of BP on HE while the keywords (mortality or outcome) were added to find studies examining the impact of HE on outcome after ICH.

Results

Incidence of Hematoma Expansion

The results of the four included prospective studies are show in Table 13.1. Over 70% of these 467 patients in the first three studies had some degree of ICH enlargement (this data was not available in the fourth study). The prospective study from Cincinnati, which imaged patients at 1 h after admission head CT and again at 20 h, found that HE mostly occurred early and was associated with a decline in Glasgow Coma Scale (GCS) and NIH stroke scale (NIHSS), but not admission BP.

Association of HE with Admission Blood Pressure

While some retrospective studies found high systolic BP associated with HE [12], the prospective cohorts described above found no association between BP and HE [11, 13]. Consistent predictors of HE in the first rFVIIa study included shorter time from onset to baseline CT and larger volume of ICH [14]. Retrospective studies enrolling patients at varying times after ICH have further demonstrated that HE occurs early with a frequency that falls dramatically as time increases [12, 15].

Association Between HE and Outcome

A pooled analysis of placebo patients from three randomized trials of rFVIIa as well as the Cincinnati cohort assessed this association [16]. Hematoma growth predicted higher mortality (OR 1.05 per 10% increase, $p < 0.0001$) and lower chance of independent recovery (OR 0.84, $p < 0.0001$), adjusting for initial ICH size, age, GCS on presentation, and presence of intraventricular hemorrhage (IVH). This corresponded to a 3% higher mortality and 7% lower chance of good outcome per milliliter increase in volume at 24 h.

Clinical Bottom Lines

1. Over 70% of patients presenting in the first 3 h after ICH have enlargement of their hematoma by 24 h (mean increase of 6–9 ml). Most of this growth occurs early.
2. One in three patients with ICH experiences significant (>33%) growth often associated with neurological deterioration.
3. Admission blood pressure does not consistently predict HE.
4. Hematoma growth independently confers worse prognosis after ICH with a 7% reduction in odds of good recovery per milliliter increase in ICH volume.

Clinical Case

Review of the patient's initial head CT (including a CT angiogram) reveals a single focus of contrast extravasation (CE) on postcontrast images.

Background

Given the compelling association between HE and poor outcome, predictors of ongoing bleeding after ICH have been sought. Extravasation of radiographic contrast into the hematoma during CT angiography (often performed concurrent with routine head CT) could be interpreted as such a sign and potentially define a subgroup at high risk for HE.

Clinical Question

1. Does the presence of *contrast extravasation* predict the occurrence of HE after ICH?

Search Strategy

We searched PubMed from its inception to October 21, 2010, using the MeSH term "Cerebral hemorrhage" combined with the keywords contrast extravasation or "spot sign." Limiting to adults and human studies, we found 18 citations. Five of these were studies evaluating CE, three with HE as their end point, and the other two only assessing mortality. All but one of these studies was retrospective, hampered by selection bias, whereby patients not receiving a CT angiogram (CTA) on presentation were excluded. To detect HE, patients must have received a follow-up head CT, further introducing selection bias unless the study is performed prospectively with all patients receiving admission CTA and 24-h head CT to uniformly assess for CE and HE. Only one of the five studies examining CE (described in the Table 13.2) met these criteria [20].

Results

Table 13.2.

Clinical Bottom Line

1. One-third of patients presenting with spontaneous ICH within 3 h of ictus demonstrate extravasation of contrast (the "spot sign") on admission CT angiography. These patients have a higher incidence of hematoma expansion with PPV of 77% and NPV of 96%.

Summary

This test may identify patients with ICH at risk for further deterioration from hematoma expansion. These patients might benefit more from aggressive therapies while those without CE are very unlikely to have HE, and so the risks of such therapies may not be warranted.

Table 13.2 Studies evaluating contrast extravasation in acute intracerebral hemorrhage

Study	Number	Study design (% ICH included)	Time to CT	Contrast extravasation	Hematoma enlargement	Sens/Spec PPV/NPV
Becker [17]	113	Retrospective (only those with CTA on admission)	4.6±19 h if CE+ vs. 6.6±28 h if CE absent	52 (46%) on postcontrast CT	N/A	77%/73% 63%/84% (for death)
Goldstein [18]	104	Retrospective (only 21% included)	No association between time to CT and CE	58 (56%) on CTA source	14 (13%)[a]	93%/50% 24%/98% (for HE)
Kim [19]	56	Retrospective (only 7% included)	13 h (10.6±13 h if CE+ vs. 37.6±53 h if CE absent)	15 (27%) on postcontrast CT or CTA	N/A[b]	50%/83% 53%/80% (for death)
Wada [20]	39	Prospective (nine patients excluded)	<3 h	13 (33%) Spot Sign on CTA source	11 (28%)[c]	91%/89% 77%/96% (for HE)
Delgado [21]	367[d]	Retrospective (45% included)	5.5 h	71 (19%) on CTA source	56 (15%)[c]	88%/93% 69%/98% (for HE)

Notes: *Sens* sensitivity, *Spec* specificity, *PPV* positive predictive value, *NPV* negative predictive value

[a]>33% increase from baseline

[b]Increase in ICH volume was 13.5 ml in CE group and only 1.4 ml in group without CE

[c]>30% increase in volume from baseline or increase by 6 ml

[d]Includes 61 of the patients from Goldstein study who were reanalyzed

A prospective, randomized, NIH-funded trial is set to begin enrolling (*The Spot Sign for Predicting and Treating ICH Growth Study* (STOP-IT); NCT00810888). Patients with ICH determined to be at high risk for HE based on the presence of the CTA "spot sign" (within 5 h of ictus) are randomized to either rFVIIa or placebo.

Treatment

Background

The recognition that hematoma expansion was a common phenomenon contributing to neurological deterioration, death, and worsening of functional outcome prompted interest in the ability of hemostatic agents, like recombinant factor VIIa (rFVIIa), to arrest bleeding when given very early after ICH onset. While the efficacy of blood pressure control in the chronic stage after ICH was clearly demonstrated in the PROGRESS trial [22, 23], whether lowering BP acutely could reduce ongoing bleeding remained uncertain.

Clinical Questions

1. Does the administration of rFVIIa prevent HE and improve outcome after spontaneous ICH?
2. Does aggressive hyperacute management of hypertension prevent HE and improve outcome?

Search Strategy

rFVIIa

PubMed was searched from inception to October 21, 2010, combining the MeSH term "Cerebral hemorrhage/drug therapy" and keyword "Factor VII." Limiting to RCTs, four studies were found. These were also incorporated into an updated Cochrane Library review [24].

The Cochrane review evaluated the evidence for hemostatic therapies, specifically rFVIIa [24]. Three phase II industry-sponsored trials were included as well as a phase III study (FAST trial) all using rFVIIa within 4 h of ICH onset. The phase II studies showed that drug therapy reduced HE by 15% (or 4.5 ml) and the risk of death or dependence (mRS 4–6) with a relative risk (RR) of 0.79 (95% CI 0.67–0.93). The FAST trial was designed to confirm these promising early results [10]. Eight hundred and forty-one patients with ICH were randomized to rFVIIa at two doses (20 or 80 µg/kg) or placebo within 4 h of onset. The primary outcome was mRS 5–6 at 90 days. Mean increase in ICH volume at 24 h was 26% in the placebo group and 11% in the high-dose rFVIIa group, corresponding to 3.8 ml less growth ($p = 0.009$). However, there was no change in mortality or functional outcome in the rFVIIa-treated groups. This study was incorporated into the Cochrane meta-analysis, resulting in rFVIIa treatment having an overall nonsignificant reduction in death or dependency (OR 0.91, 95% CI 0.72–1.15). While rFVIIa treatment did not result in an excess of venous thromboembolic events, the high-dose arm in FAST had a higher risk of arterial events, including myocardial infarction (OR 2.14, 95% CI 1.09–4.41).

Blood Pressure

PubMed was searched from inception to October 21, 2010, combining the MeSH term "Cerebral hemorrhage" with keywords (hypertension or "blood pressure"). Limiting to RCTs yielded 57 citations of which two acute BP management trials were found [25, 26].

The INTERACT study was a feasibility trial of intensive BP lowering conducted mainly in China [25]. It randomized 404 patients with spontaneous ICH and SBP 150–220 mm Hg to two treatment arms within 6 h of ictus. Patients were either treated based on "guidelines" to an SBP goal of 180 mm Hg or to an intensive SBP goal of 140 mm Hg. This goal was to be achieved within 1 h of randomization and maintained for 1 week. The primary outcome was HE (increase in ICH volume >33% or >12.5 ml within 24 h) which was seen in 23% of the guideline group vs. 15% of the intensive treatment arm ($p = 0.05$). The absolute difference in growth, however, was only 1.7 ml. Death or dependency occurred at equal rates in both groups and neurologic deterioration was also unchanged (15% in both groups). A larger phase 3 trial (INTERACT2) examining functional recovery is currently enrolling (NCT00716079).

The ATACH trial was a multicenter, open-label, phase II trial determining the tolerability and safety of three escalating levels of antihypertensive treatment goals (as low as SBP 110–140 mm Hg) in 60 patients with ICH [27]. Blood pressure was controlled using intravenous nicardipine started within 6 h of ictus (mean 4.2 h), if baseline SBP ≥ 170 mm Hg, and continued for 24 h after ICH onset. Although BP was significantly different between arms, treatment failure (inability to attain BP goals) was frequent in the lowest BP group (41% vs. none in other arms). Early neurological deterioration occurred in 4 of 22 patients in the lowest BP arm (18%) vs. 2 (10%) in the 140–170 mm Hg tier and 1 (6%) in the 170–200 mm Hg tier. This was due to HE in almost all patients. Mortality was unchanged, although the study was not powered to show a difference [26]. Phase III studies are planned.

Clinical Bottom Lines

1. Recombinant factor VIIa reduces hematoma expansion when given within 4 h of spontaneous ICH, but does not improve functional outcome.

2. Early blood pressure reduction in hypertensive patients after spontaneous ICH minimally reduces hematoma expansion, but does not appear to improve functional outcome.

Summary

The ability of both hemostatic and antihypertensive therapy to reduce HE was demonstrated in the above trials. However, neither intervention appears to improve clinical outcomes (contrary to the clear association between greater HE and worse outcome). This may be explained by the relatively small effect on HE (only 2–4 ml) that may be insufficient to produce an observable clinical result. Greater clinical benefit has been suggested if either treatment is started even earlier, when more HE is likely to occur. Furthermore, benefits of both therapies on HE might be offset by risks, including thromboembolism with rFVIIa and precipitating ischemia and neurological deterioration at low BP. The FAST trial also had some imbalances in randomization, with the treatment arm having larger hemorrhages with more IVH.

Surgery

Clinical Case

Given the patient's deteriorating neurologic status, the family asks whether surgery to evacuate the ICH would be beneficial.

Clinical Question

1. Does surgery for patients with spontaneous ICH improve functional outcome?

Search Strategy

The Cochrane Library was searched using the term "Intracerebral Hemorrhage." A recently updated review on surgery for ICH was found. No additional studies not included in that meta-analysis were found by searching PubMed using the MeSH term "Cerebral hemorrhage" (Surgery OR Craniotomy OR Evacuation), limiting to RCTs. Evidence-based guidelines from the *American Heart Association* (AHA) were also reviewed for concordance [28].

Results

The Cochrane review from 2008 included 10 trials with 2,059 ICH patients [29]. It found that surgery performed within 24–72 h was associated with a reduction in death or dependence (OR 0.71, 95% CI 0.58–0.88). The NNT, assuming a control event rate of 70%, would be 14 (95% CI 9–37). This effect was larger when examining studies that used stereotactic or endoscopic techniques (OR 0.66, 95% CI 0.46–0.95) and nonsignificant if only examining studies utilizing craniotomy (OR 0.82, 95% CI 0.59–1.15).

Most of the data for this meta-analysis comes from a large multicenter study (STICH) that randomized 1,033 patients to surgery or conservative therapy within 72 h. Patients were eligible if there was clinical equipoise (i.e., uncertainty whether surgery was beneficial) in the mind of the neurosurgeon. A significant proportion (26%) in the medical arm crossed over to surgery usually for deteriorating GCS, although analysis remained intention-to-treat. This study found no significant benefit to surgical evacuation with favorable outcome in 26% compared to 24% in the conservative group (OR 0.89, 95% CI 0.66–1.19). However, benefit was seen in those with lobar ICH within 1 cm of the surface, a prespecified subgroup (OR 0.69, 0.47–1.01).

Clinical Bottom Line

1. Surgery may reduce the risk of death and dependence (OR 0.71, 95% CI 0.58–0.88) in patients with ICH, with suggestion of greater benefit with noninvasive techniques or with craniotomy if ICH is within 1 cm of the cortical surface.

Summary

Despite the findings of the Cochrane meta-analysis, the benefit of routine surgery in ICH remains controversial. Many studies utilizing different surgical techniques were combined with the results of the largest trial showing no benefit. The AHA guidelines assign a strong recommendation against routine evacuation of ICH while assigning a weak recommendation for evacuation of lobar clots within 1 cm of the surface by craniotomy. STICH II is currently underway, evaluating patients with lobar ICH (without IVH) evacuated principally by craniotomy within 60 h of ictus (ISRCTN22153967).

Prognosis

Clinical Question

1. What is the best validated prognostic scale for functional outcome in patients with ICH?

Search Strategy

PubMed was searched from inception to October 21, 2010, combining the MeSH terms "Cerebral hemorrhage" and prognosis with keywords (score or scale), limiting to adult, human studies in English. Of 522 citations, two prognostic scales were found (the Essen ICH score and the ICH score), both validated for functional outcome.

Results

Essen ICH Score

A group of investigators developed a logistic regression model for predicting complete recovery (Barthel index ≥ 95) after ICH using the German Stroke Foundation data bank [30]. They included patients admitted within 24 h with 100-day follow-up. There were 340 patients in their development cohort and 371 in a subsequent validation cohort. In-hospital mortality was 20–27%, and 26–33% made a full recovery. Variables predicting outcome were age, NIHSS score, and level of consciousness (from the NIHSS). Performance of this new model in the validation cohort was compared to the established ICH score [31] and a modified ICH score [32] (Table 13.3).

A subsequent study validated the Essen ICH score using a large external (clinical trials) database [33]. The model was applied to 564 ICH patients of whom 171 (30%) recovered and 107 (19%) died. Prediction of outcome was correct in 76%, working better to predict those not recovering than full recovery, with area under curve of 0.79, PPV 64%, NPV 80%.

ICH Score

The ICH score had been repeatedly validated as a predictor of short-term mortality, but only recently tested as a model for long-term functional recovery after ICH [34]. The scale had a c-statistic (testing concordance between the prediction and actual outcome) of 0.81 (i.e., 81% correct prediction for mRS ≤ 1). None of those with score of four or greater recovered to this level of eventual (minimal) disability.

Clinical Bottom Line

1. The Essen ICH score incorporating patient's age, level of consciousness, and NIHSS score predicts recovery after ICH. The ICH score incorporates volume and location of hematoma, but does not appear to provide any greater predictive utility.

Table 13.3 Comparison of prognostic scales for intracerebral hemorrhage

Predictors	Essen ICH score	ICH score	Modified ICH score
Age	<60=0	<80=0	<80=0
	60–69=1	≥80=1	≥80=1
	70–79=2		
	≥80=3		
NIHSS	0–5=0		0–10=0
	6–10=1		11–20=1
	11–15=2		≥20=2
	16–20=3		
	>20 or coma=4		
NIHSS level of consciousness (or Glasgow coma scale)	Alert=0	GCS 3–4=2	
	Drowsy=1	GCS 5–12=1	
	Stupor=2	GCS 13–15=0	
	Coma=3		
Hemorrhage volume (ml)		≥30=1	≥30=1
		<30=0	<30=0
Infratentorial origin		Yes=1	Yes=1
		No=0	No=0
Intraventricular hemorrhage		Yes=1	Yes=1
		No=0	No=0
Maximum score	10	6	6
Death predicted	>7	≥3	≥3
Good outcome predicted	<3	<3	<3
Prediction of complete recovery (PPV/NPV)	70%/87%	N/A	N/A
Area under curve (95% CI)	0.88 (0.84–0.91)	0.78 (0.73–0.82)	0.81 (0.77–0.86)
Prediction of death (PPV/NPV)	89%/81%	78%/85%	65%/86%
Area under curve (95% CI)	0.83 (0.78–0.88)	0.83 (0.78–0.88)	0.84 (0.79–0.88)

Summary

Based on the initial presentation of our patient (young, alert, NIHSS 9), he would be predicted to have an excellent prognosis with PPV of complete recovery 70%. However, the occurrence of HE, not incorporated into any of the above prognostic scales, contributed to worsening of his neurological status and has been shown to reduce the chance of recovery. This may need to be studied in further cohorts and incorporated into future prognostic models. Furthermore, patients with do-not-resuscitate (DNR) orders documented within the first day of admission had a significantly worse prognosis than predicted by typical models [35]; this may also need to be taken into account when applying models to individual patients.

Subarachnoid Hemorrhage

Introduction

Subarachnoid hemorrhage (SAH) usually results from rupture of an intracranial aneurysm. The major sources of morbidity and mortality after SAH are rebleeding and delayed cerebral ischemia (DCI) associated with vasospasm.

Epidemiology/Diagnosis

Clinical Case

A 42-year-old woman presents to a small ER at 10 p.m. with sudden onset of severe headache and is found to have extensive SAH on head CT. CT angiography reveals an 8-mm anterior communicating artery aneurysm. She is transferred to a tertiary neurosurgical center for definitive treatment of her aneurysm, planned for the following day.

Clinical Questions

1. What is the incidence of early aneurysmal *rebleeding* after SAH?
2. Does the administration of antifibrinolytic drugs (AFDs) reduce this risk?

Search Strategy

PubMed was searched from inception to October 22, 2010. The MeSH term "subarachnoid hemorrhage" was combined with keywords (rebleed OR rebleeding or rehemorrhage) AND (aneurysm or aneurysmal) AND (acute or early) AND incidence. This was limited to human studies and then trials or reviews, yielding 30 final citations. Three contemporary series were selected for analysis (including one randomized trial comparing aneurysm therapies).

To evaluate AFDs, the MeSH terms "antifibrinolytic agents" and "subarachnoid hemorrhage" were combined, limiting to adult human RCTs. A number of trials were found, all but one contained within a Cochrane Library review [36].

Results

Incidence of Rebleeding After SAH

Rebleeding is typically defined as neurological deterioration associated with CT or autopsy evidence of increased hemorrhage. The three series of patients with aneu-

Table 13.4 Incidence of rebleeding in acute aneurysmal subarachnoid hemorrhage

Study	Population	Number	Time to admit	Rebleed rate	Outcome if rebleed
Ohkuma [37]	Single-center consecutive series	273	50% <2 h 75% <6 h	13.6% within 24 h	51% death, 30% severe disability
ISAT [38]	Multicenter trial	2,143	Median 2 days	1.7% prior to treatment	62% mortality
Citerio [39]	Multicenter prospective cohort	350	Unclear	8%	57% poor outcome

rysmal SAH (see Table 13.4) differed in time to enrolment; the first study found that most rebleeds occurred in the ambulance or outside hospital, half before the initial diagnosis of SAH was even made; 92% occurred within 6 h of initial ictus. Rebleeding was consistently associated with mortality in excess of 50% and few survivors had good outcomes (Table 13.4).

Antifibrinolytic Drugs to Reduce Rebleeding

A 2003 Cochrane meta-analysis reviewed 9 trials randomizing 1,399 patients to AFDs (tranexamic acid in all except one small study) vs. placebo or control therapy [36]. Many studies were performed over 20 years ago prior to the routine use of nimodipine to ameliorate DCI. Most used AFDs for a prolonged duration (till aneurysm surgery, which was often delayed for weeks). The rate of rebleeding in the control group was 26%. AFD therapy reduced rebleeding in blinded studies (OR 0.49, 95% CI 0.37–0.65), driven largely by benefit seen in two larger RCTs. However, the benefit from reduced rebleeding was offset by an increased risk of cerebral ischemia (OR 1.39, 1.07–1.82); this risk was not seen in the only study performed using a contemporary management approach, including nimodipine, early surgery, and aggressive therapies to minimize DCI. Overall, there was no effect of treatment on mortality or poor outcome (OR 1.12, 0.88–1.43).

A more recent RCT studied short-duration AFD treatment to prevent early rebleeding in 505 patients [40]. Treatment was started immediately after diagnosis (e.g., at the local hospital prior to transfer) and continued for a maximum of 72 h until the aneurysm was secured. Treatment reduced CT-confirmed rebleeding from 10.8 to 2.4% (NNT 12, 95% CI 7.9–24.2). Short-term treatment in this study did not increase the risk of stroke, permanent ischemic deficits, or TCD-related vasospasm; there was no difference in functional outcome. A more recent study with historical controls found similar results but an increased incidence of deep venous thromboses (19% vs. 4.6%, NNH 7, 95% CI 4–20) [41].

Clinical Bottom Lines

1. Rebleeding occurs most commonly early after aneurysmal SAH with a rate as high as 14% in the first day.
2. Prolonged administration of AFDs reduces rebleeding but increases DCI, and so does not improve outcome after SAH.
3. The use of AFDs in the hyperacute period for a short duration (till early surgery) reduces aneurysmal rebleeding without an increase in cerebral ischemia. DVTs may be increased.

Summary

Rebleeding is a common and frequently lethal complication of SAH. Recent studies have renewed interest in the ability of hyperacute administration of AFDs to significantly reduce this risk. Large, controlled studies are required to confirm this benefit and evaluate its impact on mortality and outcome.

Treatment: Prevention of Vasospasm

Background

Once the aneurysm has been secured (by surgical or endovascular means), the major source of neurological morbidity for patients with SAH is DCI associated with vasospasm. Prevention of DCI has been the focus of significant research efforts.

Clinical Case

She is admitted to the neurointensive care unit after clipping of her aneurysm (see Neurosurgery chapter for evidence on aneurysm management) and is started on nimodipine. The neurosurgeon also wants to initiate therapy with simvastatin to prevent vasospasm.

Clinical Questions

1. Does nimodipine reduce the incidence of DCI and improve outcome after SAH?
2. Does statin therapy reduce vasospasm, DCI, and improve outcome after SAH?

Search Strategy

The Cochrane Library was searched using the term, "Subarachnoid Hemorrhage," yielding a review of calcium antagonists (including nimodipine) updated in 2006. No more recent studies were found with a broad PubMed search from 2006 onward. PubMed was searched using the MeSH terms "Subarachnoid hemorrhage" and "Hydroxymethylglutaryl-CoA Reductase Inhibitors" or any of the keywords (statin, simvastatin, pravastatin). This search was limited to RCTs and meta-analysis. Of 29 studies retrieved, four small phase 2 RCTs were found, as well as three recent meta-analyses [42–44].

Results: Nimodipine

The Cochrane review included 16 RCTs (involving 3,361 patients), where nimodipine was used in aneurysmal SAH [45]. Treatment reduced poor outcome with RR 0.81 (95% CI 0.72–0.92), ARR of 5.3%, and NNT of 19 (1–51). Nimodipine also reduced DCI (RR 0.66, 0.59–0.75, ARR 14%, NNT 7, 6–10) and cerebral infarcts (RR 0.78, 0.70–0.87, ARR 11%, NNT 9, 6–15).

Results: Statins

The four published RCTs are summarized below. All trials started therapy within 48–96 h of SAH onset and are all single-center studies (Table 13.5).

One hundred and ninety patients from these four trials were included in a meta-analysis of DCI (vs. 151 patients in three studies for TCD vasospasm and poor outcome as end points) [44]. DCI was not reduced by statin treatment (pooled RR 0.57, 95% CI 0.29–1.13, $p = 0.1$). TCD vasospasm and poor outcome occurred at the same rate in treated and untreated patients (RR 0.99 for vasospasm, RR 0.92 for poor outcome). RR mortality was 0.37 (95% CI 0.13–1.10, $p = 0.07$). An even more recent meta-analysis included two additional trials (both pseudorandomized) available only in abstract form, raising the number of patients analyzed to 309 [43]. A fixed-effects model was used to combine the data (in contrast to the more conservative random-effects model used in the other meta-analysis), and this yielded a pooled OR for DCI of 0.38 (95% CI 0.23–0.65). Effect of treatment on mortality was 0.51 (95% CI 0.25–1.02, $p = 0.06$).

Clinical Bottom Lines

1. Nimodipine reduces the incidence of DCI, infarction, and poor outcome (OR 0.81, 95% CI 0.72–0.92) after aneurysmal SAH.
2. It is unclear whether statin therapy reduces DCI or improves outcome. Data for small trials is inconclusive and larger RCTs are required before recommendations can be made.

Table 13.5 Studies evaluating the effect of statin therapy on subarachnoid hemorrhage

Study	N	Statin	Duration	Vasospasm (TCD)[a]	DID[b]	Poor outcome	Mortality
Tseng [46]	80	Pravastatin (40 mg)	14 days or discharge	43 vs. 63% (p=0.006)	5% vs. 30% (p<0.001)	43% vs. 53% (p=0.7)	5% vs. 20% (p=0.04)
Lynch [47]	39	Simvastatin (80 mg)	14 days	N/A	26% vs. 60% (p=0.03)	N/A	N/A
Chou [48]	39	Simvastatin (80 mg)	Max 21 days (or ICU discharge)	68% vs. 50% (p=0.24)	37% vs. 50% (p=0.41)	63% vs. 50% (p=0.41)	0 vs. 15% (p=0.23)
Vergouwen [49]	32	Simvastatin (80 mg)	15 days	75% vs. 69% (p=0.024)	38% vs. 31% (p=0.71)	56% vs. 69% (p=0.63)	13% in both

[a]*TCD* Transcranial Doppler
[b]*DID* Delayed ischemic deficits

Summary

The use of nimodipine has become standard care for patients with SAH, and is effective in reducing ischemia and poor outcome. Statins are emerging as a promising therapy to prevent vasospasm, but small studies have revealed conflicting findings. Large phase III trials are planned, including the STASH trial from Cambridge, set to randomize 1,600 patients to simvastatin or placebo and evaluate disability at 6 months (NCT00731627).

Treatment: Delayed Cerebral Ischemia

Clinical Case

On the seventh day after presentation, she develops increasing confusion and left arm weakness. Angiogram reveals severe bilateral anterior cerebral artery and right middle cerebral artery vasospasm. She is currently receiving maintenance intravenous fluids and has a blood pressure of 145/88 (mean arterial pressure, MAP 107) mm Hg.

Clinical Questions

1. Do prophylactic hypervolemia and/or hypertension prevent the development of DCI?
2. Does induced hypertension, hypervolemia, and hemodilution (i.e., *Triple H Therapy*) prevent infarction from DCI and improve outcome?

Search Strategy

PubMed was searched from inception to October 22, 2010. The MeSH term "Subarachnoid hemorrhage" was combined with keywords (vasospasm, cerebral ischemia, ischemic deficits) and (hypervolemia, hypervolemic, hypertension, hypertensive, hemodilution). This search was limited to adult human studies (233 citations). These results were combined with the keywords (prevent, prevention, preventative, prophylactic) and limited to clinical trials/RCTs, from which two randomized trials and one systematic review were found [50–52]. A Cochrane review was also found, last updated in 2004, which analyzed the same two trials and another quasi-randomized study from the 1980s [53]. No RCTs were found evaluating the efficacy of hemodynamic therapies in the treatment of DCI. Reviewing the original 233 citations, a number of case series were found. We selected prospective series with clinical reversal as the end point as none were found that used functional outcomes compared to untreated controls. Initial search found only one clinical trial [54]. Further review found three additional series [55–57].

Results: Hemodynamic Therapy for Prevention of DCI

The largest truly randomized study compared postoperative normovolemia to hypervolemia until SAH day 14 in 82 patients [52]. Albumin boluses were given if filling pressures fell below targets for each group (CVP 5 vs. 8 mm Hg). Symptomatic vasospasm occurred in eight patients in each group with no difference in rates of cerebral infarction or need for hypertensive therapy. Functional independence was identical in the two groups. The other randomized trial enrolled only 16 patients in each arm, evaluating prophylactic "Triple H" therapy in good-grade patients (Hunt and Hess I to III) after surgical clipping. The intervention consisted of fluid titration to CVP of 8–12 mm Hg (including colloids), hematocrit target 30–35%, and postoperative MAP 20 mm Hg higher than preoperative MAP (typically, accomplished using dopamine infusion). Patients in the control group received intravenous fluids titrated to neutral fluid balance (2 l/day) without colloids. Hyperdynamic therapy did not result in any reduction in mortality, poor outcome, or signs of delayed ischemia. There was a higher rate of complications in the intervention group, including congestive heart failure and coagulopathy.

Results: Hemodynamic Therapy for Treatment of DCI

No randomized or even controlled studies have evaluated the efficacy of "Triple H" therapy to improve outcomes from symptomatic vasospasm (i.e., DCI). After early series showed impressive anecdotal efficacy, this paradigm was rapidly adopted as standard care for ischemic neurological deficits after SAH. A recent series examined 24 patients who developed delayed ischemic deficits and were treated with volume expansion to achieve a PCWP of 14–18 mm Hg (or whatever level optimized cardiac index). If prompt neurological improvement did not result after fluid bolus, phenylephrine was infused to increase at least MAP 20–25% above baseline. Twenty-one of twenty-four patients (88%) demonstrated improvement in neurological status with hypertensive hypervolemic therapy (HHT). Eight patients did also receive infusions of papaverine along with HHT that may have contributed to clinical improvement.

Clinical Bottom Lines

1. Prophylactic hypervolemia (± hypertensive) therapy after SAH does not reduce vasospasm, DCI, or poor outcome, and may expose patients to increased iatrogenic complications.
2. There is strong uncontrolled evidence that HHT reverses ischemic neurological deficits associated with vasospasm. However, no controlled evidence exists to prove that these treatments prevent infarction or improve outcomes after SAH.

Prognosis

Clinical Question

1. What is the rate of disability in those developing DCI and how does it compare to those without symptomatic vasospasm?

Search Strategy

PubMed was searched from inception to October 22, 2010. The MeSH term "Subarachnoid hemorrhage" was combined with keywords (Vasospasm, cerebral ischemia, ischemic deficits, infarct, infarction) and (mortality, disability, prognosis, outcome, Rankin, Barthel). This was limited to English language studies in human adults and further restricted to clinical trials or meta-analyses. Of the 169 citations, three large series were found addressing this question.

Results

An Italian multicenter study found vasospasm (based on TCD or angiography) in 30% of a prospective cohort of 350 SAH patients [39], but cerebral ischemia (defined by clinical deterioration) in only 26%. While vasospasm did not increase the odds of unfavorable outcome, patients with ischemia had a 60% chance of poor outcome (GOS 1–3) compared to 35% in those without DCI ($p = 0.02$). A second study incorporated 3,567 patients entered into four RCTs and examined the significance of cerebral infarcts on CT imaging after SAH. Infarcts were found in 27% of patients, and presence of infarction was the strongest predictor of poor outcome in multivariate analysis (OR 5.89, 95% CI 4.24–6.82).

Clinical Bottom Line

1. While the occurrence of angiographic vasospasm does not increase the risk of disability, symptoms of cerebral ischemia and especially the development of infarction confer greater risk of poor outcome.

Summary

It appears that vasospasm itself does not worsen the outcome after SAH, likely as angiographic changes even with clinical deficits can often now be reversed with aggressive hemodynamic and endovascular therapies. However, if DCI progresses to cerebral infarction, patients are much more likely to do poorly. Preventing permanent infarction, therefore, should be the ultimate goal of all interventions aimed at DCI after SAH.

References

1. Broderick JP, Brott T, Tomsick T, Huster G, Miller R. The risk of subarachnoid and intracerebral hemorrhages in blacks as compared with whites. N Engl J Med. 1992;326(11):733–6.
2. Ariesen MJ, Claus SP, Rinkel GJ, Algra A. Risk factors for intracerebral hemorrhage in the general population: a systematic review. Stroke. 2003;34(8):2060–5.
3. Furlan AJ, Whisnant JP, Elveback LR. The decreasing incidence of primary intracerebral hemorrhage: a population study. Ann Neurol. 1979;5(4):367–73.
4. Lovelock CE, Molyneux AJ, Rothwell PM. Change in incidence and aetiology of intracerebral haemorrhage in Oxfordshire, UK, between 1981 and 2006: a population-based study. Lancet Neurol. 2007;6(6):487–93.
5. Flaherty ML, Kissela B, Woo D, et al. The increasing incidence of anticoagulant-associated intracerebral hemorrhage. Neurology. 2007;68(2):116–21.
6. Woo D, Sauerbeck LR, Kissela BM, et al. Genetic and environmental risk factors for intracerebral hemorrhage: preliminary results of a population-based study. Stroke. 2002;33(5):1190–5.
7. Woo D, Flaherty ML, Sekar P, et al. Race-specific attributable risks for intracerebral hemorrhage. Stroke. 2009;40(4):6 (Abstract #24).
8. Brott T, Broderick J, Kothari R, et al. Early hemorrhage growth in patients with intracerebral hemorrhage. Stroke. 1997;28(1):1–5.
9. Mayer SA, Brun NC, Begtrup K, et al. Recombinant activated factor VII for acute intracerebral hemorrhage. N Engl J Med. 2005;352(8):777–85.
10. Mayer SA, Brun NC, Begtrup K, et al. Efficacy and safety of recombinant activated factor VII for acute intracerebral hemorrhage. N Engl J Med. 2008;358(20):2127–37.
11. Ji N, Lu JJ, Zhao YL, Wang S, Zhao JZ. Imaging and clinical prognostic indicators for early hematoma enlargement after spontaneous intracerebral hemorrhage. Neurol Res. 2009;31(4):362–6.
12. Kazui S, Minematsu K, Yamamoto H, Sawada T, Yamaguchi T. Predisposing factors to enlargement of spontaneous intracerebral hematoma. Stroke. 1997;28(12):2370–5.
13. Jauch EC, Lindsell CJ, Adeoye O, et al. Lack of evidence for an association between hemodynamic variables and hematoma growth in spontaneous intracerebral hemorrhage. Stroke. 2006;37(8):2061–5.
14. Broderick JP, Diringer MN, Hill MD, et al. Determinants of intracerebral hemorrhage growth: an exploratory analysis. Stroke. 2007;38(3):1072–5.
15. Fujii Y, Takeuchi S, Sasaki O, Minakawa T, Tanaka R. Multivariate analysis of predictors of hematoma enlargement in spontaneous intracerebral hemorrhage. Stroke. 1998;29(6):1160–6.
16. Davis SM, Broderick J, Hennerici M, et al. Hematoma growth is a determinant of mortality and poor outcome after intracerebral hemorrhage. Neurology. 2006;66(8):1175–81.
17. Becker KJ, Baxter AB, Bybee HM, Tirschwell DL, Abouelsaad T, Cohen WA. Extravasation of radiographic contrast is an independent predictor of death in primary intracerebral hemorrhage. Stroke. 1999;30(10):2025–32.
18. Goldstein JN, Fazen LE, Snider R, et al. Contrast extravasation on CT angiography predicts hematoma expansion in intracerebral hemorrhage. Neurology. 2007;68(12):889–94.
19. Kim J, Smith A, Hemphill III JC, et al. Contrast extravasation on CT predicts mortality in primary intracerebral hemorrhage. Am J Neuroradiol. 2008;29(3):520–5.
20. Wada R, Aviv RI, Fox AJ, et al. CT angiography "spot sign" predicts hematoma expansion in acute intracerebral hemorrhage. Stroke. 2007;38(4):1257–62.
21. Delgado Almandoz JE, Yoo AJ, Stone MJ, et al. Systematic characterization of the computed tomography angiography spot sign in primary intracerebral hemorrhage identifies patients at highest risk for hematoma expansion: the spot sign score. Stroke. 2009;40(9):2994–3000.
22. Chapman N, Huxley R, Anderson C, et al. Effects of a perindopril-based blood pressure-lowering regimen on the risk of recurrent stroke according to stroke subtype and medical history: the PROGRESS Trial. Stroke. 2004;35(1):116–21.

23. Randomised trial of a perindopril-based blood-pressure-lowering regimen among 6,105 individuals with previous stroke or transient ischaemic attack. Lancet. 2001;358(9287):1033–41.
24. Al-Shahi R. Haemostatic drug therapies for acute spontaneous intracerebral haemorrhage. Cochrane Database Syst Rev. 2009; 4:CD005951. doi: 10.1002/14651858.CD005951.pub3.
25. Anderson CS, Huang Y, Wang JG, et al. Intensive blood pressure reduction in acute cerebral haemorrhage trial (INTERACT): a randomised pilot trial. Lancet Neurol. 2008;7(5):391–9.
26. Antihypertensive Treatment of Acute Cerebral Hemorrhage (ATACH) Investigators. Antihypertensive treatment of acute cerebral hemorrhage. Crit Care Med. 2010;38(2):637–48.
27. Qureshi AI. Antihypertensive treatment of acute cerebral hemorrhage (ATACH): rationale and design. Neurocrit Care. 2007;6(1):56–66.
28. Broderick J, Connolly S, Feldmann E, et al. Guidelines for the management of spontaneous intracerebral hemorrhage in adults: 2007 update: a guideline from the American Heart Association/American Stroke Association Stroke Council, High Blood Pressure Research Council, and the Quality of Care and Outcomes in Research Interdisciplinary Working Group. Stroke. 2007;38(6):2001–23.
29. Prasad K, Mendelow AD, Gregson BA. Surgery for primary intracerebral haemorrhage. Cochrane Database Syst Rev. 2008;4:CD000200. doi: 10.1002/14651858.CD000200.pub2.
30. Weimar C, Benemann J, Diener HC. Development and validation of the Essen Intracerebral Haemorrhage Score. J Neurol Neurosurg Psychiatry. 2006;77(5):601–5.
31. Hemphill III JC, Bonovich DC, Besmertis L, Manley GT, Johnston SC. The ICH score: a simple, reliable grading scale for intracerebral hemorrhage. Stroke. 2001;32(4):891–7.
32. Cheung RT, Zou LY. Use of the original, modified, or new intracerebral hemorrhage score to predict mortality and morbidity after intracerebral hemorrhage. Stroke. 2003;34(7):1717–22.
33. Weimar C, Ziegler A, Sacco RL, Diener HC, Konig IR. Predicting recovery after intracerebral hemorrhage–an external validation in patients from controlled clinical trials. J Neurol. 2009;256(3):464–9.
34. Hemphill III JC, Farrant M, Neill Jr TA. Prospective validation of the ICH Score for 12-month functional outcome. Neurology. 2009;73(14):1088–94.
35. Zahuranec DB, Morgenstern LB, Sanchez BN, Resnicow K, White DB, Hemphill III JC. Do-not-resuscitate orders and predictive models after intracerebral hemorrhage. Neurology. 2010;75(7):626–33.
36. Roos YB, Vermeulen M, Algra A, van Gijn J. Antifibrinolytic therapy for aneurysmal subarachnoid hemorrhage. Cochrane Database Syst Rev. 2003;2:CD001245. doi:10.1002/14651858. CD001245.
37. Ohkuma H, Tsurutani H, Suzuki S. Incidence and significance of early aneurysmal rebleeding before neurosurgical or neurological management. Stroke. 2001;32(5):1176–80.
38. Molyneux AJ, Kerr RS, Yu LM, et al. International subarachnoid aneurysm trial (ISAT) of neurosurgical clipping versus endovascular coiling in 2143 patients with ruptured intracranial aneurysms: a randomised comparison of effects on survival, dependency, seizures, rebleeding, subgroups, and aneurysm occlusion. Lancet. 2005;366(9488):809–17.
39. Citerio G, Gaini SM, Tomei G, Stocchetti N. Management of 350 aneurysmal subarachnoid hemorrhages in 22 Italian neurosurgical centers. Intensive Care Med. 2007;33(9):1580–6.
40. Hillman J, Fridriksson S, Nilsson O, Yu Z, Saveland H, Jakobsson KE. Immediate administration of tranexamic acid and reduced incidence of early rebleeding after aneurysmal subarachnoid hemorrhage: a prospective randomized study. J Neurosurg. 2002;97(4):771–8.
41. Starke RM, Kim GH, Fernandez A, et al. Impact of a protocol for acute antifibrinolytic therapy on aneurysm rebleeding after subarachnoid hemorrhage. Stroke. 2008;39(9):2617–21.
42. Sillberg VA, Wells GA, Perry JJ. Do statins improve outcomes and reduce the incidence of vasospasm after aneurysmal subarachnoid hemorrhage: a meta-analysis. Stroke. 2008;39(9):2622–6.
43. Kramer AH, Fletcher JJ. Statins in the management of patients with aneurysmal subarachnoid hemorrhage: a systematic review and meta-analysis. Neurocrit Care. 2010;12(2):285–96.
44. Vergouwen MD, de Haan RJ, Vermeulen M, Roos YB. Effect of statin treatment on vasospasm, delayed cerebral ischemia, and functional outcome in patients with aneurysmal subarachnoid hemorrhage: a systematic review and meta-analysis update. Stroke. 2010;41(1):e47–52.

45. Dorhout Mees S, Rinkel GJ, Feigin VL et al. Calcium antagonists for aneurysmal subarachnoid haemorrhage. Cochrane Database Syst Rev. 2007;3:CD000277. doi: 10.1002/14651858. CD000277.pub3.

46. Tseng MY, Czosnyka M, Richards H, Pickard JD, Kirkpatrick PJ. Effects of acute treatment with pravastatin on cerebral vasospasm, autoregulation, and delayed ischemic deficits after aneurysmal subarachnoid hemorrhage: a phase II randomized placebo-controlled trial. Stroke. 2005;36(8):1627–32.

47. Lynch JR, Wang H, McGirt MJ, et al. Simvastatin reduces vasospasm after aneurysmal subarachnoid hemorrhage: results of a pilot randomized clinical trial. Stroke. 2005;36(9):2024–6.

48. Chou SH, Smith EE, Badjatia N, et al. A randomized, double-blind, placebo-controlled pilot study of simvastatin in aneurysmal subarachnoid hemorrhage. Stroke. 2008;39(10):2891–3.

49. Vergouwen MD, Meijers JC, Geskus RB, et al. Biologic effects of simvastatin in patients with aneurysmal subarachnoid hemorrhage: a double-blind, placebo-controlled randomized trial. J Cereb Blood Flow Metab. 2009;29(8):1444–53.

50. Treggiari MM, Walder B, Suter PM, Romand JA. Systematic review of the prevention of delayed ischemic neurological deficits with hypertension, hypervolemia, and hemodilution therapy following subarachnoid hemorrhage. J Neurosurg. 2003;98(5):978–84.

51. Egge A, Waterloo K, Sjoholm H, Solberg T, Ingebrigtsen T, Romner B. Prophylactic hyperdynamic postoperative fluid therapy after aneurysmal subarachnoid hemorrhage: a clinical, prospective, randomized, controlled study. Neurosurgery. 2001;49(3):593–605.

52. Lennihan L, Mayer SA, Fink ME, et al. Effect of hypervolemic therapy on cerebral blood flow after subarachnoid hemorrhage: a randomized controlled trial. Stroke. 2000;31(2):383–91.

53. Rosenwasser RH, Delgado TE, Buchheit WA, Freed MH. Control of hypertension and prophylaxis against vasospasm in cases of subarachnoid hemorrhage: a preliminary report. Neurosurgery. 1983;12(6):658–61.

54. Miller JA, Dacey Jr RG, Diringer MN. Safety of hypertensive hypervolemic therapy with phenylephrine in the treatment of delayed ischemic deficits after subarachnoid hemorrhage. Stroke. 1995;26(12):2260–6.

55. Otsubo H, Takemae T, Inoue T, Kobayashi S, Sugita K. Normovolaemic induced hypertension therapy for cerebral vasospasm after subarachnoid haemorrhage. Acta Neurochir (Wien). 1990;103(1–2):18–26.

56. Kassell NF, Peerless SJ, Durward QJ, Beck DW, Drake CG, Adams HP. Treatment of ischemic deficits from vasospasm with intravascular volume expansion and induced arterial hypertension. Neurosurgery. 1982;11(3):337–43.

57. Awad IA, Carter LP, Spetzler RF, Medina M, Williams Jr FC. Clinical vasospasm after subarachnoid hemorrhage: response to hypervolemic hemodilution and arterial hypertension. Stroke. 1987;18(2):365–72.

Part III
The Evidence-Based Neurology Curriculum

Chapter 14
The Evidence-Based Neurology Curriculum

Lawrence Korngut and Miguel Bussière

Keywords Evidence-based neurology • Education • Best practice • Curriculum

Introduction

Clinical training in neurology is a lengthy and complicated process that requires integration of multiple fundamental skills that coalesce into sound clinical decision making. Beyond the obvious knowledge of anatomy, physiology, and the medical sciences, there is an essential requirement for the trainee in the era of evidence-based clinical practice to acquire skills and experience in the process of critical appraisal and have a working knowledge of the best current evidence from the diverse spectrum of subspecialties that comprise neurology today. Maintaining competence in the current best evidence over a clinician's career is essential to providing high-quality medical care and choosing appropriate investigations and treatments. Evidence-based clinical practice is also becoming increasingly important from a medicolegal perspective.

Developing critical appraisal skills is a difficult process, particularly when compiled with the significant demands of a residency program. An evidence-based curriculum allows for time dedicated to teaching of critical appraisal fundamentals and engagement of discussion of current questions, topics, and controversies. Fostering an understanding of what comprises an appropriate literature search, the levels of available evidence, and the different types of studies and methodologies is difficult to consolidate outside of a formalized curriculum or graduate level training.

In this chapter, we discuss the development of an evidence-based curriculum.

M. Bussière (✉)
Neurology and Interventional Neuroradiology, The Ottawa Hospital, Civic Campus, C-2174, 1053 Carling Avenue, Ottawa, ON K1Y 4E9, Canada
e-mail: mbussiere@toh.on.ca

J.G. Burneo et al. (eds.), *Neurology: An Evidence-Based Approach*, 347
DOI 10.1007/978-0-387-88555-1_14, © Springer Science+Business Media, LLC 2012

Table 14.1 Summary of EBN curriculum objectives

1. Trainees should develop critical appraisal skills to:
   a. Formulate answerable questions based on clinical uncertainty
   b. Perform an appropriate literature search
   c. Identify the best-quality evidence from the studies identified
   d. Critically appraise the identified studies to answer the original clinical question
   e. Be familiar with the different types of clinical studies (e.g., prognosis, diagnosis, therapy, or harm) and the key methodological and statistical questions that should be addressed in each type of study
   f. Determine whether the study findings are worth considering given the methodological quality of the study and its applicability to their patient population
2. Trainees should develop a working understanding of the importance of high-quality evidence, but also realize its limitations
3. Trainees should accumulate knowledge about best current evidence practices

Objectives

Acquisition of critical appraisal skills is the primary objective of an evidence-based clinical practice curriculum. Key critical appraisal skills include: formulation of answerable questions based on clinical uncertainty, performance of an appropriate literature search, identification of the best-quality evidence from the studies returned from the search, and critical appraisal of the studies to answer the original clinical question. Trainees should become familiar with the different types of clinical studies (e.g., prognosis, diagnosis, therapy, or harm) and the key methodological and statistical questions that should be addressed in each type of study. They should also be able to determine whether the study findings are worth considering given the methodological quality of the study and its applicability to their patient population.

Trainees should develop an understanding of the importance of high-quality evidence, but also realize its limitations. Emphasis should remain on high-quality patient care and the use of the best current evidence to guide clinical judgment within the context of the patient's wishes. It should be emphasized that lack of evidence for efficacy does not necessarily mean lack of benefit with treatment, and vice versa for lack of evidence against certain treatments or investigations.

Through the evidence-based curriculum, knowledge about best current evidence practices is accumulated. Through the discussion of common clinical scenarios and review of the relevant evidence, the trainees develop a working knowledge of the current evidence (Table 14.1).

The following sections describe an example of an evidence-based neurology (EBN) curriculum based on two well-developed and highly successful programs targeting clinical neurology residents, the EBN curriculum from the University of Western Ontario in London, Canada [1–4], and the Mayo Clinic Evidence Based Clinical Practice, Research, Informatics, and Training (MERIT) Curriculum, Mayo

Table 14.2 PICO acronym for developing focused clinical questions [8]

*P*atient or population
*I*ntervention, prognostic factor, or exposure
*C*omparison or intervention
*O*utcome to measure or achieve

Clinic, Scottsdale, AZ [5, 6]. Another resource designed to help educators teach trainees to understand and use evidence-based medicine is the Web-based American Academy of Neurology Evidence-Based Curriculum [7].

Pretutorial Topic/Question Selection and Preparation

Generating the Clinical Questions

Once per year, curriculum facilitators survey all neurology trainees and faculty members to generate a list of important neurological clinical questions for potential review. These clinical questions are then rank ordered by the trainees and facilitators according to multiple factors, including clinical importance, relevance, frequency of occurrence, and interest. The highest ranked questions are reviewed in the upcoming year. The topics are screened to ensure that they are congruent with the educational recommendations of the training program (postgraduate education committee), Royal College of Physicians and Surgeons of Canada Advisory Committee, and/or Accreditation Council for Graduate Medical Education – Neurology Residency and American Board of Psychiatry and Neurology [1–6].

Flexibility is available to adjust the clinical topics to suit the needs and training level of the trainees. Semiannual meetings of the curriculum trainees and facilitators allow for appropriate curriculum content changes and adjustment of group discussion objectives to cover specific epidemiological or biostatistical topics.

Preparing for the Tutorial Session

Trainees each select one or two clinical questions per year and prepare their topic for general discussion with the group. For each clinical topic, a clinical scenario and a focused clinical question are formulated. A focused clinical question should include considerations of the specific patient group, intervention or exposure, method of comparison, and outcome measures. The acronym PICO can serve as a helpful reminder [8] (Table 14.2).

Sample Clinical Scenario and Focused Clinical Question (Modified from 9)

Clinical Problem

A 79-year-old gentleman presented with a 4-week history of left-sided weakness. A CT head demonstrated a chronic right frontoparietal subdural hematoma. He denied any history of recent head injury or head trauma. He was not taking antiplatelet agents or anticoagulants. No surgical intervention was recommended. He was started on prednisone 20 mg by mouth twice a day. The following day, a repeat CT scan was performed, which showed no change.

Clinical Question

1. Does corticosteroid therapy in patients presenting with symptomatic chronic subdural hematomas improve clinical outcome or avoid the need for surgical intervention?

Search Strategy

For a given clinical question, the presenting trainee performs a literature search and identifies studies representing the highest level of evidence [9]. Expert librarians and informatics specialists can be called upon to assist in efficient and comprehensive literature searching. Studies are evaluated according to the generally accepted hierarchy of clinical evidence. High-quality meta-analyses, systematic reviews, and randomized clinic trials are preferred over observational studies and case reports. One to four studies are selected for critical appraisal and discussion. A summary of this information is prepared in advance of the discussion in the form of a critically appraised topic (CAT) as described below. One week prior to the session, the presenting trainee circulates copies of the clinical scenario, focused clinical question, search strategy, and articles for review to the participants. The pretutorial process is supervised by one of the facilitators. The faculty often provides instruction and advice on the search strategy and reasons for inclusion or exclusion of studies. Trainees are introduced to different search engines (e.g., PubMed [10], SUMSearch [11], Cochrane Library [12]). Discussions on Medical Subject Headings (MeSH), keywords, and their uses are helpful.

Sample Literature Search (Modified from [9])

– Ovid MEDLINE database was searched for the time period from 1950 to May week 4 2009.

- The MeSH terms "hematoma, subdural, chronic" and the text words "chronic subdural hematoma" OR "subdural hematoma" OR "CSDH" were combined by the Boolean operator "OR" yielding 6,426 articles.
- The MeSH term "steroids" was exploded for comprehensive retrieval and combined using the Boolean "OR" with the text words "non-surgical" OR "nonsurgical" OR "non-operative" OR "nonoperative" yielding 623,237 articles.
- The two resulting sets were combined using the Boolean "AND" and limited to English and humans with a result of 75 articles. A search filter for therapy emphasizing relevance was applied but found to be too restrictive, so the search filter for therapy emphasizing comprehensive retrieval was applied resulting in a final set of 40 articles.
- The EMBASE database and Cochrane Library databases were also searched for relevant articles.
- Several professional organization Web sites (American Heart Association, American Stroke Association, American Academy of Neurology, Society of Critical Care Medicine, and the National Guideline Clearinghouse) were searched to determine whether practice guidelines were published for this topic.

No randomized controlled trials were found after an extensive literature search.

The final article was selected as it represented the only study investigating the role of corticosteroids in chronic subdural hematoma.

Tutorial

Each tutorial session focuses on a trainee presenting one clinical question. The session begins with a 5-min description of the clinical scenario and focused clinical question. This is followed by a 10-min presentation of the topic background, including clinical information about the condition, treatment, or diagnostic test. The trainee then presents and discusses the search strategy for 5 min. The following 45 min are dedicated to critical appraisal of the evidence.

The study type is identified (e.g., prognosis, diagnosis, therapy, or harm), the appropriate rating scale or worksheet is utilized to assist the presenting trainee, and faculty members guide the group through the critical appraisal process. Sample worksheets are available through the University of Western Ontario Evidence Based Neurology Web site [4]. These worksheets were derived from the "Users' guide to the medical literature" [13] and relevant articles contained therein. The rating scales are generally divided into three sections: (1) analysis of the study methodology to determine its validity; (2) assessment of the final results, including accuracy and clinical importance; and (3) appraisal of the applicability of these results to the target patient or patient population.

To engage the audience, it is helpful to divide into smaller groups of three or more participants (depending on the number of trainees) to each complete assigned portions of a worksheet. For example, for a therapeutic article, one group can determine whether the study addressed a focused clinical question, whether treatment allocation was randomized, and whether the randomization list was concealed. A second group could discuss the length of patient follow-up and whether an intention-to-treat analysis was employed. The whole group then discusses the interpretation of results and their applicability to the focus clinical question (5 min). The final conclusions of the group are summarized as "clinical bottom lines" (5 min). The presenting trainee's draft CAT is then reviewed, discussed, and edited. The final CAT reflects the opinion of the entire group.

Posttutorial

The presenting trainee completes final revisions of the CAT based on the suggestions of the group at the tutorial and submits it for final review to the facilitators. The final CAT is collected and made available for review either in hard copy format or posted to a central repository on the Internet.

All trainees are encouraged to utilize their evidence-based skills during their clinical rotations and in teaching sessions. Trainees are encouraged to ask about the evidence underlying their supervising faculty's medical decisions in a collegial manner and to review the literature as appropriate to enhance everyone's knowledge base.

The Critically Appraised Topic

The CAT begins with a short summary of the clinical scenario and focused clinical question. The literature search is briefly outlined. The clinical bottom lines are highlighted followed by the most relevant data, typically in table form, and the relevant references. The objective of the CAT is to summarize the tutorial topic and conclusions in a concise manner for future reference. The University of Western Ontario EBN Program maintains an online archive of CATs that assist in clinical decision making and implementation of evidence-based clinical practice [4]. Both the Mayo Clinic MERIT and UWO EBN programs have published CATs in peer-reviewed print journals [6, 14–26].

Resources

Faculty

Two full-time neurologists with expertise in evidence-based medicine, clinical epidemiology, and biostatistics are responsible for coordinating the tutorials and teaching evidence-based care principles. All Neurology and Neurosurgery faculty are invited to attend tutorials, and special invitations are extended to faculty with particular interest or expertise on the topic of discussion at a given session. Teaching faculty from other departments at the University of Western Ontario or other academic institutions are occasionally invited to participate or teach on specific evidence-based medicine topics. Neurosurgery residents attend EBN tutorials when topics relevant to neurosurgical practice are discussed. Neurology residents have graded responsibilities and assume a greater teaching role as they gain experience and skill in EBN. Neurology trainees vary in total number from 10 to 14 per year.

Medical Librarians and Informatics Experts

If available, expert librarians and informatics specialists can be called upon to assist in the literature search. They may identify more useful or encompassing search terms, suggest additional specialized databases to search, and help finalize a list of relevant articles.

Time

EBN tutorial sessions are 75–90 min in duration and held monthly throughout the 5-year neurology residency training program. Sessions are scheduled into protected educational time for neurology trainees, thus ensuring mandatory participation. Topics for discussion are decided upon early in the academic year, and therefore there is ample informal research and preparatory time.

Space

EBN tutorials are held in an available small auditorium within the hospital. Evidence-based medicine reference material is made available in the departmental library. Several computers with links to electronic databases are readily available.

Educational Material

It is helpful to provide an introductory reference book on evidence-based medicine to each new resident [27]. Other evidence-based references and educational material can be made available in the departmental library. A compilation of all CATs reviewed is made available in print format or as a Web-based searchable database [4].

Computer and Informatics

A laptop computer and digital projection unit are readily available for presentations and tutorials. Several computers with Internet access and links to commonly used searchable databases of evidence-based literature are available in the departmental library.

The Evidence for an Evidence-Based Neurology Curriculum

An increasing number of medical residency training programs devote formal educational time to developing evidence-based clinical practice knowledge and skills. Do these curricula improve knowledge of evidence-based medicine concepts and critical appraisal skills? Do they result in a change in clinical practice and patient health outcomes? Many primarily nonrandomized studies conducted over the past decade have attempted to address these questions. High-quality evidence is limited due to heterogeneity of the teaching method or intervention assessed, small sample sizes, heterogeneity of the outcome instruments or measures, and variability in the duration of the study or timing of the outcome assessment [28–30]. Systematic reviews of the available evidence suggest that postgraduate evidence-based medicine education results in improvements in a participant's knowledge, but data is lacking that it alters clinical decision making or patient outcomes [28–30].

References

1. Burneo JG, Jenkins ME. Teaching evidence-based clinical practice to neurology and neurosurgery residents. Clin Neurol Neurosurg. 2007;109:418–21.
2. Burneo JG, Jenkins ME, Bussière M, the UWO Evidence-based neurology group. Evaluating a formal evidence-based clinical practice curriculum in a neurology residency program. J Neurol Sci 2006;250:10–9.
3. Demaerschalk BM, Wiebe S. Evidence based neurology: an innovative curriculum for postgraduate training in the neurological sciences. 2001. http://www.uwo.ca/cns/ebn. Accessed 21 Sept 2009.
4. University of Western Ontario's Evidence Based Neurology. 2001. http://www.uwo.ca/cns/ebn. Accessed 21 Sept 2009.
5. Demaerschalk BM, Wingerchuk DM. The MERITs of evidence-based clinical practice in neurology. Semin Neurol. 2007;27(4):303–11.
6. Wingerchuk DM, Demaerschalk BM. The evidence-based neurologist: criticallyappraised topics. The Neurologist. 2007;13:1.
7. American Academy of Neurology Evidence Based Medicine Toolkit. http://www.aan.com/education/ebm/. Accessed 21 Sep 2009.
8. Richardson WS, Wilson MC, Nishikawa J, Hayward RS. The well-built clinical question: a key to evidence-based decisions. ACP J Club. 1995;123:A12–3.
9. University of Oxford Centre for Evidence-Based Medicine. http://www.cebm.net/levels_of_evidence.asp. Accessed 23 Feb 2009.

10. U.S. National Library of Medicine PubMed. http://www.ncbi.nlm.nih.gov/sites/entrez. Accessed 23 Feb 2009.
11. University of Texas Health Science Centre SUMSearch engine. http://sumsearch.uthscsa.edu/. Accessed 23 Feb 2009.
12. The Cochrane Collaboration. http://www.cochrane.org/index.htm. Accessed 23 Feb 2009.
13. Guyatt GH, Rennie D. Users' guides to the medical literature. A manual for evidence-based clinical practice. Chicago: AMA; 2002.
14. Zarkou S, Aguilar MI, Patel NP, Wellik KE, Wingerchuk DM, Demaerschalk BM. The role of corticosteroids in the management of chronic subdural hematomas: a critically appraised topic. Neurologist. 2009;15:299–302.
15. Wingerchuk DM, Spencer B, Dodick DW, Demaerschalk BM. Migraine with aura is a risk factor for cardiovascular and cerebrovascular disease: a critically appraised topic. Neurologist. 2007;13:231–3.
16. Demaerschalk BM, Wingerchuk DM. Treatment of vascular dementia and vascular cognitive impairment. Neurologist. 2007;13:37–41.
17. Hickey MG, Demaerschalk BM, Caselli RJ, Parish JM, Wingerchuk DM. "Idiopathic" rapid-eye-movement (REM) sleep behavior disorder is associated with future development of neuro-degenerative diseases. Neurologist. 2007;13:98–101.
18. Halker RB, Barrs DM, Wellik KE, Wingerchuk DM, Demaerschalk BM. Establishing a diagnosis of benign paroxysmal positional vertigo through the dix-hallpike and side-lying maneuvers: a critically appraised topic. Neurologist. 2008;14:201–4.
19. Hoerth MT, Wellik KE, Demaerschalk BM, Drazkowski JF, Noe KH, Sirven JI, et al. Clinical predictors of psychogenic nonepileptic seizures: a critically appraised topic. Neurologist. 2008;14:266–70.
20. Khoury JA, Hoxworth JM, Mazlumzadeh M, Wellik KE, Wingerchuk DM, Demaerschalk BM. The clinical utility of high resolution magnetic resonance imaging in the diagnosis of giant cell arteritis: a critically appraised topic. Neurologist. 2008;14:330–5.
21. Capampangan DJ, Wellik KE, Aguilar MI, Demaerschalk BM, Wingerchuk DM. Does prophylactic postoperative hypervolemic therapy prevent cerebral vasospasm and improve clinical outcome after aneurysmal subarachnoid hemorrhage? Neurologist. 2008;14:395–8.
22. Almaraz AC, Bobrow BJ, Wingerchuk DM, Wellik KE, Demaerschalk BM. Serum neuron specific enolase to predict neurological outcome after cardiopulmonary resuscitation: a critically appraised topic. Neurologist. 2009;15:44–8.
23. Khoury J, Wellik KE, Demaerschalk BM, Wingerchuk DM. Cerebrospinal fluid angiotensin-converting enzyme for diagnosis of central nervous system sarcoidosis. Neurologist. 2009;15(2):108–11.
24. Capampangan DJ, Wellik KE, Bobrow BJ, Aguilar MI, Ingall TJ, Kiernan TE, et al. Telemedicine versus telephone for remote emergency stroke consultations: a critically appraised topic. Neurologist. 2009;15:163–6.
25. Jenkins ME, Burneo JG. The return of evidence-based neurology to the Journal: it's all about patient care. Can J Neurol Sci. 2008;35:273–5.
26. Tartaglia MC, Pelz DM, Burneo JG, University of Western Ontario Evidence Based Neurology Group. Cerebral angiography and diagnosis of CNS vasculitis. Can J Neurol Sci. 2009;36:93–4.
27. Sackett DL, Strauss SE, Richardson, WS. Evidence-based medicine: How to practice and teach EBM. 2nd ed. London: Churchill Livingstone; 2000.
28. Parkes J, Hyde C, Deeks J, Milne R. Teaching critical appraisal skills in health care settings. Cochrane Database Syst Rev. 2001;3:CD001270. doi:10.1002/14651858.CD001270.
29. Coomarasamy A, Khan KS. What is the evidence that postgraduate teaching in evidence based medicine changes anything? A systematic review. BMJ. 2004;329:1–5.
30. Flores-Mateo G, Argimon JM. Evidence based practice in postgraduate healthcare education: a systematic review. BMC Health Serv Res. 2007;7:119–27.

Index